Wáng Zhízhōng's 王執中

針 灸 資 生 經

The Classic of Supporting Life with Acupuncture and Moxibustion

Zhēn Jiǔ Zī Shēng Jīng

Volumes I - III

Dr. Yue Lu, L.Ac., Dipl.Ac.

Lorraine Wilcox L.Ac., Ph.D.

The Chinese Medicine Database
www.cm-db.com
Portland, Oregon

The Classic of Supporting Life with Acupuncture and Moxibustion

針灸資生經

Zhēn Jiǔ Zī Shēng Jīng

Volume I - III

Yue Lu

Lorraine Wilcox

Copyright © 2014 The Chinese Medicine Database

1017 SW Morrison #306
Portland, OR 97205 USA

COMP designation original Chinese work and English translation

Cover Design by Jonathan Schell L.Ac.
Library of Congress Cataloging-in-Publication Data:

Zhízhōng, Wáng, fl. 1140-1207
    [The Classic of Supporting Life with Acupuncture and Moxibustion. English]
    Zhen Jiu Zi Sheng Jing = The Classic of Supporting Life with Acupuncture and Moxibustion/ translation Yue Lu, edit Lorraine Wilcox
        p.   cm.
    Includes Index.
    ISBN 978-0-9799552-1-1 (alk. paper)
    Medicine, Chinese   I. Lu, Yue. II. Title: The Classic of Supporting Life with Acupuncture and Moxibustion
    III. Title: Vol. I - III

International Standard Book Number (ISBN): 978-0-9799552-1-1
Printed in the United States of America

Contents

Translation

Volume I

Volume VI   560

Volume VII

Appendices

Indices

Illustrations

Foreword

The Life-Promoting Classic of Acupuncture and Moxibustion

The *Sòng* Dynasty (960-1279) was a time when China was finally able to shake off the political upheaval of the Five Dynasties and forge ahead to rediscover the sophistication and glory last seen in the *Táng* Dynasty. Wood block printing had already been invented, and a publishing boom ensued to complement the explosion in the newly found confidence of a flourishing, cultured society. There was new hope in the air, science, philosophy, literature, art and medicine advanced with renewed vigour and purpose. It was into this world that Wáng Zhízhōng was born. A humble tutor, he made a living by teaching in schools at provincial level in Húnán 湖南 and Húběi 湖北 provinces. Due to a combination of ill health and an inquisitive nature, he developed a keen and life long interest in medicine, that led to him setting up practise to treat patients himself, gaining inspiration and insights from the classical texts available to him at the time such as the *Bronze Statue Illustrated Classic of Acupuncture Points, Prescriptions Worth a Thousand Pieces of Gold* and the *Sage-like Prescriptions of the Tài Píng Era* to name a few.

During his studies of these exalted works, he discovered certain errors that inspired him to embark upon compiling his own magnum opus, the *Life-Promoting Classic of Acupuncture and Moxibustion*, today considered amongst a dozen or so of the most important and influential of classical texts on acupuncture & moxibustion. To do this he did not confine himself solely to studying scholarly works however, but pursued his own investigations by questioning many doctors of his age, and testing his knowledge by applying what he learned in actual clinical practice. In the process he cleared up many inconsistencies in point identification, and established standardised ways of locating points on the body as well as fixing more accurately proportional measurements (including the middle joint of the middle finger cùn measurement). He included illustrations of channels along with detailed instructions on how to locate, needle and apply moxibustion to each point. Subsequently those amended guiding notes were incorporated in to the Míng and Qīng Dynasty bronze man models that formed the basis of the point locations that we use today.

Another fascinating aspect of his work that made it so well thought of and studied by later generation is its insightful and detailed case histories. These were not only derived from his own experiences (including interestingly details of his as well as members of his own family's ill health), but also from the historical sources he studied. He crystallised a wealth of clinical experience along with hundreds of appropriate acupuncture point combinations into an accessible and well-structured treatise. In it he instructs us how to treat the broadest range of diseases, covering the widest spectrum of specialities from gynaecology and gastroenterology, to dermatology and urinary disorders.

Not only did he include the tried and tested formulae that had been passed down through the ages, as was the standard approach in classical writings, but he also put forward and commented upon numerous original and innovative combinations that he developed in the course of his own practice or heard of during his studies.

In some instances he urges the reader to rely on the miraculous efficacy of prescriptions that he himself has successfully used, whilst in others, where he freely admits to only having heard of the value of a particular combination, he encourages the need to verify effectiveness by personal experience. Many of these combinations have proved their worth and are still studied and used today.

Although the *Life-Promoting Classic of Acupuncture and Moxibustion* is a product of one man's tireless efforts, dedication and scholarship, and gives us a fascinating window into the art of acupuncture and moxibustion of the *Sòng* Dynasty, it is much more than just an historical record worthy of study for the snap shot it gives us of those ancient times. This quintessentially classical work forms a significant part of a jigsaw of medical delights that create a rich backdrop of all that we apply and practice in the modern era of Chinese medicine.

The legacy of Wáng Zhízhōng and his work the *Life-Promoting Classic of Acupuncture and Moxibustion* is without question secure. Now we must be grateful to Dr. Yue Lu for her masterful translation and for making this book available to the emerging Chinese medicine community that would not otherwise have access to this foundational masterpiece. With such a celebrated classic now available for all non-Chinese readers to scrutinise, acupuncture is truly on the path to coming of age in the West.

Mazin Al-Khafaji,

Brighton, UK 2014

Introduction to

Zhēn Jiǔ Zī Shēng Jīng 《針灸資生經》

Zhēn Jiǔ Zī Shēng Jīng 《針灸資生經》 Life-Promoting Classic of Acupuncture and Moxbustion was written by Wáng Zhízhōng 王執中 during the *Sòng* Dynasty, approximately between 1180-1195. It has seven volumes.

The author, Wáng Zhízhōng (c. 1140-1207) was from Ruìʼān 瑞安, (modern-day Wēnzhōu 温州 in Zhèjiāng 浙江 province), but he was posted as a low ranking officer in Húnán 湖南 and Húběi 湖北 where he taught in schools at the provincial level. Because he was often ill, Wáng treated himself and so began gathering medical information. In his research, he focused on the classics of acupuncture-moxibustion but collected prescriptions from the practices of the common people (including acupuncture, moxibustion, dietary, and miscellaneous treatments). He also visited local doctors and herb stores. Wáng was obviously very well-educated; in his book, he frequently cited historical cases, philosophical texts, or ancient poetry. Wáng practiced medicine himself, testing whatever he learned. He recorded what he found to be effective.

The title of the book - 'Life-Promoting' (*Zī Shēng* 資生) is a reference to people's reliance on stomach qì for life. In Volume 3, Wáng wrote, "人仰胃氣為主 。是人資胃氣以生矣 。 People rely on stomach qì as the governing principle; this means people should *promote* stomach qì in order to *live*."

Volume 1 describes the location and acupuncture techniques for 365 points. The information about the points is mainly quoted from *The Bronze Statue Illustrated Classic of Acupuncture Points* and from Volumes 99 and 100 of *Sage-like Prescriptions of Tài Píng Era*.

Earlier sources often disagreed on the location of certain points. In Volume 1, Wáng compared the location from different sources and tried to verify the proper position of these points. He especially investigated the location of abdominal points and the distance of their channels from the midline. This had great influence in later generations.

Volume 2 discusses various issues, including contraindications for acupuncture, the distance between points, proportional measurement (using same-body cùn), similarities and differences in the names of points, how to locate points, and moxibustion (the number and size of cones, how to treat moxa sores, etc.). It is a general introduction to acupuncture-moxibustion. Although Wáng frequently used passages from earlier texts, most of the text of Volume 2 is Wáng's own opinion. He presented some new ideas by researching information from many different books and combining this with his own experience.

Volumes 3 through 7 provide point indications and point prescriptions arranged according to categories of disorder. Those volumes cite the many earlier texts including *Sage-like Prescriptions of Tài Píng Era, Prescriptions Worth a Thousand Piece of Gold* and *Supplement to Prescriptions Worth a Thousand Piece of Gold*, and *The Bronze Statue*. As in the earlier volumes, Wáng compared similar passages from these books, noting and differences.

Throughout the book, Wáng is quite concerned with comparing words and phrases from various sources, trying to parse out which is correct. This was not only an issue for Wáng, but it is also an issue in translation. Because Wáng used so many different sources, both ancient and contemporary, terminology was inconsistent. Various sources may have used different terms for the same thing (point names, symptoms, diseases, and so forth) or the same term for different things. Wáng wrote many paragraphs musing over this and it was also an issue for the translator. Footnotes have been added to clarify, when possible.

Wáng included many case studies in the later volumes. Some are historical, some from people he knew or had treated, and many were about himself or his mother. Through these cases, we see glimpses of what treatment actually looked like during the *Sòng* Dynasty. We also get to know a little of Wáng Zhízhōng's personality, which is especially evident in the cases. These case studies and 'secret' formulas that were recorded made *Zī Shēng Jīng* popular in later generations.

Although acupuncture and moxibustion are both in the title of the book, it is obvious that Wáng gave as much or more respect to moxibustion as to acupuncture. He also often described herbal treatment in his own comments or in the case studies.

Zī Shēng Jīng influenced authors for hundreds of years, even up to the present. Here are some of the contributions that are still used today:

- Wáng gave references for all his sources and also made it obvious when he himself was commenting. This was quite unusual at the time.

- Wáng promoted proportional measurement, especially the use of the middle joint of the middle finger as one cùn.

- Wáng organized indications and point formulas according to category of disorder, so the book was easy to use in the clinic.

- Wáng corrected the location of many points, especially those on the abdomen. Many later books followed his point locations, including Huá Shí's *Sì Jīng Fā Huī* 滑壽《十四經發揮》, Gāo Wǔ's *Zhēn Jiǔ Jù Yīng* 高武《針灸聚英》, Xú Fèng's *Zhēn Jiǔ Dà Quán* 徐鳳《針灸大全》, and Yáng Jìzhōu's *Zhēn Jiǔ Dà Chéng* 楊繼洲《針灸大成》.

- Wáng discussed various types of contraindications. At that time, it was popular to calculate certain days when acupuncture was prohibited. Wáng was not opposed to this in principle, but felt that in urgent cases, the prohibitions could be ignored. Besides this, some points had contraindications, for example moxibustion might be forbidden on a particular point. But if moxibustion seemed to be indicated, especially in an urgent case, the contraindication need not be followed. See Xīn Shù 心俞 (UB 15) and Tiān Yǒu 天牖 (SJ 16) in Volume 1.

- In Volume 2, Wáng discussed *ā shì* points or treatment of the affected area. Sūn Sīmiǎo 孫思邈 had mentioned *ā shì* points earlier, but Wáng contributed to the theory, and added specific examples in the volumes on treatment. He suggested pressing Fèi Shù 肺俞 (UB 13) for wheezing and asthma, Dàn Zhōng 膻中 (Rèn 17) for cough, Tiān Shū 天樞 (UB 25) for intestinal abscess, Dài Mài 帶脈 (GB 26) for abnormal vaginal discharge, and so forth. If these points were found to be sore, they would be effective.

Overall, having a translation *Zhēn Jiǔ Zī Shēng Jīng* is a great contribution to the community of English-speaking practitioners of Chinese medicine.

Acknowledgements

I would like to express my appreciation to Lorraine Wilcox. I thank her for encouraging my work. Her comments and suggestions on the translation have been priceless. Without her help, this book would not have been possible.

I would also like to thank Jerome Jiang for his help during the translation. His knowledge of ancient literature is impressive.

A special thanks also goes to Jonathan Schell for introducing this ancient Chinese acupuncture classic to the English-speaking world.

Finally, I would like to express appreciation to my family. Your support is what has sustained me thus far and given me incentive to work towards my goal.

Publisher's Note

A few small things about this book:

1) Notes in the lateral margin. These are the Chinese characters for the section headings which Wáng included in the text, for example: （ 見尸厥 ） which means (see the section on deathlike reversal). In the lateral margin, you will see the Chinese character for 尸厥 and underneath it, a number. This is the page number for this section. We hope that by including these, it makes the book more usable, and let's the reader quickly check Wáng's reference. For the sake of brevity, if the reference appears twice on a single page, it is only displayed once in the lateral margin, in the order with which it appears in the Chinese text on that page.

2) On a page by page basis, when characters were repeated, such as with point names, we have chosen not to repeat them in the second instance. Thus, under the Chinese passage, in the English translation, if Pū Cān 僕參 (UB 61) is mentioned, then on the second reference on the same page, it will appear as Pū Cān (UB 61). This is the same with book titles, so if on the first instance it reads (*Qiān* 《 千 》), then on the second instance for that page it will read (*Qiān*). These are not mistakes, only an effort to save space. It was apparent from the outset that this was going to be a very large, and very dense book, therefore we instigated methods from the beginning to try to keep the size of the book manageable.

3) We have chosen to break this book into two volumes, even though in its original state it would have comprised a single book of seven volumes. For this material we decided it was better to have two 400+ page books, then it would to be have one 1,000 page book. The book you hold in your hands, has the full Table of Contents for all seven volumes with accurate page numbers, and an index for only this book. The second volume will contain the full Table of Contents, as well as a master index for both books. The page numbers of the two books are sequential from the end of chapter 3, to the beginning of chapter 4 of the next book. At the end of this book, the page numbers of the appendix and indices begin at page A-1. This represents that these sections will not be considered part of the final page numbering of the complete two volumes.

Zhēn Jiǔ Zī Shēng Jīng

《針灸資生經·第一》

1.01
Yǎn Fú Tóu Bù Zhōng Háng Shí Xué

[偃伏]頭部中行十穴

[Prone or supine position] midline of the head, ten points

神庭一穴，在鼻直入髮際五分 。灸二七壯，止七七壯 。岐伯曰：凡欲療風，勿令灸多 。緣風性輕，多即傷 。惟宜灸七壯，止三七壯 。禁針，針即發狂 。忌生冷，雞、豬、羊、酒、面動風等物 。《明堂》云：舉火之時忌熱食，不宜熱衣 。

Shén Tíng 神庭 (Dū 24) one point[1]: It is located directly above the nose, 5 fēn[2] within the [anterior] hairline. Burn two times seven cones of moxibustion; stop at seven times seven cones. Qíbó said: When you want to treat wind [using this point], do not apply a lot of moxibustion. Because wind is light in its nature, a lot of moxibustion damages [the body]. It is appropriate to apply only seven cones, up to three times seven cones of moxibustion. Needling is contraindicated, as needling will immediately cause mania. Raw cold [food], chicken, pork, lamb, liquor, flour, etc. are also contraindicated, as they can stir up the wind. *Míng Táng* 明堂 (Bright Hall)[3] says: Hot food is contraindicated when applying fire [moxibustion]; hot clothing is also not recommended.

上星（自此以下不言一穴），在鼻直上入髮際一寸陷中（《明堂》云：容豆是）。以細三稜針刺之，即宣洩諸陽熱氣，無令上衝頭目 。可灸七壯，不宜多 。若頻灸，即拔氣上，令目不明 。忌同 。《甲乙經》、《熱穴論注》並刺三分 。

Shàng Xīng 上星 (Dū 23) (I will not state 'one point' from now on)[4]: It is located directly above

---

1. One point: This means it is a point on the midline, not a bilateral point.

2. *Fēn* 分 is a unit of measurement. One *fēn* equals 0.1 *cùn*.

3. For information about the various sources cited in the text, please see the *Appendix on Book References*.

4. In Chinese, the points have names, but the channel affiliation is not part of the name. Points on the midline (Dū and Rèn) only have one point as they are not bilateral. Points of the twelve main channels are bilateral (two points). Ancient Chinese books usually state whether there are one or two points, but here the author or editor says he will not do this. He thinks his readers already know if the point is bilateral or on the midline.

the nose in the depression 1.0 cùn within the [anterior] hairline. (*Míng Táng* 《 明堂 》 says it is where [the depression] could hold a bean). Prick it with a thin three-edged needle to drain all yáng and hot qì, so it cannot surge up to the head and eyes. Burn seven cones of moxibustion; more is not recommended. If moxibustion is frequently applied, it pulls qì upward and causes dim vision. Follow the same contraindications [as Shén Tíng 神庭 (Dū 24)]. *Jiǎ Yǐ Jīng* 《 甲乙經 》 (The Systematized Classic of Acupuncture and Moxibustion) and *Rè Xué Lùn Zhù* 《 熱穴論注 》 (Annotations on the Treatise on Points for Heat)[5] both say to prick three fēn deep.

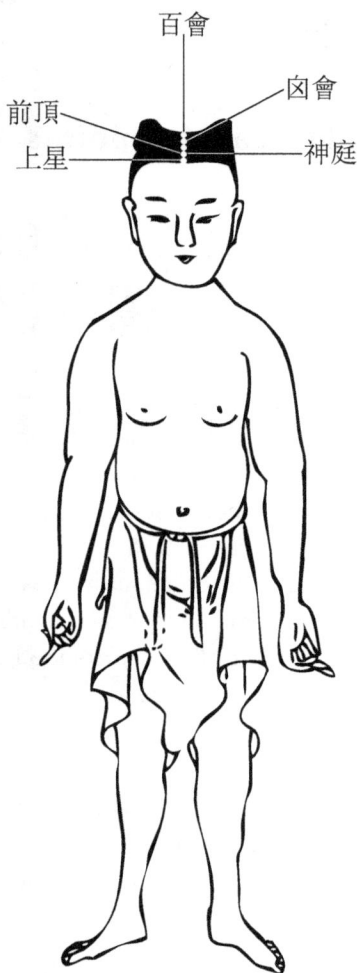

百會
囟會
前頂
神庭
上星

Fig. 1.1

囟會，在上星後（ 《明堂》云上星上 ）一寸陷中 。可灸二七壯，至七七壯 。初灸即不痛，病去即痛，痛即罷灸 。針入二分（ 此後去入字 ），留三呼，得氣即瀉 。若八歲以下不得針，緣囟門未合，刺之不幸，令人夭 。忌同 。《 素問 》注云：刺四分 。

Xìn Huì 囟會 (Dū 22): It is located in the depression 1.0 cùn posterior to Shàng Xīng 上星 (Dū 23) (*Míng Táng* says: above Shàng Xīng (Dū 23)). Burn two times seven cones of moxibustion up to seven times seven cones. If there is no pain when you begin the moxibustion, the disease will be removed when pain occurs; stop the moxibustion when [the patient] feels pain. Needle two fēn deep (from now on, the character *rù* 入 will be removed);[6] retain the needle for three respirations;[7] drain [the point] as soon as qì arrives. Do not needle if [the patient is] under eight years of age because the fontanels are not yet closed. If, unfortunately, you pierce [too deeply when the fontanels are open], the person will die. Follow the same contraindications [as Shén Tíng (Dū 24)]. The Annotation to *Sù Wèn* 《 素問 》 (Plain Questions) says to needle four fēn deep.

---

5. This is Wáng Bīng's annotations for *Sù Wèn* 《 素問 》 (Plain Questions), Chapter 61. For more details, see the *Appendix on Book References*.

6. The author wanted to phrase the text a little differently than his source. This note is of little importance for the English reader.

7. The original word here is *hū* 呼 (exhalation), but it actually refers to a whole cycle of inhalation and exhalation, one respiration. Therefore, *hū* 呼 will be translated as respiration throughout this volume.

予少刻苦，年逾壯則腦冷，或飲酒過多則腦疼如破。後因灸此穴，非特腦不復冷，他日酒醉，腦亦不疼矣。凡腦冷者灸之。

[Author's note[8]:] I worked hard when I was young, so when I passed my vigorous age [30 or 40 years old], I suffered cold in the brain, with pain in the brain, as if it would break when I drank too much liquor. Later, because I applied moxibustion on this point, I did not get cold in the brain except under very special conditions. The other day I was drunk, but there was still no brain pain. It is appropriate to apply moxibustion to it for those who have cold in the brain.

前頂在囟會後寸半骨陷中。甄權云是一寸，今依《素問》寸半為定。針一分，灸三壯，止七七。忌同。《素注》云：刺四分（此後去問字）。

Qián Dǐng 前頂 (Dū 21): It is located 1.5 cùn posterior to Xìn Huì 囟會 (Dū 22), in the depression of the bone. Zhēn Quán[9] said it is 1.0 cùn, but now it is determined to be 1.5 cùn according to *Sù Wèn* 《素問》. Needle 1.0 fēn deep; burn three cones of moxibustion; stop at seven times seven cones. Follow the same contraindications [as Shén Tíng 神庭 (Dū 24)]. *Sù Zhù* 《素注》 (Annotation to the Plain Questions) says to needle 4 fēn deep. (From now on, the character *wèn* 問 (questions) will be removed.)[10]

百會，一名三陽五會，在前頂後寸半，頂中央旋毛中，可容豆。灸七壯，止七七。凡灸頭頂不得過七壯，緣頭頂皮薄，灸不宜多。針二分，得氣即瀉。唐秦鳴鶴刺微出血，頭痛立愈。《素注》云刺四分。

Bǎi Huì 百會 (Dū 20), another name is Sān Yáng Wǔ Huì 三陽五會 (three yáng and fivefold convergence): It is located 1.5 cùn posterior to Qián Dǐng 前頂 (Dū 21), in the spinning hair [cowlick] at the center of the vertex, [in the depression] which can hold a bean. Burn seven cones of moxibustion; stop at seven times seven cones. Do not burn more than seven cones when applying moxibustion on the vertex because the skin of the vertex is thin, so more moxibustion is not recommended. Needle 2 fēn deep; drain [the point] as soon as qì arrives. Qín Mínghè[11] of the *Tàng* Dynasty pricked and bled it a little, and the headache was immediately gone. *Sù Zhù* says to needle 4.0 fēn deep.

---

8. This is a note by the author of the *Classic of Supplementing Life*, Wáng Zhízhōng 王執中. To make it clear, [Author's note:] will be added to such entries.

9. Zhēn Quán 甄權 (540-643) was a famous doctor in *Táng* (唐) Dynasty.

10. The note in parenthesis tells us that Wáng Zhízhōng 王執中 will abbreviate *Sù Wèn Zhù* 《素問注》 as *Sù Zhù* 《素注》 from now on.

11. Qín Mínghè 秦鳴鶴 was the personal doctor of Emperor Gāozōng in the *Táng* Dynasty. He was an expert in acupuncture.

舊伝秦鳴鶴針高宗頭風，武後曰：豈有至尊頭上出血之理？已而刺之，微出血，頭疼立止。後亟取金帛賜之。是知此穴能治頭風矣。《明堂經》治中風，言語寒澀，半身不遂，凡灸七處，亦先於百會。北人始生子則灸此穴，蓋防他日驚風也。予舊患心氣，偶睹《陰陽書》有云：人身有四穴最急應，四百四病皆能治之。百會蓋其一也，因灸此穴而心氣愈。後閱《灸經》，此穴果主心煩，驚悸，健忘，無心力。自是間或灸之，百病皆主，不特治此數疾而已也。（一名天滿）

[Author's note:] It is said that when Qín Mínghè needled Emperor Gāozōng [the third emperor of the *Táng* Dynasty] for head wind, Empress Wǔ said: It is ridiculous to bleed the head of His Majesty! After it was pricked and bled a little, the headache stopped right away. The Empress granted Qín gold and silks. Thus it became known that this point could be used to treat head wind. *Míng Táng Jīng*《明堂經》uses it in the treatment of wind stroke, sluggish speech, and hemiplegia by applying moxibustion on seven locations, starting with Bǎi Huì 百會 (Dū 20). People who live in the north apply moxibustion to this point right after childbirth to prevent fright wind in the future. I suffered heart qì in the past and by chance read what is in *Yīn Yáng Shū*《陰陽書》(Book of Yīn and Yáng); it says: There are four points on the human body which have the quickest response; they can treat all of the 440 disorders. Bǎi Huì (Dū 20) is one of them, because moxibustion on it can cure heart qì. Later I read in *Jiǔ Jīng*《灸經》(The Classic of Moxibustion) that this point can really treat vexation of the heart, fright palpitations, forgetfulness, and weakness of the heart. Because of this I apply moxibustion to it occasionally, and the hundred diseases are all governed, not just those several disorders listed above. (Another name is Tiān Mǎn 天滿.)

神聰四穴，在百會四面各相去一寸。理頭風目眩，狂亂風癇。左主如花，右主如果。針三分。

Shén Cōng 神聰, four points: They are located 1.0 cùn from the four sides [anterior, posterior and lateral] of Bǎi Huì (Dū 20). They regulate head wind, dizzy vision, mania, and wind epilepsy.

[The point on] the left side governs like a flower; [the point on] the right side governs like a fruit.[12] Needle 3 fēn deep.

《明堂》有此四穴，而《銅人》無之。其穴治頭風目眩，狂亂風癇，亦所不可廢者，故附入於此。

[Author's note:] These four points are described in *Míng Táng*《明堂》, but are not in *Tóng Rén*《銅人》(The Bronze Statue Illustrated Classic of Acupuncture Points). What these points treat – head wind, dizzy vision, mania and wind epilepsy – cannot be abandoned, so they should still be appended here.

---

12. This means the results of the point on the right side are better than those of the left side.

明堂一穴，在鼻直上入髮際一寸。理頭風，多鼻涕，鼻塞。三日一報，針二分。

Míng Táng 明堂, one point: It is directly above the nose, 1.0 cùn within the [anterior] hairline. It regulates head wind, profuse nasal mucus, and nasal congestion. Repeat moxibustion once every three days; needle 2 fēn deep.

按《銅人》、《明堂》及諸家針灸經，鼻直上入髮際一寸皆云上星穴。《明堂經》於此復云明堂穴，不知何所據？且附入於此，所謂疑以傳疑也。（◎今以諸經校勘，上星穴者是。）

> Note: According to *Tóng Rén* 《銅人》, *Míng Táng* 《明堂》 and all the other acupuncture-moxibustion classics, the point that is located directly above the nose, 1.0 cùn within the [anterior] hairline is Shàng Xīng 上星 (Dū 23). *Míng Táng Jīng* 《明堂經》 also states that the Míng Táng 明堂 point is here, but there is no evidence of this anywhere. What is appended here is doubtful and I pass on the doubt. ([*13] Now corrected by comparing it with all the other classics, this should be called Shàng Xīng (Dū 23).)

後頂一名交衝，在百會後寸半枕骨上。灸五壯，針二分。《明》云：四分（後凡云《明》云者，《明堂經》云也）。

Hòu Dǐng 後頂 (Dū 19), also named Jiāo Chōng 交衝: It is located 1.5 cùn posterior to Bǎi Huì 百會 (Dū 20), above the occipital bone. Burn five cones of moxibustion; needle 2 fēn deep. *Míng* 《明》 says: 4 fēn deep. (From now on, whenever it says *Míng*, it indicates *Míng Táng Jīng*.)

強間一名大羽，在後頂後寸半。針二分，灸七壯。《明》云：五壯。

Qiáng Jiān 強間 (Dū 18), also named Dà Yǔ 大羽: It is located 1.5 cùn above Hòu Dǐng (Dū 19). Needle 2 fēn deep; burn seven cones of moxibustion. *Míng* says: Five cones.

腦戶一名合顱，在枕骨上強間後寸半。禁針，針令人啞。可灸七壯，亦不可妄灸，令人夭。《明》云：灸令人失音，針三分。《素注》云：四分，《甲乙》云：不可灸。

---

13. According to *Zhēn Jiǔ Míng Zhù Jí Chéng* 《針灸名著集成》 (Grand Compendium of Famous Works on Acupuncture and Moxibustion), edited by Huáng Lóngxiáng 黃龍祥 and published in 1996, any notes with * were not written by the author Wáng Zhízhōng. They were added by an unknown later editor.

Nǎo Hù 腦戶 (Dū 17), another name is Hé Lú 合顱: It is located 1.5 cùn above Qiáng Jiān 強間 (Dū 18). Needling is contraindicated; it makes people mute. Seven cones of moxibustion are allowed; improper moxibustion is prohibited; it makes people die young. *Míng* 《明》 says: Moxibustion makes people lose their voice; needle 3 fēn deep. *Sù Zhù* 《素注》 says: Needle 4 fēn deep. *Jiǎ Yǐ* 《甲乙》 says: Moxibustion cannot be used.

《銅人》云：禁針，《素問》、《明堂》乃云針入三分、四分，亦可疑矣，不如不針為穩。《素問》蓋云刺腦戶，入腦立死故也。

[Author's note:] *Tóng Rén* 《銅人》 says: Needling is contraindicated. *Sù Wèn* 《素問》 and *Míng Táng* 《明堂》 say to needle 3 or 4 fēn deep; this is also doubtful; it is safer not to needle it. *Sù Wèn* says if the needle enters the brain when needling Nǎo Hù (Dū 17), [the patient] will immediately die.

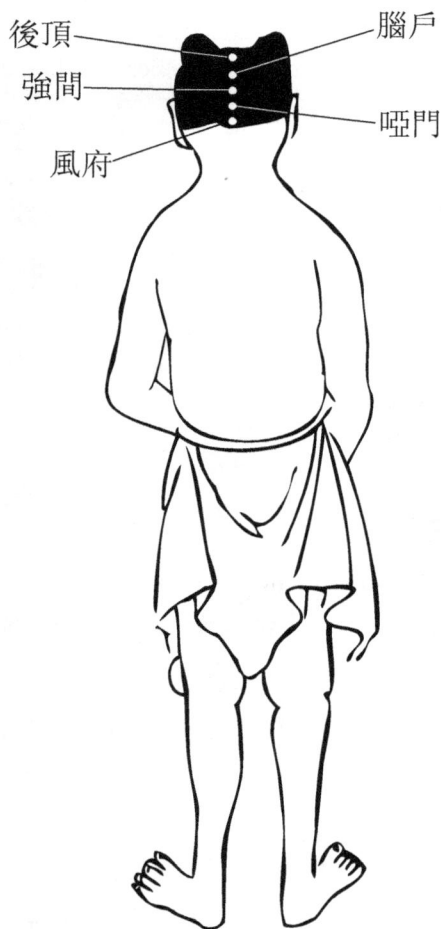

Fig. 1.2

風府一名舌本，在頂後髮際上一寸大筋內宛宛中。疾言其肉立起，言休立下。禁灸，使人失音，針三分。《明》云：四分，留三呼。又云：舌緩針風府。（見下）

Fēng Fǔ 風府 (Dū 16), another name is Shé Běn 舌本: It is located 1.0 cùn above the hairline at the nape of the neck, in the depression medial to the big sinew [the trapezius]. The flesh rises up when one speaks fast and goes down right away when one stops talking. Moxibustion is contraindicated; it makes people lose their voice. Needle 3 fēn deep. *Míng* says: Needle 4 fēn deep; retain the needle for three respirations. It also says: Needle Fēng Fǔ (Dū 16) for slack tongue. (See below)

岐伯對黃帝傷寒之問曰：巨陽者、諸陽之屬也。其脈連於風府，故為諸陽主氣也。然則風府者，固傷寒所自起也，北人皆以毛裹之，南人怯弱者，亦以帛護

其項，俗謂三角是也。予少怯弱，春冬須數次感風，自用物護後無比
患矣。凡怯弱者須護項後可也。（今婦人用帛蔽項，名護項，乃云蔽
垢膩。其名雖存，其義亡矣。）

[Author's note:] Qí Bó replied to a question from Huáng Dì on cold damage: Supreme yáng [Jù Yáng] is ascribed to all yáng. Its vessel connects with Fēng Fǔ 風府 (Dū 16), so [this point] governs the qì of all yáng. But cold damage starts from Fēng Fǔ (Dū 16), so everyone who lives in the north wraps [the region of Fēng Fǔ] with fur, while southerners who are weak cover their necks with silk; this [area of the neck] is commonly called the triangle. I was weak when I was young, so I contracted wind several times during the spring and winter, but I never had this problem after I began protecting it with something. So any weak person should protect their nape. (Nowadays ladies use silk to cover their nape, which they call neck protection; they say it covers dirt and grease.[14] The name [still] exists, but the meaning is lost.

啞門（一作瘂），一名舌橫，一名舌厭，在項中央入髮際五分宛宛中。督
脈、陽維之會，入繫舌本，仰頭取之。禁灸，令人啞。針三分。《素注》
云：在項後髮際宛中。去風府一寸。《明》云：舌急不言如何治？答曰：舌
急針瘂門，舌緩針風府，得氣即瀉。可小繞針，入八分，留三呼，瀉五吸，
瀉盡更留針取之，得氣即瀉。

Yǎ Mén 啞門 (Dū 15) (also known as Yīn 瘂 (loss of voice)), another name is Shé Héng 舌橫, another name is Shé Yàn 舌厭: It is located in the depression in the center, 0.5 cùn above the hairline at the nape of the neck. It is the meeting point of the dū mài 督脈 and yáng wéi 陽維. It connects with the root of the tongue. Locate the point with the patient looking up. Moxibustion is contraindicated; it makes people mute. Needle 3 fēn deep. *Sù Zhù* 《素注》 says: It is in the depression above the hairline at the nape of the neck, 1.0 cùn from Fēng Fǔ (Dū 16). *Míng* 《明》 says: How can we treat hypertonicity of the tongue with inability to talk? The answer is: Needle Yīn Mén 瘂門[15] for hypertonicity of the tongue; needle Fēng Fǔ (Dū 16) for slack tongue; drain [the point] as soon as qì arrives. You also can rotate the needle slightly [or gently]; enter 8 fēn deep; retain the needle for three respirations; drain for five respirations;[16] when draining is complete, retain the needle again; then drain [the point] as soon as qì arrives.

---

14. The ladies use it to protect the neck of their clothing from stains, not to protect themselves from wind.

15. Yīn Mén 瘂門 is another name for Yǎ Mén 啞門 (Dū 15) according the text.

16. The original word here is *xī* 吸 (inhalation), but it actually means respiration. The same is true for other occurrences in this volume.

1.02
Yǎn Fú Dì Èr Háng Zuǒ Yòu Shí Sì Xué

[偃伏]第二行左右十四穴

[Prone or supine position] the second line, 14 bilateral points [seven on each side]

曲差二穴，在神庭兩旁寸半入髮際。針三分，灸三壯。

Qū Chā 曲差 (UB 4), bilateral point: It is located 1.5 cùn lateral to Shén Tíng 神庭 (Dū 24), within the [anterior] hairline. Needle 3 fēn deep; apply three cones of moxibustion.

五處二穴，在上星兩旁寸半。針三分，留七呼，灸三壯。《明》云：五壯止。

Wǔ Chù 五處 (UB 5), bilateral point: It is located 1.5 cùn lateral to Shàng Xīng 上星 (Dū 23). Needle 3 fēn deep; retain the needle for seven respirations. Burn three cones of moxibustion. *Míng* 《明》 says: Stop at five cones.

承光二穴，在五處後寸半。針三分，禁灸。忌同。《明》云：在五處後二寸。《素注》云：一寸。

Chéng Guāng 承光 (UB 6), bilateral point: It is located 1.5 cùn posterior to Wǔ Chù (UB 5). Needle 3 fēn deep. Moxibustion is contraindicated. Follow the same contraindications [as Shén Tíng (Dū 24)]. *Míng* says: It is located 2 cùn posterior to Wǔ Chù (UB 5). *Sù Zhù* 《素注》 says: It is 1 cùn [posterior to Wǔ Chù (UB 5)].

通天二穴，在承光後寸半。針三分，留七呼，灸三壯。

Tōng Tiān 通天 (UB 7), bilateral point: It is located 1.5 cùn posterior to Chéng Guāng (UB 6). Needle 3 fēn deep; retain the needle for seven respirations; apply 3 cones of moxibustion.

絡卻二穴，一名強陽，又名腦蓋，在通天後寸半。灸三壯。《素注》云：針三分，留五呼。

Luò Què 絡卻 (UB 8) bilateral point, another name is Qiáng Yáng 強陽, also known as Nǎo Gài 腦蓋: It is located 1.5 cùn posterior to Tōng Tiān 通天 (UB 7). Burn three cones of moxibustion. *Sù Zhù*《素注》says: Needle 3 fēn deep; retain the needle for five respirations.

玉枕二穴，在絡卻後寸半（《明》上、下云：七分半）。夾腦戶（腦戶在強間後寸半）旁寸三分起肉，枕骨入髮際上三寸。灸二壯。《明》云：針三分。《素注》云：留三呼，《甲乙》云：二分。

Yù Zhěn 玉枕 (UB 9), bilateral point: It is located 1.5 cùn posterior to Luò Què (UB 8) (Upper and Lower *Míng*《明》say: 7.5 fēn). It is 1.3 cùn lateral to Nǎo Hù 腦戶 (Dū 17) (Nǎo Hù (Dū 17) is located 1.5 cùn posterior to Qiáng Jiān 強間 (Dū 18)), on the fleshy protuberance above the occipital bone, 3 cùn within hairline. Burn 2 cones of moxibustion. *Míng*《明》says: Needle 3 fēn deep. *Sù Zhù* says: Retain the needle for three respirations. *Jiǎ Yǐ*《甲乙》says: Needle 2 fēn deep.

《銅人》云：玉枕在絡卻後一寸半，《明堂》上、下經皆云七分半。若以《銅人》為誤，則足太陽穴亦同。若以《明堂》為誤，不應上、下經皆誤也（小本《明堂》亦同）。予按《素問注》云：玉枕在絡卻後七分，則與《明堂》之七分半相去不遠矣。固當從《素問》為準。然而玉枕二穴既夾腦戶矣，不應止七分則至於腦蓋也。《銅人》之一寸半蓋有說焉，識者當有以辨之。（◎今以諸經校勘，在絡卻後寸半者是。）

[Author's note:] Tóng Rén《銅人》says: Yù Zhěn (UB 9) is located 1.5 cùn posterior to Luò Què (UB 8). Míng Táng《明堂》(Upper and Lower Canon) both say it is 7.5 fēn. If Tóng Rén is wrong, then the [other]

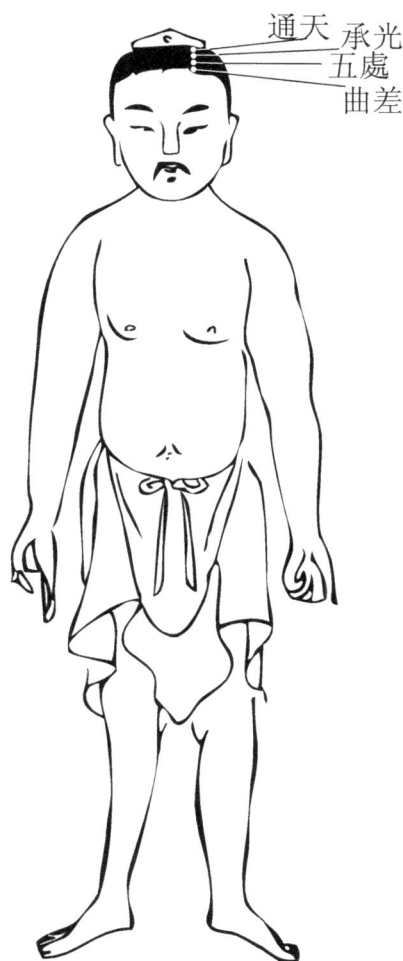

Fig. 1.3

9

points of the foot tàiyáng channel[17] are also wrong. If *Míng Táng* 《 明堂 》 is incorrect, both The Upper and Lower Canon should not be wrong. (The small [edition of] *Míng Táng* also agrees.) I note that when *Sù Wèn Zhù* 《 素問注 》 says: Yù Zhěn 玉枕 (UB 9) is located 7 fēn posterior to Luò Què 絡卻 (UB 8), there is not a big difference with the 7.5 fēn of *Míng Táng*. So we should follow *Sù Wèn* 《 素問 》. But since the bilateral point of Yù Zhěn (UB 9) is on both sides of Nǎo Hù 腦戶 (Dū 17), it should not be located just 7 fēn from Nǎo Gài 腦蓋 (UB 8). So the 1.5 cùn mentioned in *Tóng Rén* 《 銅人 》 should be discussed, and knowledgeable people should make their own differentiation. (*Now corrected by comparing with all the other classics, it should be located 1.5 cùn posterior to Luò Què (UB 8).)

絡卻 ——
玉枕 ——
天柱 ——

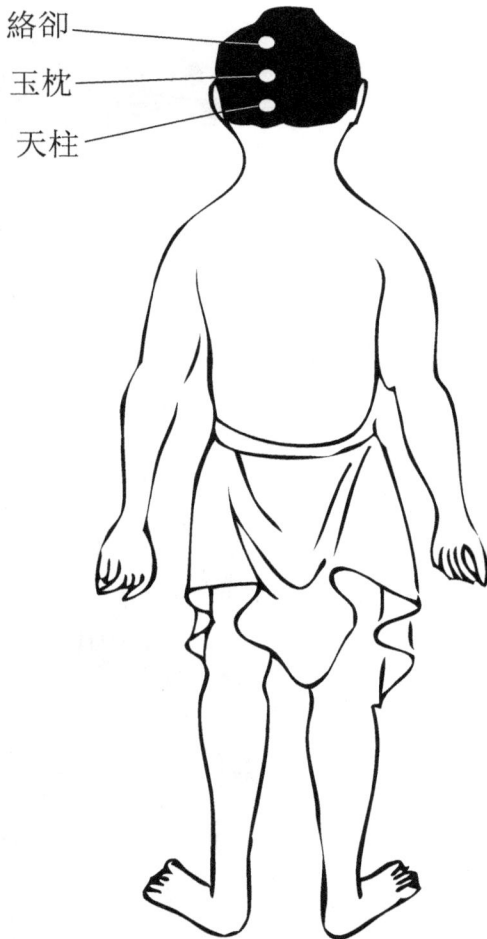

Fig. 1.4

天柱二穴，夾項後髮際，大筋外廉
陷中 。針五分，得氣即瀉 。《 明 》
云：二分，留三呼，瀉五吸，灸不
及針，日七壯，至百五 。忌同 。《
下 》云：三壯 。《 素注 》云：刺二
分 。

Tiān Zhù 天柱 (UB 10), bilateral point: It is located in the depression on the outside of big sinew, within hairline at the nape of the neck. Needle 5 fēn deep; drain [the point] as soon as qì arrives. *Míng* 《 明 》 says: Needle 2 fēn deep; retain for three respirations; drain for five respirations. Moxibustion is not as good as needling; burn seven cones of moxibustion daily, up to one hundred and fifty cones. Follow the same contraindications [as Shén Tíng 神庭 (Dū 24)]. *Xià* 《 下 》 says: Burn three cones. *Sù Zhù* 《 素注 》 says: Needle 2 fēn deep.

眉衝二穴，一名小竹，當兩眉頭直
上入髮際是 。療目五般癇，頭痛鼻
塞 。不灸，通針三分（ 《 明上 》 ）
。

---

17. Foot tàiyáng channel here refers to the chapter in Volume 1 of *Tóng Rén Shū Xué Zhēn Jiu Tú Jīng* 《 銅人腧穴針灸圖經 》 (The Bronze Statues Illustrated Classic of Acupuncture Points). In Volume 1, each chapter describes the pathway, pathological manifestation and point location of a particular channel.

Méi Chōng 眉衝 (UB 3), bilateral point, another name is Xiǎo Zhú 小竹 (Small Bamboo): It is located right above the [medial] end of the two eyebrows, within the hairline. It treats eye disorders, the five types of epilepsy, headaches, and nasal congestion. Do not apply moxibustion; needle 3 fēn deep generally. (*Míng Shàng*《明上》)

《明堂》上經有眉衝穴，而《銅人經》無之。理目五般癇，頭痛鼻塞等疾所不可廢者，其穴與曲差相近，故附於此。

[Author's note:] *Míng Táng*《明堂》 Upper Canon lists Méi Chōng 眉衝 (UB 3), but *Tóng Rén Jīng*《銅人經》 does not. It regulates – eye disorders, the five types of epilepsy, headaches, and nasal congestion – cannot be abandoned. This point is close to Qū Chā 曲差 (UB 4), so it is attached here.

1.03
Yǎn Fú Dì Sān Háng Zuǒ Yòu Shí Èr Xué

[偃伏]第三行左右十二穴

[Prone or supine position] the third line, 12 bilateral points [six on each side]

臨泣二穴，在目上直入髮際五分陷中。針三分，留七呼，得氣即瀉。忌同。《素注》云：灸五壯。

Lín Qì 臨泣 (GB 15), bilateral point: It is located directly above the eyes in the depression 5 fēn within the hairline. Needle 3 fēn deep; retain the needle for seven respirations; drain [the point] as soon as qì arrives. Follow the same contraindications [as Shén Tíng 神庭 (Dū 24)]. *Sù Zhù*《素注》 says: Burn five cones of moxibustion.

足少陽有臨泣穴矣，此亦有之，蓋此乃頭臨泣穴也。

[Author's note:] There is Lín Qì 臨泣 (GB 41) on the shàoyáng channel of the foot; it is also here, so this is Head Lín Qì 臨泣 (GB 15).

目窗二穴，在臨泣後一寸。針三分，灸五壯。今附：三度刺，目大明。

Mù Chuāng 目窗 (GB 16), bilateral point: It is located 1.0 cùn posterior to Lín Qì 臨泣 (GB 15). Needle 3 fēn deep; burn five cones of moxibustion. Appended here: Needling it three times makes the vision brighter.

正營二穴，在目窗後一寸。針三分，灸五壯。

Zhèng Yíng 正營 (GB 17), bilateral point: It is located 1.0 cùn posterior to Mù Chuāng (GB 16). Needle 3 fēn deep; burn five cones of moxibustion.

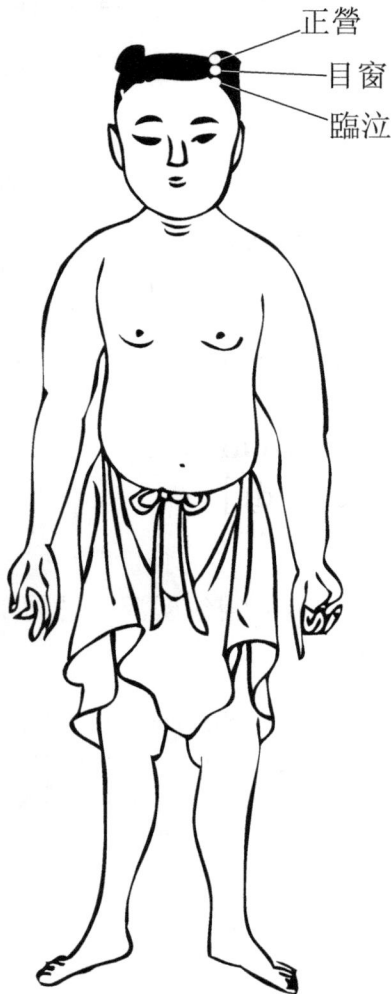

正營
目窗
臨泣

Fig. 1.5

承靈二穴，在正營後寸半。灸三壯。《素注》云：刺三分。

Chéng Líng 承靈 (GB 18), bilateral point: It is located 1.5 cùn posterior to Zhèng Yíng (GB 17). Burn three cones of moxibustion. *Sù Zhù*《素注》says: Needle 3 fēn deep.

腦空二穴，一名顳顬，在承靈後寸半，夾玉枕骨下陷中。針五分，得氣即瀉。灸三壯。曹操患頭風，發即心亂目眩，華佗針立愈。忌同。《素注》云：按腦空在完骨後，枕骨上。《甲乙經》作玉枕骨中。

Nǎo Kōng 腦空 (GB 19), bilateral point, another name is Niè Rú 顳顬: It is located 1.5 cùn posterior to Chéng Líng (GB 18), in the depression below the jade pillow bone [occipital bone]. Needle 5 fēn deep; drain [the point] as soon as qì arrives; burn three cones of moxibustion. Cáo Cāo suffered head wind; whenever it occurred he had derangement of the heart and dizzy vision. It was cured right after Huá Tuó[18] needled this point. Follow the same contraindications [as Shén Tíng 神庭 (Dū 24)]. *Sù Zhù* says: Nǎo Kōng (GB 19) is located posterior to the mastoid process and above the occipital bone. *Jiǎ Yǐ Jīng*《甲乙經》says: It is on the occipital bone.

---

18. Huá Tuó 華佗 (145-208) was a famous doctor of the Eastern *Hàn* (東漢) Dynasty.

風池二穴，在腦空後髮際中。針七分，留七呼，灸三壯。《明》云：在項後髮際陷中。《甲乙經》云：腦空後髮際陷中，針寸二分。大患風者先補後瀉，少可患者以經取之。留五呼，瀉七吸，灸不及針，日七壯，至百五。艾炷不用大。忌同。

Fēng Chí 風池 (GB 20), bilateral point: It is located within the hairline posterior to Nǎo Kōng 腦空 (GB 19). Needle 7 fēn deep; retain the needle for seven respirations; burn three cones of moxibustion. *Míng* 《明》 says: It is in the depression within hairline above nape of the neck. *Jiǎ Yǐ Jīng* 《甲乙經》 says: It is in the depression within the hairline posterior to Nǎo Kōng (GB 19). Needle 1.2 cùn deep. Use supplementation followed by draining for someone who suffers severe wind; for one with less suffering, select [points on] the channel. Retain the needle for five respirations; drain for seven respirations. Moxibustion is not as good as needling; burn seven cones of moxibustion daily up to one hundred and fifty cones. The size of the mugwort cone does not need to be large. Follow the same contraindications [as Shén Tíng 神庭 (Dū 24)].

當陽二穴，當瞳仁直上入髮際一寸。療卒不識人，風眩，鼻塞，針三分（《明下》）。

Dāng Yáng 當陽, bilateral point: It is located 1.0 cùn directly above pupil within the hairline. It treats sudden loss of consciousness, wind dizziness, and nasal congestion. Needle 3 fēn deep. (*Míng Xià* 《明下》) [19]

《銅人》無當陽穴，而《明堂下經》有之。理卒不識人，風眩，鼻塞等疾，亦不可廢者。其穴與臨泣相近，故附入於此。

[Author's note:] *Tóng Rén* 《銅人》 does not have the Dāng Yáng 當陽 point, but *Míng Táng Xià Jīng* 《明堂下經》 does. It regulates the disorders such as sudden loss of consciousness, wind dizziness, and nasal congestion, so it cannot be abandoned. This point is close to Lín Qì 臨泣 (GB 15), so it is appended here.

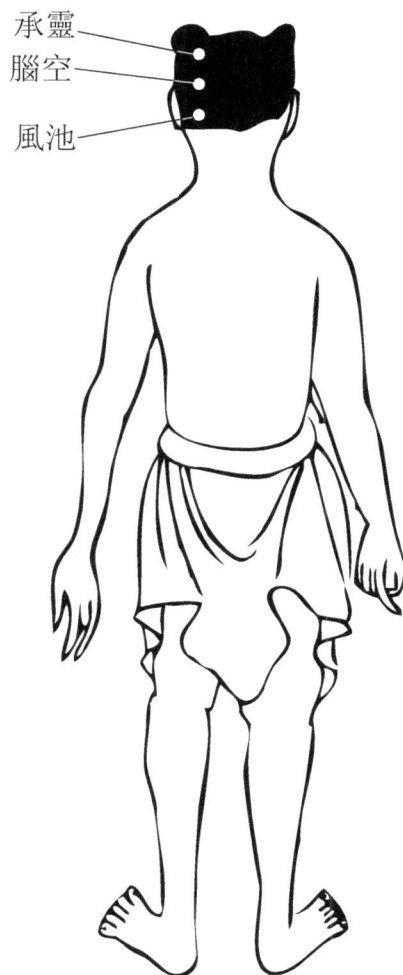

承靈
腦空
風池

Fig. 1.6

19. This section is from Volume 99 of *Tài Píng Shèng Huì Fāng* 《太平聖惠方》 (Sage-like Prescriptions of the Tài Píng Era). Volume 99 is also called *Míng Shàng* 《明上》. Volume 100 (*Míng Xià* 《明下》) is mistakenly cited here.

1.04
Cè Tóu Bù Zuǒ Yòu Èr Shí Liù Xué

側頭部左右二十六穴

Lateral side of the head,
26 bilateral points [thirteen on each side]

頷厭二穴，在曲周下（足少陽穴無下字，《明堂》同），腦空上廉。灸三
壯，針七分，留七呼。忌同。《明》云：二分。《素注》云：在曲角下，腦
空之上上廉。刺七分，若深令人耳無所聞。

Hàn Yàn 頷厭 (GB 4), bilateral point: It is located below the temporal hairline (the foot shàoyáng points [section of *Tóng Rén* 《銅人》] does not have the character *xià* 下 (below); *Míng Táng* 《明堂》 agrees), on the upper aspect of the pulsating vessel [the brain hollow].[20] Burn three cones of moxibustion; needle 7 fēn deep; retain the needle for seven respirations. Follow the same contraindications [as Shén Tíng 神庭 (Dū 24)]. *Míng* 《明》 says: 2 fēn deep. *Sù Zhù* 《素注》 says: It is below the curved corner, on the upper aspect above the pulsating vessel [the brain hollow]. Needle 7 fēn deep; it makes people deaf if needled too deeply.

懸顱二穴，在曲周上（足少陽穴同，《明堂》無上字）腦空中。灸三壯，針
三分，留三呼。《明》云：二分。《素注》云：在曲角上，腦空下廉。《
新校正》云：按後手少陽中云：角上。此云角下，必有一誤。（◎懸顱二
穴在曲角上，是。）

Xuán Lú 懸顱 (GB 5), bilateral point: It is located above the temporal hairline (The foot shàoyáng points [section of *Tóng Rén*] and *Míng Táng* do not have the word above (*shàng* 上)), on the pulsating vessel [the brain hollow]. Burn three cones of moxibustion; needle 3 fēn deep; retain the needle for three respirations. *Míng* says: 2 fēn deep. *Sù Zhù* says: It is above the curved corner, on the lower aspect of the pulsating vessel [the brain hollow]. *Xīn Jiào Zhèng* 《新校正》 (New Annotations and Corrections) says: Note that the following section on the hand shàoyáng [points] says above the corner. Here it says below the corner. One of them must be wrong. (*The bilateral point of Xuán Lú (GB 5) is definitely located above the curved corner.)

20. According to the *Sù Wèn* 《素問》 (which was annotated by Wáng Bīng 王冰) and *Tóng Rén* 《銅人》, Nǎo Kōng 腦空 should read Niè Rú 顳顬, which indicates the pulsating vessel anterior to the ear.

懸釐二穴，在曲周上（ 足少陽穴無上字 ），腦空下廉 。針三分，灸三壯 。

Xuán Lí 懸釐 (GB 6), bilateral point: It is located above the temporal hairline (The foot shàoyáng points [section of *Tóng Rén* 《 銅人 》] does not have the word above (*shàng* 上)[21]), on the lower aspect of pulsating vessel [the brain hollow]. Needle 3 fēn deep; burn three cones of moxibustion.

天衝二穴，在耳上如前三寸（ 足少陽穴同 ）。灸七壯，針三分 。

Tiān Chòng 天衝 (GB 9), bilateral point: It is located 3 cùn[22] above the ear (the foot shàoyáng points [the section of *Tóng Rén*] agrees), running anteriorly. Burn seven cones of moxibustion; needle 3 fēn deep.

率谷二穴，在耳上入髮際寸半，陷者宛宛中 。灸三壯，針三分 。《 明下 》云：嚼而取之 。

Shuài Gǔ 率谷 (GB 8), bilateral point: It is located in the depression 1.5 cùn above the ear, within the hairline. Burn three cones of moxibustion; needle 3 fēn deep. *Míng Xià* 《 明下 》 says: Locate the point while chewing.

曲鬢二穴，在耳上髮際曲隅陷中，鼓頷有空（ 《 明 》作穴 ）。針三分，灸七壯 。《 明下 》云：曲髮，灸三壯 。（ 《 指迷 》：在耳上，將耳掩前正尖上 。 ）

Qū Bìn 曲鬢 (GB 7), bilateral point: It is located in the depression on the curved corner [temporal hairline] above the ear. When chattering the jaw,[23] there is a hollow[24] (*Míng* 《 明 》 says point). Needle 3 fēn deep; burn seven cones of moxibustion. *Míng Xià* 《 明下 》 calls it Qū Fà 曲髮 (curved hair). Burn three cones of moxibustion. (*Zhǐ Mí* 《 指迷 》 (Comments on Confusion) says: It is above the ear, at the tip of the ear when it is folded forward.)

---

21. The word *shàng* 上 (above) is included in the foot shàoyáng points section in Volume 1 in *Tóng Rén* 《 銅人 》 (*Míng* Dynasty edition). It is unclear which other edition of *Tóng Rén* Wáng Zhízhōng 王執中 cited.

22. According to the five volume edition of *Tóng Rén Shū Xué Zhēn Jiǔ Tú Jīng* 《 銅人腧穴針灸圖經 》 (The Bronze Statue Illustrated Classic of Acupuncture Points), this point is located 3 fēn above the ear. But in the foot shàoyáng point section of Volume 1 of *Tóng Rén* 《 銅人 》, it is located 2 cùn posterior to the ear, within the hairline. It is not clear which book or edition Wáng Zhízhōng 王執中 cited; or perhaps he just made a mistake here.

23. Chattering of the jaws: In English, we say chattering teeth. This is due to the coldness.

24. *Kōng* 空 can be a synonym for *kǒng* 孔 which means hole or hollow.

《銅人》云：曲鬢，足少陽穴同，《素問》亦同。《明堂下經》云：
曲髮，疑髮字誤也。（◎曲鬢穴是，曲髮字誤）。

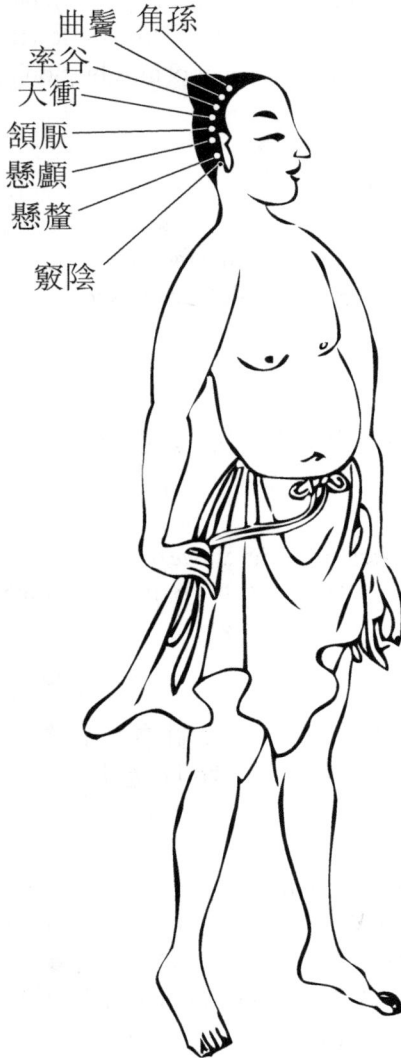

曲鬢　角孫
率谷
天衝
頷厭
懸顱
懸釐

竅陰

[Author's note:] *Tóng Rén* 《銅人》 calls [this point] Qū Bìn 曲鬢 (GB 7) in the foot shàoyáng points [section]; *Sù Wèn* 《素問》 agrees. *Míng Táng Xià Jīng* 《明堂下經》 calls it Qū Fà; *Fà* 髮 might be a typographical error.[25] (*It is Qū Bìn 曲鬢 (GB 7); Qū Fà is wrong.)

角孫二穴，在耳郭中間上，開口有空
（《明》作穴）。治目生膚翳，齒齗
腫。灸三壯。《明堂》別無療病法。
《明》云：主齒牙不嚼物，齲痛腫。
針八分。

Jiǎo Sūn 角孫 (SJ 20), bilateral point: It is located above the center of auricle, in the hollow (*Míng* says point) when the mouth is open. It treats skin screens in the eyes[26] and swollen gums. Burn three cones of moxibustion. *Míng Táng* 《明堂》 does not have [a listing of] disorders that it treats. *Míng* says: It treats inability to chew food and pain and swelling due to tooth decay. Needle 8 fēn deep.

按《明堂》云：角孫主齒牙不嚼
物，齲痛腫，則有療病法矣。《銅
人》乃云：《明堂》別無療病法，
豈後人增益之耶？將所治止此，因
謂之無療病法歟？

Fig. 1.7

[Author's note:] According to *Míng Táng*: Jiǎo Sūn (SJ 20) treats inability to chew food and pain and swelling due to tooth decay; these are the disorders that it treats. *Tóng Rén* says: *Míng Táng* does not have [a listing of] disorders that it treats. Could it have been added by later generations? How can it say there is no [listing of] disorders it can treat when the indications are right here?

---

25. *Bìn* 鬢 specifies the hair near the ear, while *fà* 髮 indicates the hair around the forehead, ears, and head. These two words look similar so they are easily substituted for each other.

26. *Fū yì* 膚翳 (Skin screens) indicate an eye disease with a thin screen like the wing of a fly over the eye.

竅陰二穴，在枕骨下（足少陽穴云在完骨上），搖動有空。針三分，灸七壯。《明》云：五壯，針四分。在完骨上，枕骨下（完骨二穴在耳後入髮際四分）。

Qiào Yīn 竅陰 (GB 11), bilateral point: It is located below the occipital bone (the foot shàoyáng points [section of *Tóng Rén*] says above the mastoid process), in the hollow when shaking [the head]. Needle 3 fēn deep; burn seven cones of moxibustion. *Míng* 《明》 says: Five cones; needle 4 fēn deep. It is located above the mastoid process and below the occipital bone. (The bilateral point of Wán Gǔ 完骨 (GB 12) is located 4 fēn posterior to the ear, within the hairline.)

此有竅陰矣，足少陽膽經亦有此穴，此當為頭竅陰也。

[Author's note:] Here, there is Qiào Yīn 竅陰 (GB 11); the section for the foot shàoyáng channel also has a point [with this name]. This one should be called Head Qiào Yīn 頭竅陰 (GB 11).

浮白二穴，在耳後入髮際一寸。針五分，灸七壯。《明》云：三壯，針三分。

Fú Bái 浮白 (GB 10), bilateral point: It is located 1.0 cùn posterior to the ear, within the hairline. Needle 5 fēn deep; burn seven cones of moxibustion. *Míng* says: Three cones; needle 3 fēn deep.

顱息二穴，在耳後間青絡脈。灸七壯，不宜針。《明》云：顱息在耳後青脈間。灸三壯，針一分，不得多出血，出血多殺人。

Lú Xī 顱息 (SJ 19), bilateral point: It is located on the green-blue network vessels in the space posterior to the ear. Burn seven cones of moxibustion; needling is not recommended. *Míng* says: Lú Xī (SJ 19) is located between the green-blue vessels posterior to the ear. Burn three cones of moxibustion; needle 1 fēn deep. Bleeding a lot is contraindicated; bleeding a lot can kill people.

瘈脈二穴，一名資脈。在耳本後雞足青絡脈。刺出血如豆汁，不宜出血多，灸三壯，針一分。《明》云：在耳內雞足青脈。

Chì Mài 瘈脈 (SJ 18), bilateral point, another name is Zī Mài 資脈. It is located in the green-blue network vessels that look like a chicken's claw, posterior to the root of the ear. Prick it to obtain blood that resembles bean juice; bleeding a lot is not recommended. Burn three cones of moxibustion; needle 1 fēn deep. *Míng* 《明》 says: It is in the green-blue network vessels that look like a chicken's-claw posterior to the ear.

完骨二穴，在耳後入髮際四分。灸七壯，針三分。《明》云：二分，灸依年
壯。

Wán Gǔ 完骨 (GB 12), bilateral point: It is located 4 fēn posterior to the ear, within the hairline. Burn seven cones of moxibustion; needle 3 fēn deep. *Míng* says: 2 fēn deep; burn the same number of cones as the age of the patient.

翳風二穴，在耳後陷中，按之引耳中。針七分，灸七壯。《明下》云：三
壯，在耳後尖角陷中。

Yì Fēng 翳風 (SJ 17), bilateral point: It is located in the depression posterior to the ear; when pressed, [a sensation] radiates into the ear. Needle 7 fēn deep; burn seven cones of moxibustion. *Míng Xià* 《明下》 says: Three cones. It is located in the depression at the pointed angle posterior to the ear.

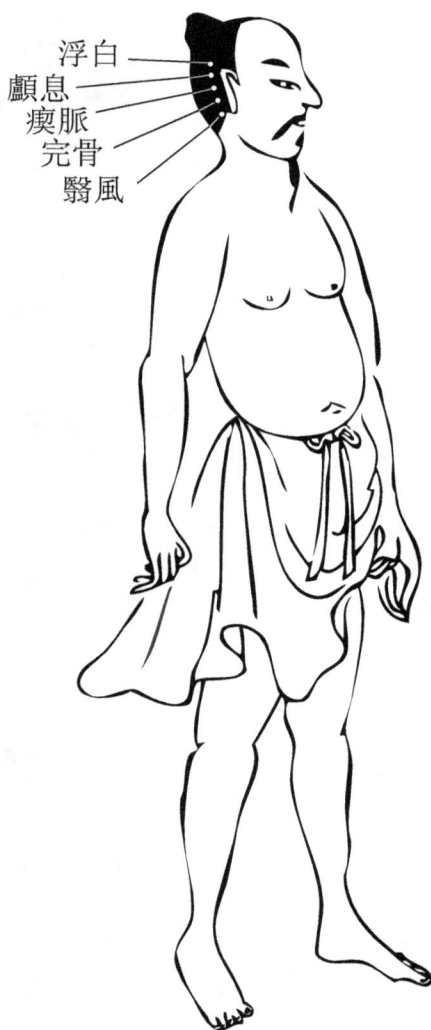

浮白
顱息
瘈脈
完骨
翳風

Fig. 1.8

1.05
Zhèng Miàn Bù Zhōng Háng Liù Xué

正面部中行六穴

6 points on the midline of the face

素髎一名面王 。在鼻柱之端 。《 外臺 》云：不宜灸，針一分 。

Sù Liáo 素髎 (Dū 25), another name is Miàn Wáng 面王. It is located on the tip of the nose pillar [stem of the nose]. *Wài Tái* 《 外臺 》 says: Moxibustion is not recommended; needle 1 fēn deep.

水溝一名人中 。在鼻柱下 。針四分，留五呼，得氣即瀉 。灸不及針，日三壯，若灸，可艾炷如小雀糞 。風水面腫，針此一穴，出水盡，頓愈 。忌同 。《 明 》云：日灸三壯，至二百罷 。若是水氣，唯得針此穴，若針餘穴，水盡即死 。《 下 》云：灸五壯 。

Shuǐ Gōu 水溝 (Dū 26), another name is Rén Zhōng 人中. It is located directly below the nose pillar [stem of the nose]. Needle 4 fēn deep; retain the needle for 5 respirations; drain [the point] as soon as qì arrives. Moxibustion is not as good as needling; burn three cones of moxibustion per day; use small mugwort cones the size of sparrow droppings. Needle this point for wind-water with facial swelling; it will discharge the water completely and bring about an immediate cure. Follow the same contraindications [as Shén Tíng 神庭 (Dū 24)]. *Míng* 《 明 》 says: Burn three cones of moxibustion daily; up to two hundred cones. If there is water qì, this is the only point to needle; needling other points makes people die when the water is completely [discharged]. *Xià* 《 下 》 says: Burn five cones of moxibustion.

兌端，在唇上端 。針二分，灸三壯，炷如大麥 。《 明下 》云：在頤前下唇下，開口取之 。

Duì Duān 兌端 (Dū 27): It is located at the tip of the [upper] lip. Needle 2 fēn deep; burn three cones of moxibustion. Use grain-of-wheat size cones. *Míng Xià* 《 明下 》 says: It is below the lip, inferior and anterior to the cheek. Locate the point with the mouth open.

齦交，在唇內齒上齗縫筋中。針三分，灸三壯。

Yín Jiāo 齦交 (Dū 28): It is located in the cleft of sinew on the upper gum inside the lip. Needle 3 fēn deep; burn three cones of moxibustion.

承漿一名懸漿。在頤前唇下宛宛中。日灸七壯，止七七。灸即血脈通宣，其風立愈。炷依小箸頭作。針三分，得氣即瀉。忌同。《明》云：頤前下唇之下。針三分半，得氣即瀉，瀉盡更留三呼，徐徐引氣而出，日灸七壯，過七七，停四五日後，灸七七。若一向灸，恐足陽明脈斷，令風不差。停息復灸，令血脈通宣，其風立愈。《下》云：下唇稜下宛中。

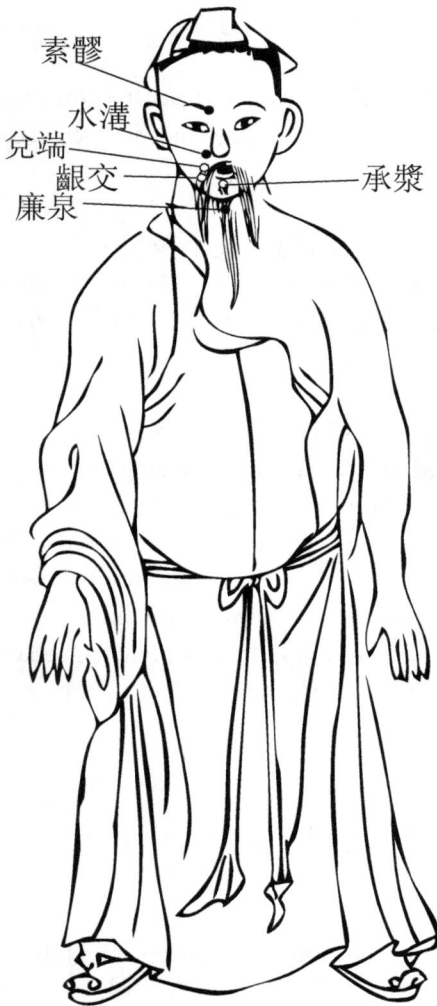

Fig. 1.9

素髎
水溝
兌端
齦交
廉泉
承漿

Chéng Jiāng 承漿 (Rèn 24), another name is Xuán Jiāng 懸漿. It is located in the depression inferior to the [lower] lip, anterior to the cheeks. Burn seven cones of moxibustion daily, up to seven times seven cones. Moxibustion can free and diffuse the blood vessels, thus immediately curing wind. Make the cones the size of the head of a small chopstick. Needle 3 fēn deep; drain [the point] as soon as qì arrives. Follow the same contraindications [as Shén Tíng 神庭 (Dū 24)]. *Míng* 《明》 says: It is below the lower lip and anterior to the cheeks. Needle 3.5 fēn deep; drain [the point] as soon as qì arrives; retain the needles for another three respirations after draining; guide the qì out slowly. Burn seven cones of moxibustion daily; stop for four or five days after seven times seven cones; then burn another seven times seven cones. If moxibustion is applied continuously, it might break the foot yángmíng vessel [channel], and the wind would not be cured. Stopping for a while, then applying moxibustion again will free and diffuse the blood vessels, thus immediately curing the wind. *Xià* 《下》 says: It is in the depression below the lower lip.

廉泉一名舌本，在頷下結喉上（《明》云：舌本間）。灸三壯，針三分，得氣即瀉。《明》云：二分。（《千》云：當頤直下骨後陷中。）

Lián Quán 廉泉 (Rèn 23), another name is Shé Běn 舌本: It is above laryngeal prominence and below the chin (*Míng* 《 明 》 says: It is on the root of the tongue). Burn three cones of moxibustion; needle 3 fēn deep. Drain [the point] as soon as qì arrives. *Míng* says: 2 fēn deep. (*Qiān* 《 千 》 (Thousand)[27] says: It is in the depression directly below the cheek and posterior to the bone.)

1.06
Miàn Dì Èr Háng Zuǒ Yòu Shí Xué

面第二行左右十穴

The second line on the face,
10 bilateral points [five on each side]

攢竹二穴，一名始光，一名光明，一名員柱 。在兩眉頭少陷宛宛中 。不宜灸，針一分，留三呼，瀉三吸，徐徐出針 。宜以細三稜針刺之，宣洩熱氣 。三度刺，目大明 。忌同 。《 明 》云：宜細三稜針，針三分，出血 。《 下 》云：灸一壯 。

Zǎn Zhú 攢竹 (UB 2), bilateral point, another name is Shǐ Guāng 始光, another name is Guāng Míng 光明, another name is Yuán Zhù 員柱. It is located in the small depression at the head [medial end] of the eyebrows. Moxibustion is not recommended; needle 1 fēn deep; retain the needle for three respirations; drain for three respirations; remove the needle slowly. It is appropriate to prick it with a thin, three-edged needle to diffuse and let out the hot qì. Needling three times makes the vision brighter. Follow the same contraindications [as Shén Tíng 神庭 (Dū 24)]. *Míng* says: It is appropriate to use a thin three-edged needle; needle 3 fēn deep; bleed it. *Xià* 《 下 》 says: Burn one cone of moxibustion.

晴明二穴，一名淚孔，在目內眥 。針寸半，留三呼 。雀目者可久留針，然後速出，禁灸 。忌同 。《 明 》云：目內眥頭外畔陷宛宛中 。針[一]分半，留三呼，補，不宜灸 。一云：在目內眥外一分 。

---

27. *Qiān* 《 千 》 (Thousand) may refer to *Qiān Jīn Yì Fāng* 《 千金翼方 》 (Appendix to Prescriptions Worth a Thousand Pieces of Gold) or *Qiān Jīn Fāng* 《 千金方 》 (Prescriptions Worth a Thousand Pieces of Gold). Here, it refers to the former.

Jīng Míng 睛明 (UB 1), bilateral point, another name is Lèi Kǒng 淚孔: It is located at the inner canthus of the eye. Needle 1.5 cùn deep; retain the needle for three respirations. Retain the needle for a long time when [the patient has] sparrow vision.[28] Then remove the needle rapidly. Moxibustion is contraindicated. Follow the same contraindications [as Shén Tíng 神庭 (Dū 24)]. *Míng* 《明》 says: It is in the depression lateral to the end of the inner canthus of the eye. Needle 1.5[29] fēn deep; retain the needle for three respirations; use supplementation. Moxibustion is not recommended. One source says: It is 1 fēn lateral to the inner canthus of the eye.

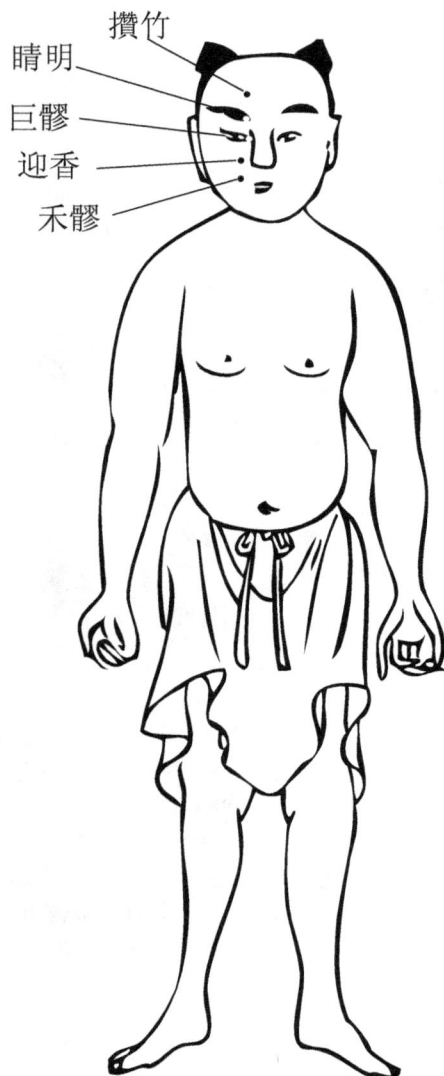

攢竹
睛明
巨髎
迎香
禾髎

Fig. 1.10

按《明堂》云：針一分半，《銅
人》乃云入一寸半，二者必有一
誤。予觀面部所針，淺者入一分，
深者四分爾。而《素問·氣府》注
亦云刺入一分，則是《銅人》誤寫
一分為一寸也。

[Author's note:] Note that *Míng Táng* 《明堂》 says: Needle 1.5 fēn deep, while *Tóng Rén* 《銅人》 says 1.5 cùn deep; one of them must be wrong. I have observed needling on the face: superficial needling is 1 fēn deep while deep needling is only 4 fēn deep. The Annotation to *Sù Wèn · Qì Fǔ*[30] 《素問·氣府》 also say to needle 1 fēn deep. So *Tóng Rén* mistakenly wrote 1 cùn instead of 1 fēn.

巨髎二穴，夾鼻孔兩旁八分，直目瞳
子。蹻脈、足陽明之會。針三分，得
氣即瀉，灸七壯。《明》云：巨窌在
鼻孔下夾水溝旁八分。蹻脈、足陽明
之會。針三分，灸七七壯。

Jù Liáo 巨髎 (ST 3), bilateral point: It is located 8 fēn to the sides of the nostrils, directly in-line

---

28. Sparrow vision indicates blurred vision in the night. It is caused by insufficiency of the prenatal source, or liver deficiency.

29. The character *yī* 一 (one) should be inserted in the Chinese text, based on *Tài Píng Shèng Huì Fāng* 《太平聖惠方》 (Sage-like Prescriptions of Tài Píng Era).

30. This is referring to *Sù Wèn* 《素問》 (Plain Questions), Chapter 59.

with the pupils. It is a meeting point of the [yáng]qiāo mài and the foot yángmíng [channel]. Needle 3 fēn deep; drain [the point] as soon as qì arrives; burn seven cones of moxibustion. *Míng* 《明》 says: Jù Liáo 巨窌 (ST 3) is located below the nostrils, 8 fēn lateral to Shuǐ Gōu 水溝 (Dū 26). It is the meeting point of the [yáng]qiáo vessel and the foot yángmíng. Needle 3 fēn deep; burn seven times seven cones of moxibustion.

迎香二穴，在禾髎上一寸，鼻下孔旁五分 。針三分，留三呼，不宜灸 。忌同 。

Yíng Xiāng 迎香 (LI 20), bilateral point: It is located 1 cùn above Hé Liáo 禾髎 (LI 19), 5 fēn lateral to the nostrils. Needle 3 fēn deep; retain the needle for three respirations; moxibustion is not recommended. Follow the same contraindications [as Shén Tíng 神庭 (Dū 24).

禾髎二穴，在鼻孔下，夾水溝旁五分 。針二分 。又手陽明穴云：禾髎，一名長頻，直鼻孔，夾水溝旁五分 。《明》云：和窌，在鼻孔下，夾水溝旁五分 。《下》云：禾窌，在鼻孔下夾水溝旁五分 。灸三壯 。

Hé Liáo 禾髎 (LI 19), bilateral point: It is located below the nostrils, 5 fēn lateral to Shuǐ Gōu (Dū 26). Needle 2 fēn deep. The hand yángmíng points [section of *Tóng Rén* 《銅人》 [31] also says: Hé Liáo (LI 19), another name is Cháng Pín 長頻: It is directly in line with the nostrils, 5 fēn lateral to Shuǐ Gōu (Dū 26). *Míng* says: Hé Liáo 和窌 (LI 19) is below the nostrils, 5 fēn lateral to Shuǐ Gōu (Dū 26). *Xià* 《下》 says: Hé Liáo 禾窌 (LI 19) is below the nostrils, 5 fēn lateral to Shuǐ Gōu (Dū 26). Burn three cones of moxibustion.

《銅人經》：禾髎，在鼻孔下，夾水溝旁五分。《明堂下經》作禾窌，窌，即髎也。《上經》乃作和窌，皆云：在鼻孔下，夾水溝旁五分，則是一穴也。而《銅人》手少陽穴復有和窌二穴，在耳前兌（《素問》作銳）髮陷中。其穴相去遠矣。恐《明堂上經》誤寫禾字作和字也。（◎今以諸經校勘，禾髎穴者是。）

[Author's note:] *Tóng Rén Jīng* 《銅人經》 says: Hé Liáo 禾髎 (LI 19) is below the nostrils, 5 fēn lateral to Shuǐ Gōu (Dū 26). *Míng Táng Xià Jīng* 《明堂下經》 says [in the point name] Hé Liáo 禾窌, *liáo* 窌 means *liáo* 髎 [the cleft of a bone]. [*Míng Táng*] *Shàng Jīng* 《上經》 calls it Hé Liáo 和窌. All of them say: It is below the nostrils, 5 fēn lateral to Shuǐ Gōu (Dū 26), so it is [all] the same point. However, there are also the bilateral points of Hé Liáo 和窌 in the hand shàoyáng points [section] of *Tóng Rén*; it is located in the depression anterior to the ear, within the

---

31. Hand yángmíng points refers to a section of *Tóng Rén Shū Xué Zhēn Jiǔ Tú Jīng* 《銅人腧穴針灸圖經》 (The Bronze Statues Illustrated Classic of Acupuncture Points) Volume 1.

tapered[32] hairline. These points are far from each other. I suspect *Míng Táng Shàng Jīng* may have accidentally written Hé 和 instead of Hé 禾. (*Now corrected by comparing it with all the other classics: Hé Liáo 禾髎 (LI 19) is correct.)

1.07
Miàn Dì Sān Háng Zuǒ Yòu Shí Xué

面第三行左右十穴

The third line on the face,
10 bilateral points [five on each side]

陽白二穴，在眉上一寸，直目瞳子。灸三壯，針入二分。

Yáng Bái 陽白 (GB 14) bilateral point: It is located 1 cùn above the eyebrows, directly above the pupil. Burn three cones of moxbustion; needle 2 fēn deep.

承泣二穴，在目下七分，直目瞳子陷中。禁針，針之令人目烏色，可灸三壯，炷如大麥。忌同。《明》云：針入四分半，得氣即瀉。特不宜灸。若灸，無問多少，三日後眼下大如拳，息肉日加長如桃大，至三十日定不見物，妨或如五升許大。

Chéng Qì 承泣 (ST 1), bilateral point: It is located 7 fēn below the eyes, in the depression directly below the pupil. Needling is contraindicated; it causes black eyes. It is appropriate to burn three grain-of-wheat size cones of moxibustion. Follow the same contraindications [as Shén Tíng 神庭 (Dū 24)]. *Míng*《 明 》says: Needle 4.5 fēn deep; drain [the point] as soon as qì arrives. In particular, moxibustion is not recommended. If you apply moxibustion to it, [the patient] will have [a bump] as big as a fist below their eyes three days later, regardless of the quantity of cones that are used, and the polyps will grow bigger each day until it is the size of a peach. [The patient] will certainly not be able to see anything by the thirtieth day when the damage may be around 5 *shēng*[33] in size.

---

32. *Tóng Rén*《 銅人 》(The Bronze Statue Illustrated Classic of Acupuncture Points) uses *duì* 兌; *Sù Wèn*《 素問 》(Plain Questions) uses *ruì* 銳. They are used as the same word in ancient literature, meaning sharp or tapered.

33. *Shēng* 升 is a unit of dry measurement for grain, equal to 1 deciliter. Here it indicates how serious the damage is.

《銅人》云：此穴可灸三壯。禁針，針之令人目烏色。《明堂》乃
云：針入四分半，特不宜灸，灸後眼下大如拳。二家必各有所據，未
知其孰是，不針不灸可也。

[Author's note:] *Tóng Rén*《銅人》says: It is appropriate to burn three cones of moxibustion, but needling is contraindicated; it causes black eyes. *Míng Táng*《明堂》says: Needle 4.5 fēn deep; in particular, moxibustion is not recommended as [the patient] will have [a bump] as big as fist below their eyes after moxibustion is applied. Both schools must have their own sources. We cannot be sure which one is correct. So it is inappropriate to needle and apply moxibustion.

四白二穴，在目下一寸。灸七壯，
針三分。凡用針，穩審方得下針，
深即令人目烏色。

Sì Bái 四白 (ST 2), bilateral point: It is located 1 cùn below the eyes. Burn seven cones of moxibustion; needle 3 fēn deep. When using acupuncture, you must insert the needle after checking properly; needling too deep will cause black eyes.

地倉二穴，夾口吻旁四分，外如近
下，有脈微微動是也。針三分（《
明》云：針三分半），留五呼，
得氣即瀉。日可灸二七壯，重者七
七。炷如粗釵腳大，炷若大，口轉
喎，卻灸承漿七七即愈。忌同。

Dì Cāng 地倉 (ST 4), bilateral point: It is located 4 fēn lateral to the corner of the mouth. There is a vessel that pulsates lightly inferior and lateral [to the mouth]. Needle 3 fēn deep (*Míng*《明》says: Needle 3.5 fēn deep); retain the needle for five respirations, drain [the point] as soon as qì arrives. Burn two times seven cones, the size of the leg of a thick hairpin daily, and seven times seven cones for

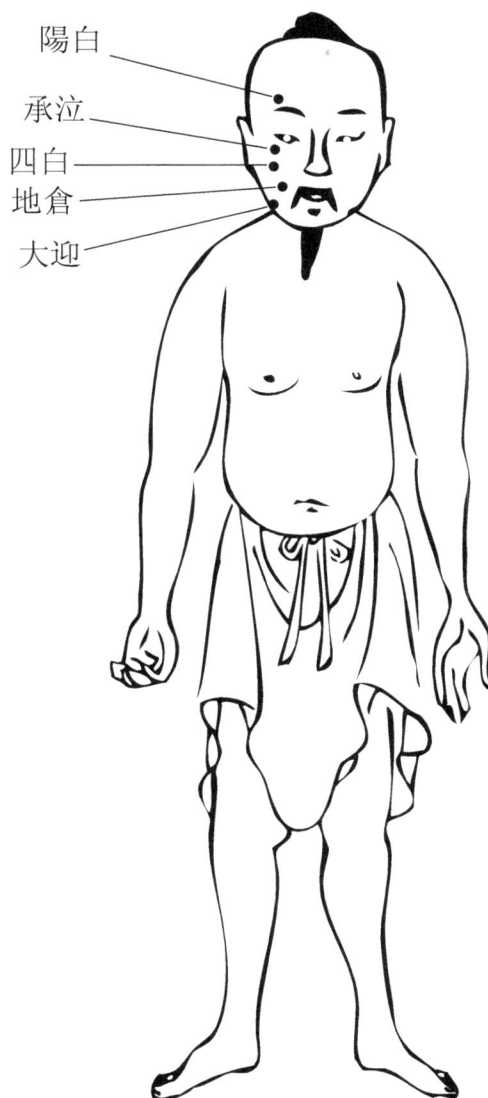

陽白
承泣
四白
地倉
大迎

Fig. 1.11

25

severe cases. [The patient will suffer] deviation of the mouth if the size of the cone is too big, but it can be cured by applying seven times seven cones of moxibustion to Chéng Jiāng 承漿 (Rèn 24). Follow the same contraindications [as Shén Tíng 神庭 (Dū 24)].

大迎二穴，在曲頷前寸二分，骨陷中動脈。又以口下當兩肩。針三分，留七呼，灸三壯。

Dà Yíng 大迎 (ST 5), bilateral point: It is located 1.2 cùn anterior to the angle of the mandible, in the depression on the bone where there is a pulsating vessel. It is below the mouth and on a line [drawn between the corner of the mouth and] the shoulder. Needle 3 fēn deep, retain the needle for seven respirations; burn three cones of moxibustion.

1.08
Miàn Dì Sì Háng Zuǒ Yòu Shí Xué

面第四行左右十穴

The fourth line on the face,
10 bilateral points [five on each side]

本神二穴，在曲差旁寸半。一云：直耳上入髮際四分。針二分，灸七壯。（二說相去遠矣，可疑。《千》云：耳正直上入髮際二分。）

Běn Shén 本神 (GB 13), bilateral point: It is located 1.5 cùn lateral to Qū Chā 曲差 (UB 4). One source says: It is 4 fēn directly above the ear, within the hairline. Needle 2 fēn deep; burn seven cones of moxibustion. (There is a big difference between the two opinions, so it is dubious. *Qiān* 《千》 says: 2 fēn directly above the ear, within the hairline.)

絲竹空二穴，一名目髎。在眉後陷中。針三分，留二呼，宜瀉不宜補。禁灸，使人目小，又令目無所見。

Sī Zhú Kōng 絲竹空 (SJ 23), bilateral point: Another name is Mù Liáo 目髎. It is located in the depression at the lateral end of the eyebrow. Needle 3 fēn deep, retain the needle for two respirations; it is appropriate to drain, but not to supplement. Moxibustion is contraindicated; it causes the eyes to become small and blind.

瞳子髎二穴，在目外眥五分 。灸三壯，針三分 。《 素注 》：在目外去眥五分 。（《 千 》注：一名太陽，一名前關 。 ）

Tóng Zǐ Liáo 瞳子髎 (GB 1), bilateral point: It is located 5 fēn lateral to the outer canthus. Burn three cones of moxibustion; needle 3 fēn deep. *Sù Zhù* 《 素注 》 says: It is on the lateral side of the eyes, 5 fēn from outer canthus. (A note in *Qiān* 《 千 》 says: Another name is Tài Yáng 太陽, another name is Qián Guān 前關).

顴髎二穴，在面頰骨下廉兌骨陷中 。針二分 。

Quán Liáo 顴髎 (SI 18), bilateral point: It is located on the lower ridge of the cheekbone, in the depression on the sharp bone. Needle 2 fēn deep.

頭維二穴，在額角入髮際本神旁寸半 。針三分，禁灸 。（ 本神在曲差旁寸半 。 ）

Tóu Wéi 頭維 (ST 8), bilateral point: It is located at the corner of forehead, within the [anterior] hairline, 1.5 cùn lateral to Běn Shén 本神 (GB 13). Needle 3 fēn deep; moxibustion is contraindicated. (Běn Shén (GB 13) is located 1.5 cùn lateral to Qū Chā 曲差 (UB 4).)

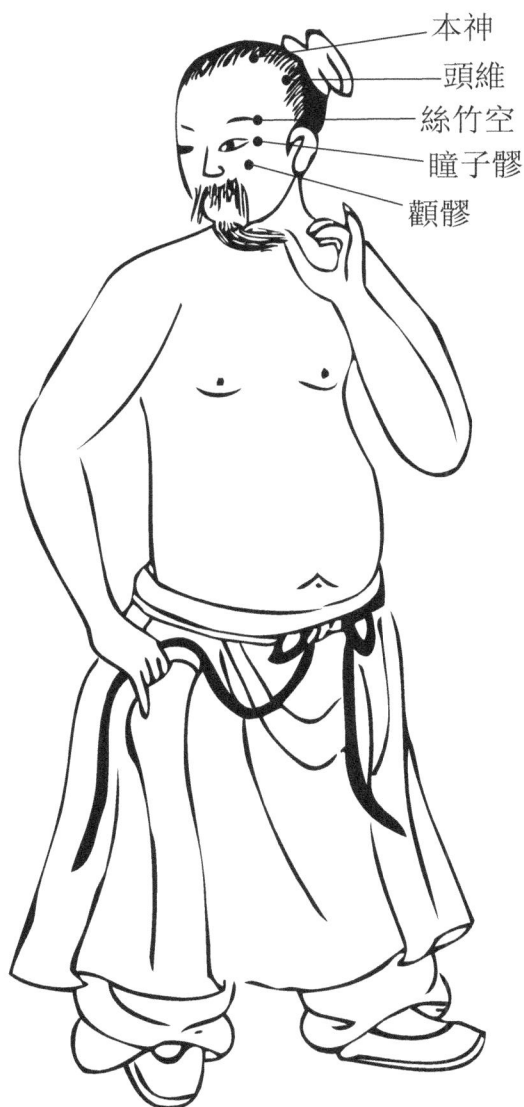

本神
頭維
絲竹空
瞳子髎
顴髎

Fig. 1.12

27

1.09
Cè Miàn Bù Zuǒ Yòu Shí Sì Xué (Gèng Èr Xué)

側面部左右十四穴（更二穴）

Lateral side of the face,
14 bilateral points [seven on each side]
(plus one more bilateral point)

上關二穴，一名客主人。在耳前起骨上廉，開口有空動脈宛宛中。灸七壯，艾炷不用大，箸頭作炷。若針，必須側臥張口取之乃得，禁針深。問曰：何以不得針深？岐伯曰：上關若刺深，令人欠而不得欯。下關久留針，即欯而不得欠，牙關急。是故上關不得刺深，下關不得久留針也。《明》云：客主二穴，針入一分留之，得氣即瀉。日灸七壯，至二百，炷不用大。其針灸之，必須側臥張口取之，乃得穴，避風。《千》云：灸一壯。

Shàng Guān 上關 (GB 3), bilateral point, another name is Kè Zhǔ Rén 客主人: It is located anterior to the ear, at the upper ridge of the protuberance of the bone. It is in the hollow when the mouth is opened; there is pulsating vessel in the depression. Burn seven cones of moxibustion; the size of the cone cannot be large; use cones the size of the head of a chopstick. If performing acupuncture, one must locate the point while [the patient] lies on his side and opens his mouth; deep needling is contraindicated. Question: Why can't it be deeply needled? Qí Bó answered: If Shàng Guān (GB 3) is needled deeply, people will yawn but cannot open their mouth. If the needle is retained in Xià Guān 下關 (ST 7) too long, people will open their mouth but cannot yawn, and they can also have clenched jaws. That's why Shàng Guān (GB 3) cannot be needled deeply and the needle cannot be retained in Xià Guān (ST 7) for a long time either. *Míng* 《 明 》 says: Needle 1 fēn deep on both points of Kè Zhǔ (GB 3) and retain the needle; drain [the point] as soon as qì arrives. Burn seven cones of moxibustion daily, up to two hundred cones; the size of the cone cannot be large. When applying acupuncture and moxibustion, find the point with the patient lying on their side with their mouth open. Wind should be avoided. *Qiān* 《 千 》 says: Burn one cone of moxibustion.

按《素問》刺禁曰：刺客主人內陷中脈，為內漏，為聾。注云：言刺太深，則交脈破決，故為耳內之漏，脈內漏則氣不營，故聾。審若是，又不止，令人欠而不得欯而已。用針者所當知也。

[Author's note:] *Sù Wèn · Cì Jìn* 《素問·刺禁》 (Plain Questions · Treatise on Needling Contraindications)[34] says: Pricking the vessel in the depression of Kè Zhǔ Rén 客主人 (GB 3) causes internal leakage[35] or deafness. [Wáng Bīng's] Annotation says: If needled too deeply, it will break the intersecting vessels and cause leakage in the ear. The internal leakage of the vessel will deplete the nourishment of qì, thus causing deafness. If that happens, and the internal leakage cannot be stopped, the person will yawn but cannot open their mouth.[36] The acupuncturist should know this.

下關二穴，在上關下，耳前動脈下廉，合口有空，開口即閉。針入四分，得氣即瀉，禁灸。又云：下關不得久留針（見上），側臥閉口取穴。

Xià Guān 下關 (ST 7), bilateral point: It is located below Shàng Guān 上關 (GB 3), on the lower aspect of the pulsating vessel anterior to the ear. There is a hollow with the mouth closed; the hollow disappears when the mouth opens. Needle 4 fēn deep, drain [the point] as soon as qì arrives. Moxibustion is contraindicated. It is also said: Do not retain the needle in Xià Guān 下關 (ST 7) for too long (see above). Locate the point while the patient lies on their side with their mouth closed.

前關二穴，在目後半寸，亦名太陽之穴。理風，赤眼頭痛，目眩目澀。不灸，針三分（《明》）。

Qián Guān 前關 (GB 1), bilateral point: It is located 0.5 cùn posterior to the eyes; it is also named Tài Yáng 太陽. It regulates wind, red eyes, headaches, dizzy vision and dry eyes. Moxibustion is contraindicated; needle 3 fēn deep. (*Míng* 《明》)

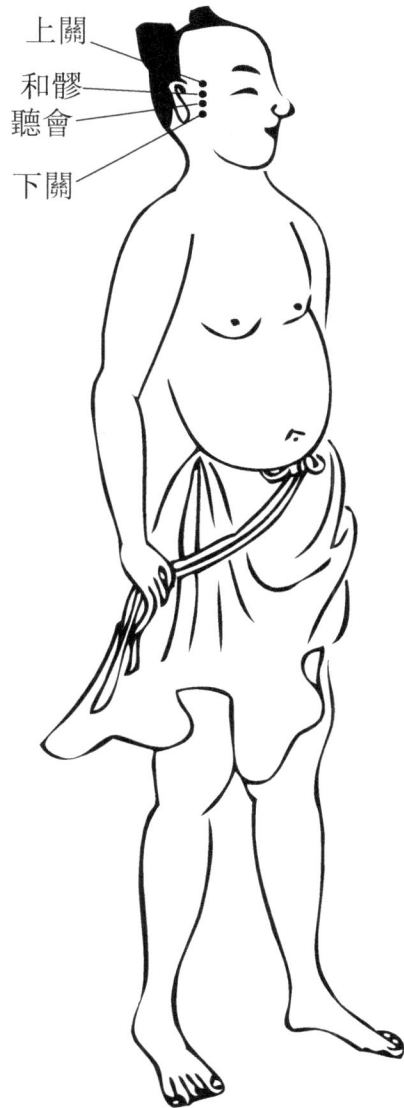

上關
和髎
聽會
下關

Fig. 1.13

---

34. This refers to *Sù Wèn* 《刺禁》 (Plain Questions), Chapter 52.

35. *Nèi lòu* 內漏 (internal leakage): after accidently puncturing the vessel, the bleeding does not stop, causing a fistula or discharge of pus.

36. Based on the text above, *yú* 歟 is a typographical error for *qū* 欼.

《銅人》有上關、下關各二穴，《素問》亦同，但《明堂》上、下經有上關，而無下關，惟上經有前關穴，又不與下關穴同，在上關之下，恐別自是。前關穴一名太陽穴，理風，赤眼頭痛，目眩澀等疾所不可廢，故附入於下關之後。

[Author's note:] *Tóng Rén* 《銅人》 and *Sù Wèn* 《素問》 both have Shàng Guān 上關 (GB 3) and Xià Guān 下關 (ST 7), each bilateral. Yet *Míng Táng Shàng* and *Xià Jīng* 《明堂上、下經》 have Shàng Guān (GB 3) but do not have Xià Guān (ST 7). Only *Shàng Jīng* 《上經》 has Qián Guān 前關 (GB 1) but it is not the same as Xià Guān (ST 7). Xià Guān (ST 7) is located below Shàng Guān (GB 3), so it must be different from this [*Qián* Guān (GB 1)]. Qián Guān 前關穴 is also named Tài Yáng 太陽. It regulates diseases such as wind, red eyes, headaches, dizzy vision and dry eyes, so it cannot be abandoned. Therefore it is appended after Xià Guān (ST 7).

和髎二穴，在耳前兌髮下橫動脈。針七分，灸三壯。《素注》：在耳前銳髮下橫動脈。

Hé Liáo 和髎 (SJ 22), bilateral point: It is located anterior to the ear, on the transverse pulsating vessel below the tapered hair. Needle 7 fēn deep; burn three cones of moxibustion. *Sù Zhù* 《素注》 says: [It is located] anterior to the ear, on the transverse pulsating vessel below the sharp hair.

和髎二穴在耳前銳髮陷中。《明堂上經》亦有和窌二穴。窌，即髎也，在鼻孔下，夾水溝旁五分，即《銅人》之禾髎，《明堂下經》之禾窌也。或者《明堂上經》誤寫"禾"字作"和"字爾，恐人以和髎、和窌為一穴，故備論之。

[Author's note:] The bilateral point of Hé Liáo 和髎 (SJ 22) is located anterior to the ear, in the depression in the tapered hair. The bilateral point of Hé Liáo 和窌 [is also listed] in *Míng Táng Shàng Jīng* 《明堂上經》. *Liáo* 窌 means *liáo* 髎 [a cleft in the bone]. It is located below the nostrils (ala nasi), 5 fēn lateral to Shuǐ Gōu 水溝 (Dū 26). This is the same as Hé Liáo 禾髎 (LI 19) in *Tóng Rén* and Hé Liáo 禾窌 in *Míng Táng Xià Jīng* 《明堂下經》. Perhaps [the author of] *Míng Táng Shàng Jīng* accidentally wrote 和 instead of 禾. I fear people might think Hé Liáo 和髎 (SJ 22) and Hé Liáo 和窌 (LI 19) are the same point, so it is discussed here.

聽會二穴，在耳微前陷中，上關下一寸動脈宛宛中，張口得之。針七分，留三呼，得氣即瀉，不須補。日灸五壯，止三七壯，十日後依前報灸。《明》云：針三分，忌冷食呵。《下》云：灸三壯（一云聽呵，前一云：後關名聽會）。一名聽呵。

Tīng Huì 聽會 (GB 2), bilateral point: It is located in the depression slightly anterior to the ear, 1 cùn below Shàng Guān 上關 (GB 3), in the depression on the pulsating vessel. Locate the point with the mouth open. Needle 7 fēn deep, retain the needle for three respirations, drain [the point] as soon as qì arrives, Supplementation is not necessary. Burn five cones of moxibustion daily, up to three times seven cones. Repeat the previously described moxibustion sessions ten days later. *Míng* 《 明 》 says: Needle 3 fēn deep. Cold food is contraindicated. *Xià* 《 下 》 says: Burn three cones of moxibustion. (One source says [this point is named] Tīng Hē 聽呵; an earlier [source] says: Hòu Guān 後關 is a name for Tīng Huì) Another name is Tīng Hē.

耳門二穴 ，在耳前起肉當耳缺者陷中 。針三
分 ，留三呼 ，灸三壯 。《 明下 》云 ：禁灸 ，有
病不過三壯 。

Ěr Mén 耳門 (SJ 21), bilateral point: It is located anterior to the supratragic notch of the ear, in the depression on the fleshy protuberance. Needle 3 fēn deep, retain the needle for three respirations; burn three cones of moxibustion. *Míng Xià* 《 明下 》 says: moxibustion is contraindicated. Do not burn more than three cones of moxibustion, even if there is disease.

聽宮二穴 ，在耳中珠子 ，大如赤小豆 。針三
分 ，灸三壯 。《 明 》云 ：針一分 。

Tīng Gōng 聽宮 (SI 19), bilateral point: It is located in the center of the ear at the 'bead' that is the size of a red bean [meaning the tragus]. Needle 3 fēn deep; burn three cones of moxibustion. *Míng* says: Needle 1 fēn deep.

頰車二穴 ，在耳下曲頰端陷中 。針四分 ，得氣
即瀉 ，日灸七壯 ，止七七 ，炷如大麥 。忌同 。
《 明下 》云 ：在耳下二韭葉陷中 。灸三壯 。又
云耳下曲頰骨後 。《 千 》云 ：一名機關 ，在耳
下八分 、小近前 。

Jiá Chē 頰車 (ST 6), bilateral point: It is located anterior to the ear, in the depression at the end of the mandible. Needle 4 fēn deep, drain [the point] as soon as qì arrives. Burn seven cones of moxibustion daily, up to seven times seven cones.

耳門
聽宮
頰車

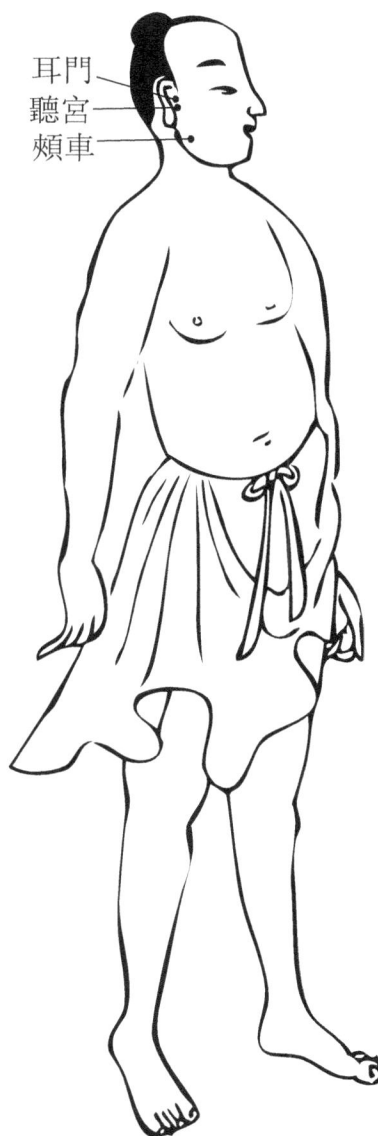

Fig. 1.14

31

Use grain-of-wheat size cones. Follow the same contraindications.[37] *Míng Xià* 《明下》 says: It is below the ear in the depression that is the width of two leek leaves. Burn three cones of moxibustion. It also says: It is anterior to the ear and posterior to the mandible. *Qiān* 《千》 says: Another name is Jī Guān 機關; it is 8 fēn below the ear, and slightly anterior.

1.10
Jiān Bó Bù Zuǒ Yòu Èr Shí Liù Xué

肩髆部左右二十六穴

Shoulder and arm section, 26 bilateral points [thirteen on each side]

肩井二穴，一名膊井，在肩上陷（《明堂》此有罅中二字）缺盆上，大骨前寸半，以三指按取之，當中指下陷中。《甲乙經》云：祇可針五分。此髆井脈，足陽明之會，乃連入五藏氣，若刺深，則令人悶倒不識人。則速須三里下氣，先補不瀉，須臾平復如故。凡針肩井，皆以三里下其氣，大良，灸七壯。《明》云：針四分，先補而後瀉，特不宜灸。針不得深，深即令人悶。若婦人胎落後微損，手足弱者，針肩井立差。灸乃勝針，日灸七壯，止一百。若針肩井，必三里下氣，如不灸三里，即拔氣上。

Jiān Jǐng 肩井 (GB 21), bilateral point, another name is Bó Jǐng 膊井: It is located in the depression on the shoulder (*Míng Táng* 《明堂》 has 'in the cleft' here), above the empty basin,[38] 1.5 cùn anterior to the large bone [scapular spine]. Press and find the point with three fingers, it is located in the depression under the tip of the middle finger. *Jiǎ Yǐ Jīng* 《甲乙經》 says: Needle only 5 fēn deep. This Bó Jǐng vessel is the confluence of the foot yángmíng; it connects the qì of five viscera. If needled too deeply, the patient feels oppression, then falls down and loses consciousness. [In that case,] quickly use Sān Lǐ 三里 (ST 36) to descend qì by supplementing first without draining; the patient will return to normal after a while. It is very good to use Sān Lǐ (ST 36) to

---

37. The first point that mentioned contraindications was Shén Tíng 神庭 (Dū 24). Therefore, everything afterwards that said to 'follow the same contraindications' must refer to Shén Tíng. Now, Tīng Huì 聽會 (GB 2) has contraindicated cold food, so it is assumed that from here until the next point listing prohibitions, 'follow the same contraindications' refers to those of Tīng Huì. Each time the text says to 'follow the same contraindications,' it is assumed that it refers to the most recently given prohibitions.

38. Quē Pén 缺盆 literally means 'the empty basin.' It refers to the supraclavicular fossa as a region and is also the name of ST 12.

descend qì when needling Jiān Jǐng 肩井 (GB 21). Burn seven cones of moxibustion. *Míng*《明》says: needle 4 fēn deep, supplement first then drain; moxibustion is especially not recommended. Do not needle deeply because it can cause oppression. If a woman has minor injury after a miscarriage with weakness of the hands and feet, needling Jiān Jǐng (GB 21) will cure the disease immediately. Moxibustion is better than needling. Burn seven cones of moxibustion daily, stopping at a hundred cones. You must use Sān Lǐ 三里 (ST 36) to descend the qì when needling Jiān Jǐng (GB 21); if moxibustion is not applied to Sān Lǐ (ST 36), it pulls qì upward.

《明堂》既云特不宜灸，又云灸乃勝針，日灸七壯，至百壯罷。則是又可灸矣，不知何自畔其說也。或者肩井不可灸，惟胎落後手足弱者可灸耶？

[Author's note:] *Míng Táng*《明堂》already said not to apply moxibustion, but it also says moxibustion is better than needling; burn seven cones of moxibustion, up to a hundred cones. This means one can apply moxibustion. Why it disputes its own opinion here is unknown. Possibly one should not apply moxibustion to Jiān Jǐng (GB 21) except after a miscarriage, when there is weakness of hands and feet.

天髎二穴，在肩缺盆中上秘骨之際陷中央。針八分，灸三壯。

Tiān Liáo 天髎 (SJ 15), bilateral point: It is located in the depression of the empty basin, on the border of the upper hidden bone [*mì gǔ* 秘骨].[39] Needle 8 fēn deep; burn three cones of moxibustion.

巨骨二穴，在肩端上行兩叉骨間陷中。灸五壯，針寸半。《明》云：巨骨一穴，在心脾骨頭，日灸三壯至七壯。禁針，針則倒懸一食頃乃得下針，針入四分，瀉之勿補，針出始得正臥。忌同。《下》云：巨骨二穴，在肩端上兩行骨陷中。灸一壯。（《銅》云：雲門在巨骨下夾氣戶旁各二寸。俞府在巨骨下璇璣旁各二寸。氣戶在巨骨下俞府兩旁各二寸。）

Jù Gǔ 巨骨 (LI 16), bilateral point: It is located in the depression at the end of the shoulder, between the junction of the bones.[40] Burn five cones of moxibustion; needle 1.5 cùn deep. *Míng* says: Jù Gǔ point is located on the heart and spleen bones.[41] Burn three to seven cones of moxibus-

---

39. *Shàng mì gǔ* 上秘骨 (upper hidden bone): *Mì* 秘 is equivalent to *Mì* 秘 hidden. The bone is hidden between the the junction of the bones of the shoulder, posterior to the empty basin (suprascapular fossa). This probably means the superior angle of the scapula.

40. *Liǎng chà gǔ* 兩叉骨 the junction of the bones here refers to the acromioclavicular joint.

41. According to the text below and an annotation in *Zhēn Jiǔ Míng Zhù Jí Chéng*《針灸名著集成》(Grand Compendium of Famous Works on Acupuncture and Moxibustion) by Huáng Lóngx-

tion daily. Needling is contraindicated. When performing acupuncture, [one] can only insert the needle after hanging upside down for the time it takes to eat a meal;[42] needle 4 fēn deep, only use draining techniques. The patient can lie face up only after the needle is removed. Follow the same contraindications [as Tīng Huì 聽會 (GB 2)].[43] *Xià* 《下》 says: The bilateral point of Jù Gǔ (LI 16) is located in the depression made by the two bones at the end of the shoulder. Burn one cone of moxibustion. (*Tóng* 《銅》 says: Yún Mén 雲門 (LU 2) is located below the great bone [clavicle], 2 cùn lateral to Qì Hù 氣戶 (ST 13). Shù Fǔ 俞府 (KI 27) is located 2 cùn lateral to Xuán Jī 璇璣 (Rèn 21), below the great bone. Qì Hù (ST 13) is located below the great bone,[44] 2 cùn lateral to Shù Fǔ (KI 27).)

《銅人》云：巨骨一穴，在肩端上兩叉骨間，《明堂下經》亦同。但《明堂上經》云巨骨一穴在心脾骨頭，不特一穴字不同，而穴在心脾骨頭亦異，豈其所謂一穴在心脾頭者，非巨骨耶？不然，即是誤寫二字作一字，肩胛為心脾也。

[Author's note:] *Tóng Rén* 《銅人》 says: The one point of Jù Gǔ 巨骨 (LI 16) is located at the end of the shoulder, between the junction of the bones. *Míng Táng Xià Jīng* 《明堂下經》 says the same thing. But *Míng Táng Shàng Jīng* 《明堂上經》 says: The one point of Jù Gǔ (LI 16) is located on the heart and spleen bones. So the discrepancy is not just the word one [*yī* 一], but also that the point is located on the heart and spleen bones. How can it be that the one point they mention is located at the end of the heart and spleen bone? This is not Jù Gǔ (LI 16). On the other hand, they may have accidentally written one [*yī* 一] instead of two [*èr* 二] as well as heart and spleen [心脾] instead of scapula [肩胛].

臑會二穴，一名臑髎。在肩前廉去肩頭三寸宛宛中。針七分，留三呼，得氣即瀉，灸七壯。（《素注》：臂前廉肩端。）

Nào Huì 臑會 (SJ 13), bilateral point, another name is Nào Liáo 臑髎: It is located on the anterior side of the shoulder, in the depression 3 cùn from the end [of the shoulder]. Needle 7 fēn deep, retain the needle for three respirations, drain [the point] as soon as qì arrives; burn seven cones

---

iáng 黃龍祥, published in 1996, *xīn pí gǔ tóu* 心脾骨頭 (heart and spleen bone) might refer to *xīn bì gǔ tóu* 心蔽骨頭 (end of the heart covering bone [the xiphoid process]). But it does not make sense for the location of Jù Gǔ 巨骨 (LI 16).

42. *Míng* 《明》 contradicts itself by saying "Needling is contraindicated," but discusses "performing acupuncture." In addition, the phrase "hanging upside down" is obscure.

43. According to *Zhēn Jiū Míng Zhù Jí Chéng* 針灸名著集成, the Jù Gǔ 巨骨 point described by *Míng* 《明》 is located 5 fēn above Jiū Wěi 鳩尾 (turtledove tail [xiphoid process] or Rèn 15). It is a different point from Jù Gǔ 巨骨 (LI 16) of the hand yángmíng channel.

44. Jù Gǔ is the name of the clavicle as well as LI 16. Here, Wáng records points that are just below the clavicle because the anatomic structure has the same name as the point.

of moxibustion. (*Sù Zhù*《素注》says: It is on the anterior aspect of the arm, at the end of the shoulder).

肩髃二穴，在髃骨頭肩端兩骨間陷宛宛中，舉臂取之。灸七壯，至二七，以差為度。若灸偏風不遂，可七七壯，不宜多，恐手臂細。若風病筋骨無力，久不差，灸不畏細也。刺即洩肩臂熱氣。唐庫秋欽患風痹，手足不得伸，甄權針此穴，令將弓箭射之如故。《明》云：針八分，留三呼，瀉五吸，灸不及針，以平手取其穴，日灸七壯，增至二七。若灸偏風不隨，可至二百，若更多灸恐手臂細。若刺風痹、風瘙、風病，當其火艾，不畏細也。忌同。（《千》云：肩頭正中兩骨間，一名中肩井。《外臺》名扁骨。）

Jiān Yú 肩髃 (LI 15), bilateral point: It is located at the shoulder-end of scapula, in the depression between the two bones. Locate the point while raising [abducting] the arm. Burn seven cones of moxibustion, up to two times seven cones; the criteria is the recovery from disease. One can apply seven times seven cones of moxa for hemilateral wind[45] and paralysis. More cones are not recommended; this might cause the arms to become thin. If the patient suffers wind with weakness of sinews and bones which has not recovered for a long time, one can apply moxibustion without caring about thinning [of the arms]. Pricking it can diffuse hot qì of the shoulder and arm. During the *Táng* Dynasty, Kù Qiūqín[46] suffered wind *bì*-impediment with inability to stretch the extremities. Zhēn Quán needled this point on him and he could shoot an arrow as before. *Míng*《明》says: Needle 8 fēn deep, retain the needle for three respirations, and drain for five respirations. Moxibustion is not as good as needling. Locate the point with the patient's arm relaxed. Burn seven cones of moxibustion daily; add up to two times seven cones. Apply up to two hundred cones for hemilateral wind with paralysis, but if even more cones are used, it could cause thinning of the arms. Do not be afraid of thinning of the arms when applying moxibustion[47] for various types of paralysis due to wind. Follow the same contraindications [as Tīng Huì 聽會 (GB 2)]. (*Qiān*《千》says: It is in the center of shoulder, between two bones; another name is Zhōng Jiān Jǐng 中肩井. *Wài Tái*《外臺》named it Biǎn Gǔ 扁骨 (flat bone)).

---

45. In *Zhū Bìng Yuán Hóu Lùn · Fēng Bìng Zhù Hóu*《諸病源候論·風病諸候》(The Origin and Indicators of Disease · Indications of All Wind Disease)：偏風者，風邪偏客於身一邊也。人體有偏虛者，風邪乘虛而傷之，故為偏風也 states: Hemilateral wind indicates that the wind evil settles on one-side of the body. When the body is deficient on one-side, the wind evil overwhelms the deficiency and damages [the side]. Therefore, this is hemilateral wind.

46. According to *Zhēn Jiǔ Míng Zhù Jí Chéng* 針灸名著集成 (Grand Compendium of Famous Works on Acupuncture and Moxibustion), Kù Qiūqín 庫秋欽 probably lived during the *Suí* (隋) Dynasty. The mistake was originally made in *Tóng Rén Shū Xué Zhēn Jiǔ Tú Jīng*《銅人腧穴針灸圖經》(The Bronze Statues Illustrated Classic of Acupuncture Points).

47. The Chinese text has *cì* 刺 (pricking), but based on the context, this is an error for *jiǔ* 灸 (moxibustion).

肩髎二穴，在肩端臑上陷中，舉臂取之。針七分。灸三壯，《明》云：五壯。

Jiān Liáo 肩髎 (SJ 14), bilateral point: It is located in the depression on the upper arm. Locate the point while raising the arm. Needle 7 fēn deep; burn three cones of moxibustion. *Míng* 《明》 says: Five cones.

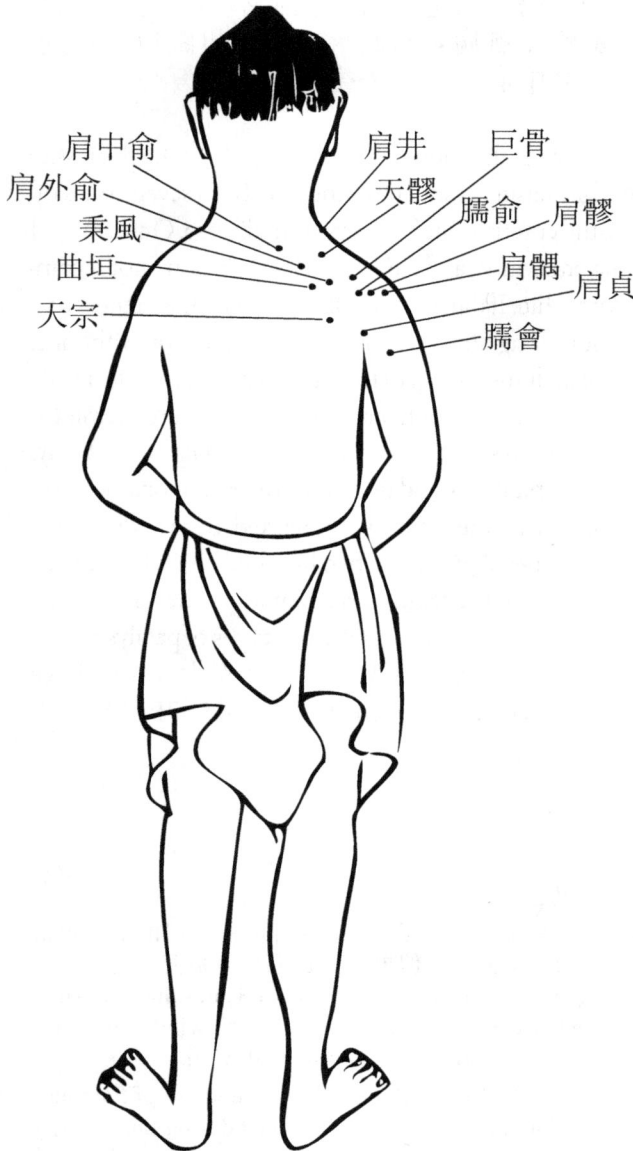

Fig. 1.15

肩貞二穴，在肩胛下兩骨解間，肩髃後陷中。針五分。

Jiān Zhēn 肩貞 (SI 9), bilateral point: It is located below the scapula, in the depression posterior to Jiān Yú 肩髃 [the acromion or LI 15] and between the two split bones [shoulder joint]. Needle 5 fēn deep.

天宗二穴，在秉風後大骨下陷中。灸三壯，針五分，留六呼。

Tiān Zōng 天宗 (SI 11), bilateral point: It is located in the depression below the large bone [scapular spine] and posterior to Bǐng Fēng 秉風 (SI 12). Burn three cones of moxibustion; needle 5 fēn deep, retain the needle for six respirations.

秉風二穴，在肩上小髃後舉臂有空。灸五壯，針五分。

Bǐng Fēng (SI 12), bilateral point: It is located on the shoulder posterior to the acromion,[48] in the depression that appears while raising the arm. Burn five cones of moxibustion; needle 5 fēn deep.

---

48. *Liáo* 髎 (bone cleft) should be *yú* 髃 (acromion) here.

臑俞二穴，在肩髎後大骨下，胛上廉陷中。針八分，灸三壯。《素》：在肩髎後，舉臂取之。

Nào Shù 臑俞 (SI 10), bilateral point: It is located below the large bone [scapular spine], posterior to Jiān Liáo 肩髎 (SJ 14), in the depression on the upper ridge of scapula. Needle 8 fēn deep; burn three cones of moxibustion. *Sù* 《素》says: It is posterior to the shoulder and upper arm. Locate the point while raising the arm.

曲垣二穴，在肩中央曲胛陷中，按之應手痛。灸三壯，針五分。《明》云：九分。

Qū Yuán 曲垣 (SI 13), bilateral point: It is located in the depression on the curve of the shoulder blade [scapular spine], in the center of the shoulder. When you press it, it responds to the hand with pain. Burn three cones of moxibustion; needle 5 fēn deep. *Míng* 《明》says: 9 fēn deep.

肩外俞二穴，在肩胛上廉，去脊骨三寸陷中。針六分，灸三壯。《明上》云：一壯。

Jiān Wài Shù 肩外俞 (SI 14), bilateral point: It is located in the depression 3 cùn from the spine, at the upper ridge of scapula. Needle 6 fēn deep; burn three cones of moxibustion. *Míng Shàng* 《明上》says: One cone.

肩中俞二穴，在肩胛內廉，去脊二寸陷中。針三分，留七呼，灸十壯。

Jiān Zhōng Shù 肩中俞 (SI 15), bilateral point: It is located in the depression 2 cùn from the spine, medial to the ridge of the scapula. Needle 3 fēn deep, retain the needle for seven respirations, and burn ten cones of moxibustion.

1.11
Bèi Yú Bù Zhōng Háng Shí Sān Xué

背俞部中行十三穴

Midline on the back, 13 points

大椎一穴，（一作剉），在第一椎上陷者宛宛中。針五分，留三呼，瀉五吸，灸以年為壯。（《明》云：日灸七壯，至七七壯）。《甲乙》云：大椎下至尾骶骨二十一椎長三尺，折量取俞穴。

Dà Zhuī 大椎 (Dū 14) one point, (Someone wrote *zhuī* 椎 as *cuò* 剉): It is located in the depression above the first vertebra.[49] Needle 5 fēn deep; retain the needle for three respirations; drain for five respirations. Burn the same number of cones of moxibustion, as the age of the patient. (*Míng* 《明》 says: Burn seven cones of moxibustion daily, up to seven times seven cones). *Jiǎ Yǐ* [*Jīng*] 《甲乙》 says: It is 3 *chǐ*[50] from Dà Zhuī (Dū 14) to the twenty-first vertebra [fourth sacral vertebra] on the sacrum-coccyx. Use this measurement to locate points.

既曰「大椎」，又曰「在第一椎上陷中」，必是二穴，非二穴則不言在第一椎上矣，此大椎、第一椎所以異也。但《銅人》云：「大椎在第一椎上陷中」，諸經皆同。惟《明堂下經》云「在第一椎下」，陶道穴既在第一椎下，不應大椎亦在一椎下，必是《下經》誤寫「上」字作「下」字也。考之《下經》，亦言陶道穴在大椎節下。與《銅人》合，足見其誤寫「上」字作「下」無疑矣。

[Author's note:] The book says Dà Zhuī (Dū 14) ['the great mallet,' a reference to the most protruding vertebra, the seventh cervical vertebra], but it also says it is in the depression above the first vertebra; so this should indicate two [different] points. If it is not two [different] points, the book should not say [the point is located] above the first vertebra.[51] This is because Dà Zhuī ('the great mallet') [C7] and the first vertebra are different. But *Tóng Rén* 《銅人》 says: Dà Zhuī (Dū 14) is

49. The first vertebra means the first thoracic vertebra. In ancient Chinese texts, the vertebrae were not divided into thoracic, lumbar, and sacral. The spine is treated as one unit counting down from the first thoracic vertebra.

50. *Chǐ* 尺 is a unit of measurement. Three *chǐ* equal about one meter.

51. Wáng is concerned that Dà Zhuī 大椎 [the great mallet] should mean C7 itself, not the depression below it.

in the depression above the first vertebra, which is the same as in other classics. Only *Míng Táng Xìa Jīng* 《 明堂下經 》 says: It is below the first vertebra. Táo Dào 陶道 (Dū 13) is located below the first vertebra, so Dà Zhuī 大椎 (Dū 14) cannot be located in the same place. *Xìa Jīng* 《 下經 》 must have erroneously written below [*xìa* 下] instead of above [*shàng* 上]. When checking *Xìa Jīng*, it also says Táo Dào (Dū 13) is located below Dà Zhuī (Dū 14) which is the same as in *Tóng Rén*. So there is no doubt that *Xìa Jīng* must have erroneously written below [*xìa* 下] instead of above [*shàng* 上].

陶道，在大椎節下間，俛而取之。灸五壯，針五分。

Táo Dào (Dū 13): It is located below Dà Zhuī ('the great mallet') [C₇ and/or Dū 14]. Locate the point with the patient in the prone position. Burn five cones of moxibustion; needle 5 fēn deep.

身柱，在第三椎節下間。針五分，灸七七壯。《明》云：五壯。《下》云：三壯。

Shēn Zhù 身柱 (Dū 12): It is located in the depression below the third vertebra. Needle 5 fēn deep; burn seven times seven cones of moxibustion. *Míng* 《 明 》 says: Five cones. *Xìa* 《 下 》 says: Three cones.

神道，在五椎節下間，俛而取之。灸七七壯，止百壯，小兒風癇，瘈瘲可灸七壯。《明》云：針五分，灸三壯。《下》云：五壯。

Shén Dào 神道 (Dū 11): It is located in the depression below the fifth vertebra. Locate the point with the patient in the prone position. Burn seven times seven cones of moxibustion, stop at a hundred cones. Burn seven cones for wind epilepsy, or tugging

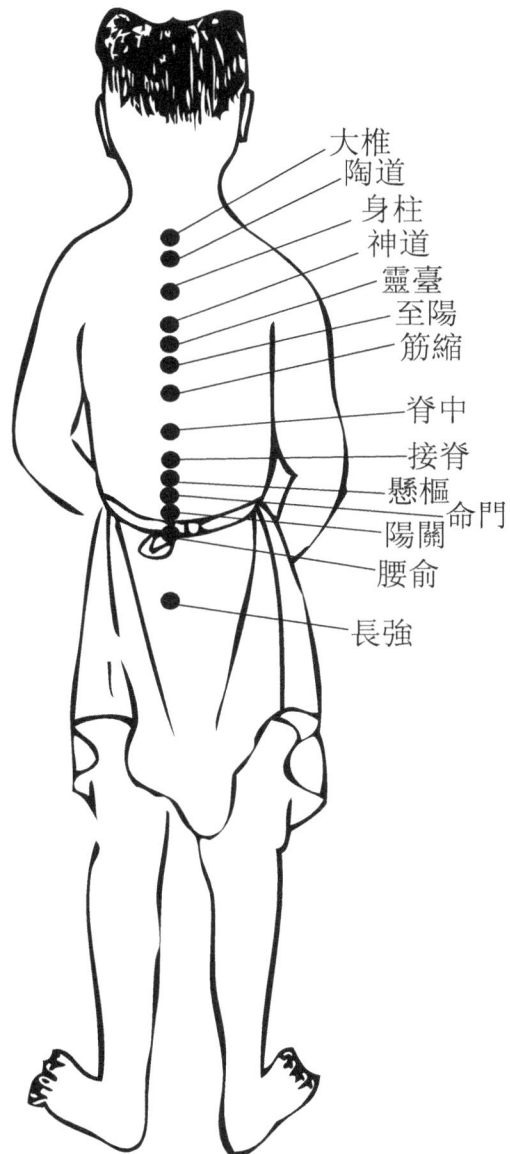

大椎
陶道
身柱
神道
靈臺
至陽
筋縮
脊中
接脊
懸樞
命門
陽關
腰俞
長強

Fig. 1.16

39

and slackening in children. *Míng*《明》says: Needle 5 fēn deep; burn three cones of moxibustion. *Xià*《下》says: Five cones.

靈臺，在六椎節下間，俛而取之。經闕療病法。出《素問》。

Líng Tái 靈臺 (Dū 10): It is located in the depression below the sixth vertebra. Locate the point with the patient in the prone position. This is from the treatment methods of the diseases using channel and points, coming from *Sù Wèn*《素問》.[52]

至陽，在七椎節下間，俛而取之。針五分，灸三壯。《明下》云：七壯。

Zhì Yáng 至陽 (Dū 9): It is located in the depression below the seventh vertebra. Locate the point with the patient in the prone position. Needle 5 fēn deep; burn three cones of moxibustion. *Míng Xià*《明下》says: Seven cones.

筋縮，在九椎節下間，俛而取之。針五分，灸三壯。《明下》云：七壯。

Jīn Suō 筋縮 (Dū 8): It is located in the depression below the ninth vertebra. Locate the point with the patient in the prone position. Needle 5 fēn deep; burn three cones of moxibustion. *Míng Xià* says: Seven cones.

脊中，一名神宗。在十一椎節下間，俛而取之。禁灸，灸令人腰背傴僂。針五分，得氣即瀉。《明堂》作：脊俞，一名脊中，在十一椎中央。

Jǐ Zhōng 脊中 (Dū 6), another name is Shén Zōng 神宗: It is located in the depression below the eleventh vertebra. Locate the point with the patient in the prone position. Moxibustion is contraindicated; it causes stooped back. Needle 5 fēn deep, drain [the point] as soon as qì arrives. *Míng Táng*《明堂》says: Another name for Jǐ Shù 脊俞 (Dū 6) is Jǐ Zhōng; it is located in the center of eleventh vertebra.

接脊，在十二椎下節間（《下經》治小兒疳，脫肛。）

Jiē Jǐ 接脊: It is located in the depression below the twelfth vertebra. (*Xià Jīng*《下經》says: it treats *gān*[53] and prolapsed rectum in children.)

---

52. It is not clear what this is referring to in *Sù Wèn*《素問》.

53. *Gān* 疳 refers to *gān jī* 疳積 (*gān* accumulation); it is usually caused by spleen damage and liver heat and often occurs in children. The symptoms include indigestion, sallow complexion, emaciation, bulging belly, tidal fever, vexation, thirst, reduced appetite, and loose stool that is sour-smelling and malodorous.

懸樞，在十三椎節下間，伏而取之 。針三分，灸三壯 。《 明 》云：在十二椎
下節間 。《 下 》云：十一椎下 。

Xuán Shū 懸樞 (Dū 5): It is located in the depression below the thirteenth vertebra [first lumbar vertebra]. Locate the point with the patient in the prone position. Needle 3 fēn deep; burn three cones of moxibustion. *Míng* 《 明 》 says: It is in the depression below the twelfth vertebra. *Xià* 《 下 》 says: It is in the depression below the eleventh vertebra.

《 銅人 》 云：懸樞在十三椎節下間， 《 明堂上經 》 作十二椎節間， 《
下經 》 作十一椎下 。脊中穴既在十一椎下， 不應懸樞又在十一椎下，
固知其誤矣。考之 《 素問 》 亦與 《 銅人 》 同， 當以 《 銅人 》 為正 。 《
明堂上經 》 亦誤三字作二字也。要之， 接脊穴在十二椎節下爾 。

[Author's note:] *Tóng Rén* 《 銅人 》 says: Xuán Shū (Dū 5) is located in the depression below the thirteenth vertebra [first lumbar vertebra]. *Míng Táng Shàng Jīng* 《 明堂上經 》 says the **twelfth vertebra** while *Xià Jīng* 《 下經 》 says: the **eleventh vertebra**. Jǐ Zhōng 脊中 (Dū 6) is located in the depression below the eleventh vertebra already, so Xuán Shū (Dū 5) cannot also be located below the eleventh vertebra. Thus we know there is mistake. Checking *Sù Wèn* 《 素問 》 and *Tóng Rén*, they are in agreement, so [we should] set *Tóng Rén* as the law. *Míng Táng Shàng Jīng* might have written two [*èr* 二] instead of three [*sān* 三] in error. The conclusion is that the Jiē Jǐ 接脊 point is located below the twelfth vertebra [see the previous entry].

命門，一名屬累 。在十四椎節下間，伏而取之（ 《 明 》作俛而取之 ）。針五
分，灸三壯 。

Mìng Mén 命門 (Dū 4), another name is Shǔ Lèi 屬累: It is located in the depression below the fourteenth vertebra [second lumbar vertebra]. Locate the point with the patient in the prone position (*Míng* uses **inclined** [*fǔ* 俛] instead of **prone** [*fú* 伏]). Needle 3 fēn deep; burn three cones of moxibustion.

陽關，在十六椎下間，伏而取之 。針五分，灸三壯 。[經]關療病法 。（ 出《
素問 》 ）。

Yáng Guān 陽關 (Dū 3), it is located in the depression below the sixteenth vertebra [fourth lumbar vertebra]. Locate the point with the patient in the prone position. Needle 5 fēn deep; burn three cones of moxibustion. This is from the treatment methods of the diseases using channel and points. (This comes from *Sù Wèn*.[54])

---

54. It is unclear what this is referring to in *Sù Wèn* 《 素問 》.

腰俞，一名背解，一名髓孔，一名腰柱，一名腰戶。在二十一椎節下間宛宛
中，以挺腹地舒身，兩手相重支額，縱四體後乃取其穴。針八分，留三呼，
瀉五吸。灸七壯，至七七壯。忌房勞、舉重強力。《甲乙》云：針二寸，留
七呼，灸七七壯。《明》云：三壯，《下》云：五壯。《素注》云：針一
分。《新校正》云：按《甲乙經》作二寸，《水熱穴》注亦可二寸。《氣府
論》注、《骨空論》注作一分。一名髓空。

Yāo Shù 腰俞 (Dū 2), another name is Bèi Jiě 背解, also named Suí Kǒng 髓孔, Yāo Zhù 腰
柱, and Yāo Hù 腰戶: It is located in the depression below the twenty-first vertebra [fourth sacral
vertebra]. Ask the patient to relax and lie down with his abdomen against the ground [face down],
placing one hand on the other to support his forehead, and letting his limbs lie loose. Then locate
the point. Needle 8 fēn deep; retain the needle for three respirations; drain for five respirations.
Burn seven cones of moxibustion, up to seven times seven cones. Sexual taxation, lifting heavy
weights and using force are contraindicated. *Jiǎ Yǐ* 《甲乙》 says: Needle 2 cùn deep; retain the
needle for seven respirations. Burn seven times seven cones of moxibustion. *Míng* 《明》 says:
Three cones. *Xià* 《下》 says: Five cones. *Sù Zhù* 《素注》 says: Needle 1 fēn deep. *Xīn Jiào
Zhèng* 《新校正》 says: According to *Jiǎ Yǐ Jīng* 《甲乙經》, needle 2 cùn deep; the Annotation to *Shuǐ Rè Xué* 《水熱穴》 also say to needle 2 cùn deep. The Annotation of *Qì Fǔ Lùn* 《
氣府論》 and *Gǔ Kōng Lùn* 《骨空論》 (Treatise on Bone Hollows)[55] both say to needle 1
fēn deep. Another name is Suí Kǒng 髓空.

長強一名氣之陰郄，督脈絡別。其穴趺地取之。《甲乙》云：在脊骶端。
針三分，轉針以大痛為度。其穴趺地取之乃得，灸不及針，日三十壯，止二
百。此痔根本是冷，忌冷食房勞。《甲乙》云：針二寸，留七呼。《明下》
云：五壯。

Cháng Qiáng 長強 (Dū 1), another name is *Xī*-cleft of the Yīn Qì: It is the diverging network of
the dū mài. Locate the point with the patient sitting on the ground with crossed legs. *Jiǎ Yǐ* [*Jīng*]
says: [It is located] at the end of the sacral spine. Needle 3 fēn deep; rotate the needle until [the
patient] feels severe pain. Locate the point with the patient sitting on the ground with crossed legs.
Moxibustion is not as good as acupuncture; burn thirty cones of moxibustion daily, stop at two
hundred cones. The root of hemorrhoids is coldness, so cold food and sexual taxation are contraindicated. *Jiǎ Yǐ* says: Needle 2 cùn deep; retain the needle for seven respirations. *Míng Xià* 《明
下》 says: Five cones.

自大椎至腰俞長同身寸三尺，折量取之。（《甲》）。

The distance from Dà Zhuī 大椎 (Dū 14) to Yāo Shù (Dū 2) is 3 *chǐ* in proportional measurement. Locate points using this measurement. (*Jiǎ* 《甲》)

---

55. These two chapters refer to *Sù Wèn* 《素問》 (Plain Questions), Chapters 59 and 60.

有里醫言，凡灸椎骨，當灸骨節突處方驗，灸節下當骨無驗。以魚肉骨參之，其言為可信，盡依其言當骨節灸之。

> [Author's note:] Some doctors say: when applying the moxibustion to the vertebra, it is effective only when the moxibustion is burned on the prominence of the bone; it is ineffective when performed below the prominence of the bone. This is believeable when examining fish bones. So moxibustion should be applied to the prominence of the bone as these doctors say.

1.12
Bèi Yú Dì Èr Háng Sì Shí Sì Xué

背俞第二行四十四穴

The second line on the back,
44 points [twenty-two on each side]

大杼二穴，在項後第一椎下，兩旁相去各寸半陷中。針五分，灸七壯。（《甲乙》同）。《明》云：禁灸。《下經》云：灸五壯。《素》同。（《難疏》：骨會大杼，骨病治此。）

Dà Zhù 大杼 (UB 11) bilateral point: It is located in the depression 1.5 cùn from the inferior aspect of the first vertebra at the nape of the neck. Needle 5 fēn deep; burn seven cones of moxibustion (*Jiǎ Yǐ* 《甲乙》 agrees). *Míng* 《明》 says: Moxibustion is contraindicated. *Xià Jīng* 《下經》 says: Burn five cones of moxibustion; *Sù* 《素》 agrees. (*Nàn Shū* 《難疏》 (Explanation and Verification of the Classic of Difficulties) says: Dà Zhù (UB 11) is the meeting [influential] point of the bones; it treats bone diseases.)

《明堂》云禁灸，而《銅人》云：可灸七壯，必有說也。要非大急，不必灸。

> [Author's note:] *Míng Táng* 《明堂》 says moxibustion is contraindicated, but *Tóng Rén* 《銅人》 says: Burn seven cones of moxibustion. There must be some theory [for that], so moxibustion is not recommended unless it is for a very urgent condition.

風門二穴，一名熱府，在二椎下兩旁相去各寸半。針五分，留七呼。今附：
若頻刺，洩諸陽熱氣，背永不發癰疽。灸五壯。

Fēng Mén 風門 (UB 12) bilateral point, another name is Rè Fǔ 熱府: It is located 1.5 cùn from the inferior aspect of the second vertebra. Needle 5 fēn deep, retain the needle for seven respirations. Appended here: Frequent needling drains all yáng and hot qì, so there will never be welling- and flat-abscesses on the [patient's] back. Burn five cones of moxibustion.

肺俞二穴，在三椎下兩旁各寸半。（ 自此後不寫相去二字 ）。針三分，留七呼，得氣即瀉。出《甲乙經》。甄權《針經》云：在三椎下兩旁，以搭手左取右，右取左，當中指末是穴。針五分，留七呼，灸百壯。《明下》云：三壯。（《千》：肺俞對乳引繩度之。 ）

Fèi Shù 肺俞 (UB 13) bilateral point: It is located 1.5 cùn lateral to the inferior aspect of the third vertebra. (From here on, I am removing the characters for away from [*xiāng qù* 相去]).[56] Needle 3 fēn deep; retain the needle for seven respirations; drain [the point] as soon as qì arrives. This comes from *Jiǎ Yǐ Jīng* 《甲乙經》. *Zhēn Jīng* 《針經》 (Copy of the Acupuncture Classic)[57] by Zhēn Quán says: It is lateral to the inferior aspect of the third vertebra. The point is located by [having the patient] reach over their right [shoulder] with their left hand and over their left [shoulder] with their right hand, similar to the method for locating flat-abscesses on the back.[58] The point is located under the tip of the middle finger. Needle 5 fēn deep; retain the needle for seven respirations. Burn a hundred cones of moxibustion. *Míng Xià* 《明下》 says: Three cones. (*Qiān* 《千》 says: Fèi Shù (UB 13) is opposite to the breast; measure with a string.)

厥陰俞二穴，在四椎下兩旁各寸半。針三分，灸七七壯。《千》：扁鵲云名
關俞。

Jué Yīn Shù 厥陰俞 (UB 14) bilateral point: It is located 1.5 cùn lateral to the inferior aspect of the fourth vertebra. Needle 3 fēn deep; burn seven times seven cones of moxibustion. *Qiān* says: Biǎn Què[59] named it Jué Shù 關俞.

---

56. The author is quoting earlier texts but wants to remove characters that are repetitive and superfluous to the meaning. This is not important to the English reader.

57. *Zhēn Jīng* 針經 refers to *Zhēn Jīng Chāo* 《針經鈔》 (Copy of the Acupuncture Classic) by Zhēn Quán 甄權 of the *Táng* (唐) Dynasty.

58. *Dā shǒu* 搭手 indicates a flat-abscess on the back, lateral to the spine where it can be reached with the hand. It is divided into upper, middle and lower types. The upper type is near Fèi Shù 肺俞 (UB 13), the middle type is near Gāo Huāng Shù 膏肓俞 (UB 43), and the lower one is near Huāng Mén 肓門 (UB 51).

59. Biǎn Què 扁鵲 is the name of an ancient doctor, who was also known as Qín Yuèrén 秦越人.

心俞二穴，在五椎下兩旁各各寸半。針三分，留七呼，得氣即瀉，不可灸。
《明下》云：灸五壯。（《千》云：第七節對心橫三間。）

Xīn Shù 心俞 (UB 15) bilateral point: It is located 1.5 cùn lateral to the inferior aspect of the fifth vertebra. Needle 3 fēn deep; retain the needle for seven respirations; drain [the point] as soon as qì arrives. Moxibustion is contraindicated. *Míng Xià* 《明下》 says: Burn five cones. (*Qiān* 《千》 says: The seventh vertebra; it is opposite to the heart and in the third [intercostal] space.

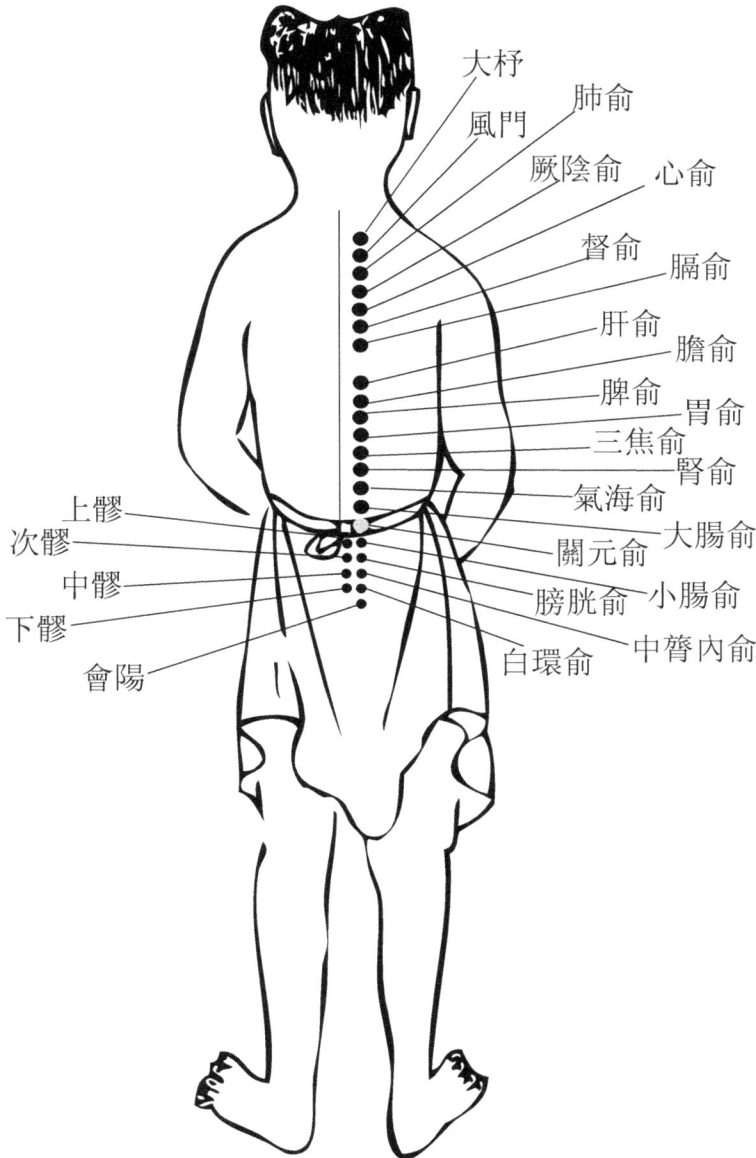

Fig. 1.17

45

《銅人》云：心俞不可灸，可針入三分。世醫因此遂謂心俞禁灸，但可針爾。殊不知刺中心一日死，乃《素問》之所戒，豈可妄針耶？《千金》言風中心，急灸心俞百壯，服續命湯。又當權其緩急可也，豈可泥不可灸之說，而坐受斃耶。

[Author's note:] *Tóng Rén* 《銅人》 says: Moxibustion is not recommended on Xīn Shù 心俞 (UB 15), but it is appropriate to needle 3 fēn deep. Based on this, doctors now say moxibustion is contraindicated on Xīn Shù (UB 15), but not acupuncture. However, what they do not know is that the patient will die in one day if the heart is punctured. That contraindication is from *Sù Wèn* 《素問》, so how can we needle it recklessly? *Qiān Jīn* 《千金》 says: to immediately burn a hundred cones of moxibustion on Xīn Shù (UB 15) for wind attacking the heart and then take *Xù Mìng Tāng* 續命湯 (Life-Prolonging Decoction). So we must evaluate the level of urgency of the situation; we cannot stick to the theory that moxibustion is contraindicated. That is what is called *sitting still and waiting for death.*

督俞二穴，一名高蓋。在六椎下兩旁各寸半。禁針，通灸。

Dū Shù 督俞 (UB 16) bilateral point, another name is Gāo Gài 高蓋: It is located 1.5 cùn lateral to the inferior aspect of the sixth vertebra. Needling is contraindicated; moxibustion is generally acceptable.

《銅人經》缺此穴，《明堂經》有之，今依《明堂》入在此，恐《銅人》本不全也。

[Author's note:] *Tóng Rén Jīng* 《銅人經》 missed this point, but *Míng Táng Jīng* 《明堂經》 has it. This point is appended here based on *Míng Táng*. I fear that *Tóng Rén* is incomplete.

膈俞二穴，在七椎下兩旁各寸半。針三分，留七呼，灸三壯。《明下》云：五壯。（《難疏》：血會膈俞，血病灸此。）

Gé Shù 膈俞 (UB 17) bilateral point: It is located 1.5 cùn lateral to the inferior aspect of the seventh vertebra. Needle 3 fēn deep; retain the needle for seven respirations. Burn three cones of moxibustion. *Míng Xià* 《明下》 says: Five cones. (*Nàn Shū* 《難疏》 says: Gé Shù 膈俞 (UB 17) is the meeting [influential] point of the blood. Apply moxibustion to this point for blood diseases.)

八椎下兩旁，《銅人》、《明堂》並缺俞穴。

> [Author's note:] *Tóng Rén* 《銅人》 and *Míng Táng* 《明堂》 both missed the point that is located lateral to the inferior aspect of the eighth vertebra.

肝俞二穴，在九椎下兩旁各寸半。針三分，留六呼，灸三壯。《明下》云：七壯。《素》云：刺中肝，五日死。

Gān Shù 肝俞 (UB 18) bilateral point: It is located 1.5 cùn lateral to the inferior aspect of the ninth vertebra. Needle 3 fēn deep; retain the needle for six respirations. Burn three cones of moxibustion. *Míng Xià* 《明下》 says: Seven cones. *Sù* 《素》 says: The patient will die in five days if the liver is punctured.

膽俞二穴，在十椎下兩旁各寸半，正坐取之。灸三壯，針五分。《明》云：三分。《下經》云：灸五壯。《素》：刺中膽，一日半死。

Dǎn Shù 膽俞 (UB 19) bilateral point: It is located 1.5 cùn lateral to the inferior aspect of the tenth vertebra. Locate the point with the patient sitting upright. Burn three cones of moxibustion; needle 5 fēn deep. *Míng* 《明》 says: 3 fēn deep. *Xià Jīng* 《下經》 says: Burn five cones of moxibustion. *Sù* says: The patient will die in one and a half days if the gallbladder is punctured.

脾俞二穴，在十一椎下兩旁各寸半。針三分，留七呼，灸三壯。《明下》云：五壯。《素》云：刺中脾，十日死。

Pí Shù 脾俞 (UB 20) bilateral point: It is located 1.5 cùn lateral to the inferior aspect of the eleventh vertebra. Needle 3 fēn deep; retain the needle for seven respirations. Burn three cones of moxibustion. *Míng Xià* says: Five cones. *Sù* says: The patient will die in ten days if the spleen is punctured.

胃俞二穴，在十二椎下兩旁各寸半。針三分，留七呼，灸隨年為壯。《明》云：三壯。《下》云：七壯。

Wèi Shù 胃俞 (UB 21) bilateral point: It is located 1.5 cùn lateral to the inferior aspect of the twelfth vertebra. Needle 3 fēn deep; retain the needle for seven respirations. Burn the same number of cones of moxibustion as the age of the patient. *Míng* says: Three cones. *Xià* 《下》 says: Seven cones.

三焦俞二穴，在十三椎下兩旁各寸半。針五分，留七呼，灸三壯。《明》云：針三分。《下》云：灸五壯。

Sān Jiāo Shù 三焦俞 (UB 22) bilateral point: It is located 1.5 cùn lateral to the inferior aspect of the thirteenth vertebra [first lumbar]. Needle 5 fēn deep; retain the needle for seven respirations. Burn three cones of moxibustion. *Míng* 《明》 says: Needle 3 fēn deep. *Xià* 《下》 says: Burn five cones of moxibustion.

腎俞二穴，在十四椎下兩旁各寸半。與臍平。針三分，留七呼，灸以年為壯。忌同。《明》云：三壯。《下》云：五壯。（刺腎，六日死。）

Shèn Shù 腎俞 (UB 23) bilateral point: It is located 1.5 cùn lateral to the inferior aspect of the fourteenth vertebra [second lumbar], level with umbilicus. Needle 3 fēn deep; retain the needle for seven respirations. Burn the same number of cones of moxibustion as the age of the patient. Follow the same contraindications [as Cháng Qiáng 長強 (Dū 1)]. *Míng* says: Three cones. *Xià* says: Five cones. (The patient will die in six days if a kidney is punctured).

氣海俞二穴，在十五椎下兩旁各寸半。通灸。

Qì Hǎi Shù 氣海俞 (UB 24) bilateral point: It is located 1.5 cùn lateral to the inferior aspect of the fifteenth vertebra [third lumbar]. Moxibustion is generally acceptable.

按《明堂》有氣海俞，而《銅人》無之。恐《銅人》本不全，故依《明堂》附入於此。

[Author's note:] Qì Hǎi Shù (UB 24) is described in *Míng Táng* 《明堂》 but not in *Tóng Rén* 《銅人》. I fear that *Tóng Rén* is incomplete, so this point is appended here based on *Míng Táng*.

大腸俞二穴，在十六椎下兩旁各寸半。針三分，留六呼，灸二壯。

Dà Cháng Shù 大腸俞 (UB 25) bilateral point: It is located 1.5 cùn lateral to the inferior aspect of the sixteenth vertebra [fourth lumbar]. Needle 3 fēn deep; retain the needle for six respirations. Burn two cones of moxibustion.

關元俞二穴，在十七椎下兩旁各寸半。針三分。

Guān Yuán Shù 關元俞 (UB 26) bilateral point: It is located 1.5 cùn lateral to the inferior aspect of the seventeenth [fifth lumbar] vertebra. Needle 3 fēn deep.

按《明堂》有關元俞，而《銅人》無之。恐《銅人》本不全，故依《明堂》附入於此。

[Author's note:] Guān Yuán Shù 關元俞 (UB 26) is described in *Míng Táng* 《明堂》 but not in *Tóng Rén* 《銅人》. I fear that *Tóng Rén* is incomplete, so this point is appended here based on *Míng Táng*.

小腸俞二穴，在十八椎下兩旁各寸半。針三分，留六呼，灸三壯。

Xiǎo Cháng Shù 小腸俞 (UB 27) bilateral point: It is located 1.5 cùn lateral to the inferior aspect of the eighteenth vertebra [first sacral vertebra]. Needle 3 fēn deep; retain the needle for six respirations. Burn three cones of moxibustion.

膀胱俞二穴，在十九椎下兩旁各寸半。針三分，留六呼，灸三壯。《明下》云：七壯。

Páng Guāng Shù 膀胱俞 (UB 28) bilateral point: It is located 1.5 cùn lateral to the inferior aspect of the nineteenth vertebra [second sacral vertebra]. Needle 3 fēn deep; retain the needle for six respirations. Burn three cones of moxibustion. *Míng Xià* 《明下》 says: Seven cones.

中膂內俞二穴，一名脊內俞。在二十椎下兩旁各寸半，俠脊起肉。針三分，留十呼，灸三壯。《明下》云：主腰痛夾脊膂痛，上下按之應者，從項後至此穴痛，皆灸之立愈。

Zhōng Lǚ Nèi Shù 中膂內俞 (UB 29) bilateral point, another name is Jǐ Nèi Shù 脊內俞. It is located 1.5 cùn lateral to the inferior aspect of the twentieth vertebra [third sacral vertebra], on the fleshy prominence lateral to the spine. Needle 3 fēn deep; retain the needle for ten respirations. Burn three cones of moxibustion. *Míng Xià* says: It treats lower back pain and pain of the muscles along the spine. When pressed from the nape of the neck to this point, the response to the hand is pain. [The pain] will be cured immediately when moxibustion is applied to this point.

白環俞二穴，在二十一椎下兩旁各寸半。《甲乙》云：針如腰戶法同，挺腹地端身，兩手相重支額，縱息令皮膚俱緩，乃取其穴。針八分，得氣即瀉，訖多補之，不宜灸。忌房勞，不得舉重。《明下》云：灸三壯。

Bái Huán Shù 白環俞 (UB 30) bilateral point: It is located 1.5 cùn lateral to the inferior aspect of the twenty-first vertebra [fourth sacral vertebra]. *Jiǎ Yǐ* 《甲乙》 says: Use the same needling technique as for Yāo Hù 腰戶 (Dū 2). Ask the patient to relax and lie down with his abdomen against the ground [face down] and place one hand on the other to support his forehead. Relax the breath to make all the the skin soft. Then locate the point. Needle 8 fēn deep; drain [the point] as soon as qì arrives; supplement after draining is complete. Moxibustion is not recommended. Sexual taxation and lifting heavy weights are contraindicated. *Míng Xià* 《 明下 》 says: Burn three cones of moxibustion.

上髎二穴，在第一空腰髁下俠脊陷中 。針三分，灸七壯 。《 千 》云：腰髁下一寸 。

Shàng Liáo 上髎 (UB 31) bilateral point: It is located in the depression lateral to the spine, in the first hollow [of the sacral foramen] below the lumbar bones. Needle 3 fēn deep; burn seven cones of moxibustion. *Qiān* 《 千 》 says: 1 cùn below the lumbar bones.

次髎二穴，在第二空俠脊陷中 。可灸七壯，針三分 。

Cì Liáo 次髎 (UB 32) bilateral point: It is located in the depression lateral to the spine, in the second hollow [of the sacral foramen] below the lumbar bones. Burn seven cones of moxibustion; needle 3 fēn deep.

中髎二穴，在第三空俠脊陷中 。針二分，留十呼，灸二壯 。

Zhōng Liáo 中髎 (UB 33) bilateral point: It is located in the depression lateral to the spine, in the third hollow [of the sacral foramen] below the lumbar bones. Needle 2 fēn deep; retain the needle for ten respirations; burn two cones of moxibustion.

下髎二穴，在第四空俠脊陷中 。針二分，留十呼，灸三壯 。

Xià Liáo 下髎 (UB 34) bilateral point: It is located in the depression lateral to the spine, in the fourth hollow [of the sacral foramen] below the lumbar bones. Needle 2 fēn deep; retain the needle for ten respirations; burn three cones of moxibustion.

會陽二穴，一名利機 。在陰尾骨兩旁 。針八分，灸五壯 。

Huì Yáng 會陽 (UB 35) bilateral point, another name is Lì Jī 利機: It is located lateral to the tailbone. Needle 8 fēn deep; burn five cones of moxibustion.

《千金》八窌在腰目下三寸，俠脊相去四寸（兩邊四穴故名八窌），
其曰夾脊四寸，是除脊各寸半也。凡大杼下穴皆當除脊各寸半。

[Author's note:] *Qian Jin* 《千金》says: The Bā Liáo 八窌 are located 3 cùn below the lumbar eyes, 4 cùn from the spine (there are four points on each side, so they are called Bā [Eight] Liáo 八窌). What it says, 4 cùn from the sides of the spine, actually should be 1.5 cùn from spine on each side. All the points below Dà Zhù 大杼 (UB 11) should be 1.5 cùn from the spine.[60]

1.13
Bèi Yú Dì Sān Háng Zuǒ Yòu Èr Shí Bā Xué

背俞第三行左右二十八穴

The third line on back,
28 bilateral points [fourteen on each side]

附分二穴，在第二椎下附項內廉兩旁，相去俠脊各三寸。灸五壯，針三分。

Fù Fēn 附分 (UB 41) bilateral point: It is located 3 cùn beside the spine, lateral to the inferior aspect of the second vertebra, on the medial aspect of the nape of the neck. Burn five cones of moxibustion; needle 3 fēn deep.

魄戶二穴，在三椎下兩旁各三寸，正坐取之。針五分，得氣即瀉，又宜久留針。日灸七壯，止百壯。忌同。《明》云：日七壯，至二百。《下》云：魄戶在三椎下兩旁各三寸，灸三壯。又云：魄戶在三椎下兩旁各三寸，灸五壯。《素注》云：魄戶上直附分。

Pò Hù 魄戶 (UB 42) bilateral point: It is located 3 cùn lateral to the inferior aspect of the third vertebra. Locate the point while the patient sits upright. Needle 5 fēn deep; drain [the point] as soon as qì arrives; it is also recommended to retain the needle for a long time. Burn seven cones of moxibustion daily; stop at a hundred cones. Follow the same contraindications [as Bái Huán Shù

---

60. The Bā Liáo 八窌 points mentioned here seem to indicate Xiǎo Cháng Shù 小腸俞 (UB 27), Páng Guāng Shù 膀胱俞 (UB 28), Zhōng Lǚ Shù 中膂俞 (UB 29) and Bái Huán Shù 白環俞 (UB 30), since it says they are all located 1.5 cùn lateral to the spine. However, earlier the author said *Liáo* 窌 means *Liáo* 髎, so this could also be an erroneous description of the location of the Eight Liáo 八髎 points (UB 31-UB 34).

白環俞 (UB 30)]. *Míng*《明》says: Burn seven cones of moxibustion daily, up to two hundred cones. *Xià*《下》says: Pò Hù 魄戶 (UB 42) is located 3 cùn lateral to the inferior aspect of the third vertebra. Burn three cones of moxibustion. It also says: Pò Hù (UB 42) is located 3 cùn lateral to the inferior aspect of the third vertebra. Burn five cones of moxibustion. *Sù Zhù*《素注》says: Pò Hù (UB 42) is directly in line with Fù Fēn 附分 (UB 41) which is above it.

《銅人》有魄戶穴，《明堂上經》亦同。而《下經》既有魄戶穴，又有魂戶穴，皆云在三椎下。若謂誤寫魄字作魂，不應兩出魄戶穴也。考之《下經》既有懸鍾矣，後又有懸鍾。既有天突矣，其治小兒，又有天突。意者，魂戶即魄戶（誤作魂）而兩出之。不然，何其穴皆在三椎旁歟？

[Author's note:] *Tóng Rén*《銅人》describes Pò Hù (UB 42), so does *Míng Táng Shàng Jīng*《明堂上經》. But *Xià Jīng*《下經》has Pò Hù (UB 42) as well as Hún Hù 魂戶, both of which are located below the third vertebra. If *hún* 魂 (ethereal soul) was erroneously written instead of *pò* 魄 (corporeal soul), Pò Hù (UB 42) should not show up twice. When checking *Xià Jīng*, it has Xúan Zhōng 懸鍾 (GB 39) and later Xúan Zhōng (GB 39) shows up again; it also has Tiān Tū 天突 (Rèn 22) which treats pediatric [diseases], and later has Tiān Tū (Rèn 22) again. So the idea here is that Hún Hù means Pò Hù (UB 42) (*hún* 魂 is a typographical error); this is why it shows up twice. If not, why are they both located lateral to the third vertebra?

膏肓俞二穴，在四椎下（《明》云：近五椎）兩旁各三寸。主無所不療，羸瘦虛損，夢中失精，上氣咳逆，發狂健忘（《明》云：狂惑忘誤）。取穴之法：令人正坐，曲脊伸兩手，以臂得動搖，從胛骨上角摸索至骨下頭。其間當有四肋三間，灸中間。從胛骨之裏去胛骨容側指許。摩膂去表肋間空處按之，自覺牽引於肩中。灸兩胛中一處至百壯，多至五百（《明》云：六百壯，多至千壯），當覺下礱礱然似流水之狀，亦當有所下出。若得痰疾，則無所不下也。如病人已困，不能正坐，當令側臥，挽上臂，令取穴灸之。又以右手從左肩上住指頭所不及者，是穴也。右取亦然。乃以前法灸之。若不能久坐，當伸兩臂，令人挽兩胛骨使相離。不爾，即胛骨覆其穴，灸之無驗。此灸訖後，令人陽氣益盛，當消息以自補養。論曰：昔在和、緩不救晉侯之疾，以其在膏之上，肓之下，針藥所不能及，即此穴是也。時人拙，不能求得此穴，所以宿病難追。若能用心，方便求得灸之，無疾不愈（出《千金》、《外臺》）。

Gāo Huāng Shù 膏肓俞 (UB 43) bilateral point: It is located 3 cùn lateral to the inferior aspect of the fourth vertebra. (*Míng* says: It is near the fifth vertebra). It treats everything: marked emaciation, vacuity detriment, seminal loss while dreaming, counterflow cough with qì ascent, mania, and forgetfulness (*Míng* says: mania and confusion).

Point location method: Ask the patient to sit upright, bend his spine and stretch his two hands, moving his arms from the upper angle of the scapula toward the lower end of the bone [scapula].[61] There are four ribs with three [intercostal] spaces between them. Apply moxibustion to the middle [intercostal space]. Locate the point a finger-breath from the medial border of the scapula. Rub the spine[62] and press the depression of the intercostal space where the patient feels a [sensation] radiating to the shoulder. Apply up to a hundred cones of moxibustion to the space between the two scapulae, up to five hundred cones. (*Míng* 《 明 》 says: six hundred, up to a thousand cones). The patient should feel a sensation of water flowing downward like something grinding, and something will come out below.[63] If [the patient] has a phlegm disease, the phlegm will descend. If the patient is sleepy and cannot sit upright, ask them to lie on their side, flex their upper arm, then locate the point and apply moxibustion. The point is located [on the back] where the the patient's finger tip cannot reach when putting their right hand over the left upper shoulder. Use the same method on the right side. Apply moxibustion as before. If the patient cannot sit for a long time, ask them to stretch their two arms, and let other people pull the two arms to separate the two scapulae. Otherwise, applying moxibustion to it will be ineffective because the scapula will cover the points.

[This method] causes the yáng qì to become exuberant after moxibustion; the patient should rest for supplementation. Some books say: In the past, Hé and Huǎn[64] did not want to treat the disease of Jìn Hóu 晉候 [the Duke of Jìn], because the disease was located above the *gāo* 膏 [the fatty area below the tip the heart] and below the *huāng* 肓 [the space below the heart and above the diaphragm]. The effects of acupuncture and herbs cannot reach this location. That [story] indicates this point [Gāo Huāng Shù 膏肓俞 (UB 43)]. The people living at that time were not clever enough, so they could not find this point. That is why chronic diseases could not be cured. If they had been attentive enough to discover this point and apply moxibustion to it, then any disease could have been cured. ([This discussion] is from *Qiān Jīn* 《 千金 》 and *Wài Tái* 《 外臺 》).

灸膏肓功效，諸經例能言之，而取穴則未也。《千金》等方之外，莊綽論之最詳，然繁而無統，不能定於一。予嘗以意取之，令病人兩手交在兩膊上（灸時亦然），胛骨遂開，其穴立見。以手指摸索第四椎下兩旁各三寸，四肋三間之中間按之，酸疼是穴。灸至千百壯，少亦七七壯。當依《千金》：立點立灸，坐點坐灸，臥點臥灸云。（若只合尒在兩膝頭中點穴，亦得。）

61. The reason for this seems to be, to open up the space between the two scapulae, not because the hand can reach this point. Above, it is stated that the place the finger can reach is Fèi Shù 肺俞 (UB 13). Below it states that the patient cannot reach this point.

62. *Lǚ* 胠 (spine) is another way of writing *lǚ* 膂 (spine). This character is corrected from *qū* 胠 (axillary fossa), based on *Tóng Rén Tú Jīng* 《 銅人圖經 》.

63. *Lóng* 礱 indicates a tool for hulling rice (as a noun) or grinding grain (as a verb). This sentence is rather obscure. It is repeated from earlier books.

64. Hé 和 and Huǎn 緩 refer to Yī Hé 醫和 and Yī Huǎn 醫緩, two famous ancient doctors. Most sources only name Yī Huǎn 醫緩 in the story that follows. The only reference to Yī Hé 醫和 was in *Qiān Jīn Yào Fāng* 《 千金要方 》. This does not match historical accounts.

[Author's note:] All the classics talk about the effects of applying moxibustion to Gāo Huāng 膏肓 (UB 43), but none of them mention how to locate the point. Besides *Qiān Jīn* 《千金》, Zhuān Chuō discussed it thoroughly, but he was too fussy so [his book] cannot be set as the standard. I tried to locate this point based on the meaning: Ask the patient to cross his two arms (including while burning moxibustion) to separate the scapulae; in this way the point appears. Use your finger to palpate the space 3 cùn lateral to the inferior aspect of the fourth vertebra, and press between the fourth rib and the third [intercostal] space. Locate the point at the site where the patient feels soreness. Burn seven times seven cones of moxibustion, up to hundreds or thousands of cones. Follow *Qiān Jīn*'s method: If locating the point in the standing postion, then apply moxibustion in the same position; if locating the point in sitting postion, then apply moxibustion in the same position; if locating the point in a reclining postion, then apply moxibustion in the same position. (It is acceptable to locate the point with the patient putting his hands between his knees.)

神堂二穴，在五椎下兩旁各三寸陷中，正坐取之。針三分，灸五壯。《明下》云：三壯。《素注》云：上直魄戶（餘同）。

Shén Táng 神堂 (UB 44) bilateral point: It is located 3 cùn lateral to the inferior aspect of the fifth vertebra. Locate the point while the patient is sitting upright. Needle 3 fēn deep; burn five cones of moxibustion. *Míng Xià* 《明下》 says: Three cones. *Sù Zhù* 《素注》 says: It is in line with Pò Hù 魄戶 (UB 42) which is above it (the others are the same).

譩譆二穴，在肩膊內廉，俠（《明堂》作在）六椎下兩旁各三寸，正坐取之，以手痛按之，病者言譩譆。針六分，留三呼，瀉五吸，灸二七壯，止百壯。忌莧菜，白酒。《明下》云：五壯。

Yī Xī 譩譆 (UB 45) bilateral point: It is located on the medial aspect of the scapular [spine], 3 cùn lateral (*Míng Táng* 《明堂》 says *zài* 在 'at') to the inferior aspect of the sixth vertebra. Locate the point with the patient sitting upright. The patient will say Yī Xī 譩譆 [sounds of exclamation] when the point is pressed aggressively. Needle 6 fēn deep; retain the needle for three respirations, and drain for five respirations. Burn two times seven cones of moxibustion, stop at a hundred cones. Amaranth and white liquor are contraindicated. *Míng Xià* says: Five cones.

膈關二穴，在七椎下兩旁各三寸陷中，正坐取之。針五分，灸五壯。

Gé Guān 膈關 (UB 46) bilateral point: It is located in the depression 3 cùn lateral to the inferior aspect of the seventh vertebra. Locate the point with the patient sitting upright. Needle 5 fēn deep; burn five cones of moxibustion.

魂門二穴，在九椎下兩旁各三寸陷中，正坐取之。灸三壯，針五分。

Hún Mén 魂門 (UB 47) bilateral point: It is located in the depression 3 cùn lateral to the inferior aspect of the ninth vertebra. Locate the point with the patient sitting upright. Needle 5 fēn deep; burn five cones of moxibustion.

陽綱二穴，在十椎下兩旁各三寸陷中，正坐闊肩取之。針五分，灸三壯。《明下》云：七壯。

Yáng Gāng 陽綱 (UB 48) bilateral point: It is located in the depression 3 cùn lateral to the inferior aspect of the tenth vertebra. Locate the point with the patient sitting upright and broadening their shoulders. Needle 5 fēn deep; burn three cones of moxibustion. *Míng Xià* 《明下》 says: Seven cones.

意舍二穴，在十一椎下兩旁各三寸陷中，正坐取之。針五分，灸五十壯至百壯。《明》云：五十壯至百二十壯。《甲乙》云：三壯，針五分。《下》云：灸七壯。《素注》：二壯。

Yì Shè 意舍 (UB 49) bilateral point: It is located in the depression 3 cùn lateral to the inferior aspect of the eleventh vertebra. Locate the point with the patient sitting upright. Needle 5 fēn deep; burn fifty, up to a hundred cones of moxibustion. *Míng* 《明》 says: Fifty to one hundred twenty cones. *Jiǎ Yǐ* 《甲乙》 says: Three cones; needle 5 fēn deep. *Xià* 《下》 says: Burn seven cones of moxibustion. *Sù Zhù* 《素注》 says: Two cones.

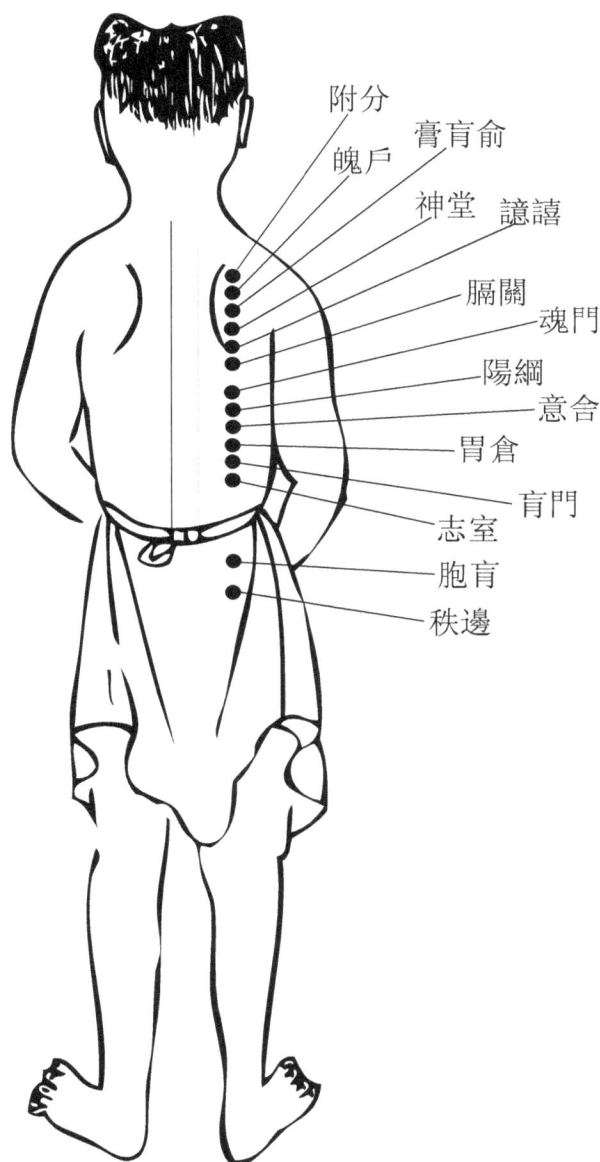

附分
魄戶
膏肓俞
神堂
譩譆
膈關
魂門
陽綱
意舍
胃倉
肓門
志室
胞肓
秩邊

Fig. 1.18

55

胃倉二穴，在十二椎下兩旁各三寸。針五分，灸五十壯。《明》云：五十壯。《甲乙》云：三壯。

Wèi Cāng 胃倉 (UB 50) bilateral point: It is located in the depression 3 cùn lateral to the inferior aspect of the twelfth vertebra. Needle 5 fēn deep; burn fifty cones of moxibustion. *Míng* 《明》 says: Fifty cones. *Jiǎ Yǐ* 《甲乙》 says: Three cones.

肓門二穴，在十三椎下兩旁各三寸叉肋間。其（《明堂》作異）經云：與鳩尾相直。灸三十壯，針五分。

Huāng Mén 肓門 (UB 51) bilateral point: It is located in the depression at the junction of the ribs [with the spine], 3 cùn lateral to the inferior aspect of the thirteenth vertebra [first lumbar vertebra]. The Classic says (*Míng Táng* 《明堂》 writes: 'A different classic says'): in line with Jiū Wěi 鳩尾 (Rèn 15). Burn thirty cones of moxibustion; needle 5 fēn deep.

志室二穴，在十四椎下兩旁各三寸陷中，正坐取之。針五分，灸三壯。《明下》云：兩旁各三寸半，灸七壯。

Zhì Shì 志室 (UB 52) bilateral point: It is located in the depression 3 cùn lateral to the inferior aspect of the fourteenth vertebra [second lumbar vertebra]. Locate the point with the patient sitting upright. Needle 5 fēn deep; burn three cones of moxibustion. *Míng Xià* 《明下》 says: 3.5 cùn lateral to [the vertebra]. Burn seven cones of moxibustion.

《明堂上經》作兩旁各三寸，與《銅人經》同，而《下經》乃作三寸半，必是分外半字也。

[Author's note:] *Míng Táng Shàng Jīng* 《明堂上經》 says: 3 cùn lateral [to the vertebra]. *Tóng Rén Jīng* 《銅人經》 says the same thing. But *Xià Jīng* 《下經》 says 3.5 cùn. Half (*bàn* 半) must be an extra word beyond the main part [3 cùn].

胞肓二穴，在十九椎下兩旁各三寸陷中，伏而取之。灸五七壯，針五分。《明》云：灸五七壯至五十壯。《甲乙》云：三壯。《下》云：五壯。

Bāo Huāng 胞肓 (UB 53) bilateral point: It is located in the depression 3 cùn lateral to the inferior aspect of the nineteenth vertebra [second sacral vertebra]. Locate the point with the patient in the prone position. Burn five times seven cones of moxibustion; needle 5 fēn deep. *Míng* says: Burn five times seven, up to fifty cones of moxibustion. *Jiǎ Yǐ* says: Three cones. *Xià* 《下》 says: Five cones.

秩邊二穴，在二十椎下兩旁各三寸陷中，伏而取之 。灸三壯，針五分 。忌
同 。《明 》云：在二十椎下兩旁各三寸，灸三壯，針三分 。

Zhì Biān 秩邊 (UB 54) bilateral point: It is located in the depression 3 lateral to the inferior aspect of the twentieth vertebra [third sacral vertebra]. Locate the point with the patient in the prone position. Burn three cones of moxibustion; needle 5 fēn deep. Follow the same contraindications [as Yì Xī 譩譆 (UB 45)]. *Míng* 《 明 》 says: It is located in the depression 3 cùn lateral to the inferior aspect of the twentieth vertebra. Burn three cones of moxibustion; needle 3 fēn deep.

《素問·氣府論》注曰：秩邊在二十一椎下兩旁，上胞肓，與《銅人經》 、《明堂經》二十椎下不同。 未知其孰是，姑兩存之。

[Author's note:] The Annotations to *Sù Wèn · Qì Fǔ Lùn* 《 素問·氣府論 》 says: Zhì Biān (UB 54) is located lateral to the inferior aspect of the twenty-first vertebra [fourth sacral vertebra], directly in the line with Bāo Huāng 胞肓 (UB 53) which is above it. This is different from the twentieth vertebra [third sacral vertebra] in *Tóng Rén Jīng* 《 銅人經 》 and *Míng Táng Jīng* 《 明堂經 》. I do not know which one is correct, so I am just keeping the [two ideas regarding location] together.

以上二十八穴，當準《千金方》除脊各三寸取穴。

We should follow *Qiān Jīn Fāng* 《 千金方 》 and locate the above 28 points [14 on each side] 3 cùn from the spine.

1.14
Cè Jǐng Xiàng Bù Zuǒ Yòu Shí Bā Xué

側頸項部左右十八穴

Lateral side of the neck and nape,
18 bilateral points [nine on each side]

天容二穴，在耳下曲頰後。灸三壯。

Tiān Róng 天容 (SI 17) bilateral point: It is located below the ear and posterior to the mandible. Burn three cones of moxibustion.

天牖二穴，在頸筋缺盆上，天容後，天柱前，完骨下，髮際上（《明》云：髮際上一寸陷中）。針一寸，留七呼，不宜補，亦不宜灸。若灸，面腫眼合。先取譩譆，後針天牖、風池即差。若不先針譩譆，即難療。《明》云：針五分，得氣即瀉，瀉盡更留三呼，瀉三吸，不宜補，亦不宜灸。《下》云：灸三壯，《素注》同。

Tiān Yǒu 天牖 (SJ 16) bilateral point: It is located on the sinew of the neck,[65] above the empty basin (supraclavicular fossa), posterior to Tiān Róng (SI 17), anterior to Tiān Zhù 天柱 (UB 10). It is below the mastoid process and above the hairline (*Míng* 《明》 says: It is in the depression 1 cùn above the hairline). Needle 1 cùn deep, retain the needle for seven respirations; supplementation and moxibustion are not recommended. Moxibution will cause the face to swell until the eyes shut. This be cured by needling Yī Xī 譩譆 (UB 45) first, then Tiān Yǒu (SJ 16) and Fēng Chí 風池 (GB 20). But if you do not needle Yī Xī (UB 45) first, it will be difficult to treat. *Míng* says: Needle 5 fēn deep; drain [the point] as soon as qì arrives; retain the needle for three respirations after draining, then drain for three [more] respirations. Supplemention and moxibustion are not recommended. *Xià* 《下》 says: Burn three cones of moxibustion. *Sù Zhù* 《素注》 agrees.

《銅人》、《明堂上經》皆云：不宜灸，《下經》、《素問》注乃云：灸三壯。恐凡禁穴許灸一壯至三壯也。

---

65. The *sinew of the neck* refers to the sternocleidomastoid muscle.

[Author's note:] *Tóng Rén* 《銅人》 and *Míng Táng Shàng Jīng* 《明堂上經》 both say: Moxibustion is not recommended. But *Xià Jīng* 《下經》 and the Annotation to *Sù Wèn* 《素問》 both say: Burn three cones of moxibustion. It might be all right to apply one to three cones of moxibustion on the contraindicated points.

天窗二穴，一名窗籠。在頸大筋
前，曲頰下扶突後，動脈應手陷
中。灸三壯，針三分。

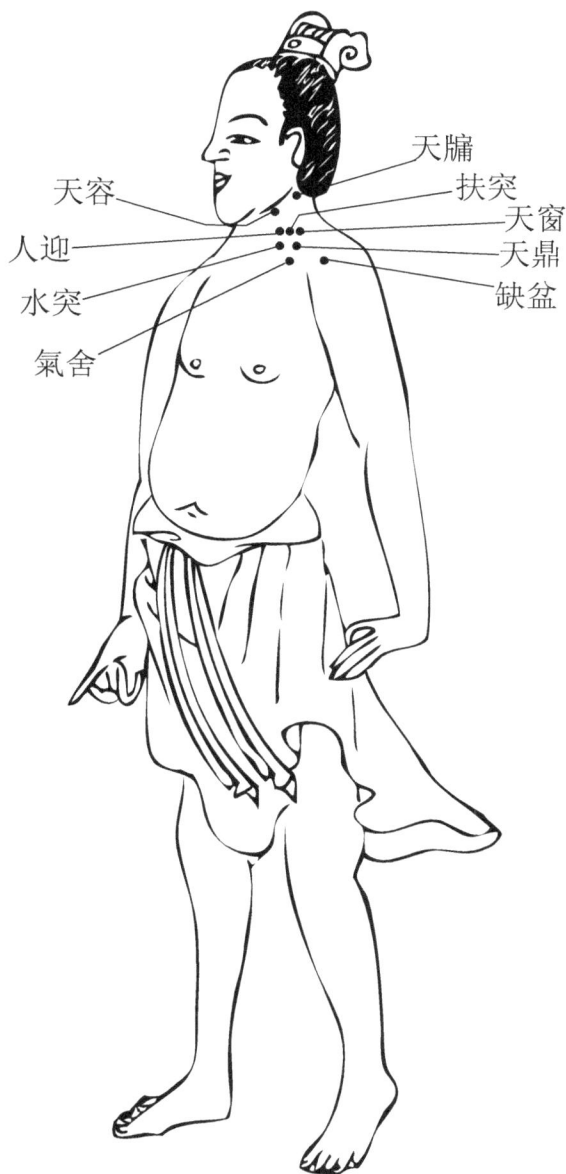

Tiān Chuāng 天窗 (SI 16) bilateral point, another name is Chuāng Lóng 窗籠: It is located anterior to the big sinew on the neck, posterior to Fú Tū 扶突 (LI 18), in the depression where the pulsating vessel responds to the hand. Burn three cones of moxibustion; needle 3 fēn deep.

天鼎二穴，在頸缺盆直扶突後一
寸。灸三壯，針三分。忌同。《
明下》云：天頂在項缺盆直扶
突，氣舍後一寸陷中。灸七壯。
《素·氣府論》注云：天鼎在頸
缺盆上直扶突，氣舍後同身寸之
半。按《甲乙經》作寸半。

Tiān Dǐng 天鼎 (LI 17) bilateral point: It is located in the empty basin,[66] directly in line with and 1 cùn posterior to Fú Tū (LI 18). Burn three cones of moxibustion; needle 3 fēn deep. Follow the same contraindications [as Yì Xǐ 譩譆 (UB 45)]. *Míng Xià* 《明下》 says: Tiān Dǐng 天頂 (LI 17) is located in the empty basin, in the line with Fú Tū (LI 18), in the depression 1 cùn posterior to Qì Shè 氣舍 (ST 11). Burn seven cones of moxibustion. The Annotation to *Sù [Wèn] · Qì Fǔ Lùn* 《素·氣府論》 says: Tiān Dǐng (LI 17) is

Fig. 1.19

---

66. The *empty basin* is the supraclavicular fossa.

located on the neck, above the empty basin, in line with Fú Tū 扶突 (LI 18) and 0.5 cùn posterior to Qì Shè 氣舍 (ST 11), using proportional measurements. *Jiǎ Yǐ Jīng*《甲乙經》says 1.5 cùn.

扶突二穴，一名水穴。在人迎後寸半。灸三壯，針三分。《素注》：在頸當曲頰下一寸人迎後，仰而取之。

Fú Tū (LI 18) bilateral point, another name is Shuǐ Xué 水穴: It is located 1.5 cùn posterior to Rén Yíng 人迎 (ST 9). Burn three cones of moxibustion; needle 3 fēn deep. *Sù Zhù*《素注》says: It is on the neck, 1 cùn below the mandible, posterior to Rén Yíng (ST 9). Locate the point with the patient in a supine position.

缺盆二穴，一名天蓋。在肩下橫骨陷中。灸三壯，針三分（《素》云：二分），不宜刺太深，使人逆息也。《明》云：肩上橫骨陷中（《素》同），一名天蓋，肩上是穴。

Quē Pén 缺盆 (ST 12) bilateral point, another name is Tiān Gài 天蓋: It is located in the depression on the transverse bone [clavicle] below the shoulder. Burn three cones of moxibustion; needle 3 fēn deep (*Sù*《素》says: 2 fēn deep). It is not appropriate to needle too deeply; it causes counterflow of breath [difficulty breathing]. *Míng*《明》says: It is in the depression on the transverse bone above the shoulder (Same as in *Sù*). Another name is Tiān Gài, which is a point above the shoulder.

《銅人》云：在肩下橫骨陷中，《明堂》乃云：在肩上橫骨陷中，又云：肩上是穴，恐《銅人》誤下字也。

[Author's note:] *Tóng Rén*《銅人》says: It is in the depression on the transverse bone [clavicle] below the shoulder. *Míng Táng*《明堂》says: in the depression on the transverse bone [clavicle] above the shoulder; it also says: it is a point above the shoulder. So *Tóng Rén* may have made a mistake with the word *xià* 下 (below).

人迎二穴，一名五會。在頸大脈，動脈應手，俠結喉旁，仰而取之。以候五臟氣，足陽明脈氣所發。禁灸，灸之不幸傷人，針四分。

Rén Yíng (ST 9) bilateral point, another name is Wǔ Huì 五會: It is located lateral to the laryngeal prominence [Adam's apple], on the big vessel in the neck where the pulsating vessel responds to the hand. Locate the point with the patient in a supine position. [This point] reflects the qì of the five viscera; it is also a point where the qì of the foot yángmíng vessel comes out. Moxibustion is contraindicated; it will hurt people. Needle 4 fēn deep.

水突二穴，一名水門。在頸大筋前，直人迎下，氣舍上。針三分，灸三壯。

Shuǐ Tū 水突 (ST 10) bilateral point, another name is Shuǐ Mén 水門: It is located anterior to the big sinew of the neck, directly below Rén Yíng 人迎 (ST 9) and above Qì Shè 氣舍 (ST 11). Needle 3 fēn deep; burn three cones of moxibustion.

氣舍二穴，在頸直人迎，俠天突陷中。針三分，灸三壯。

Qì Shè (ST 11) bilateral point: It is located on the neck, in the depression lateral to Tiān Tū 天突 (Rèn 22), directly below Rén Yíng (ST 9). Needle 3 fēn deep; burn three cones of moxibustion.

1.15
Yīng Yú Bù Zhōng Háng Qī Xué

膺俞部中行七穴

7 points on the midline of chest

天突在結喉下一夫宛宛中。針五分，留三呼，得氣即瀉。灸亦得，即不及針。其下針直橫下，不得低手，即五藏之氣傷，人短壽。忌同。《明下》云：在結喉下五分中央宛宛中，灸五壯。《素·氣穴》注云：在結喉下四寸中央宛宛中，刺一寸，灸三壯。《甲乙》云：在結喉下五寸。《明下》灸小兒云：結喉下三寸兩骨間（《千》名天瞿。◎今校勘，在結喉下五寸是穴）。

Tiān Tū (Rèn 22): It is located in the depression one hand [width] inferior to the laryngeal prominence [Adam's apple]. Needle 5 fēn deep; retain the needle for three respirations; drain [the point] as soon as qì arrives. Moxibustion is recommended, but is not as good as needling. When needling, prick transversely downward without lowering the hand; otherwise, it will damage the qì of five viscera and shorten the lifespan. Follow the same contraindications [as Yì Xī 譩譆 (UB 45)]. *Míng Xià* 《 明下 》 says: It is in the depression 5 fēn deep below the laryngeal prominence. Apply five cones of moxibustion. The Annotation of the *Sù [Wèn]·Qì Xuè* 《 素·氣穴 》 says: It is in the central depression, 4 cùn below the laryngeal prominence. Needle 1 cùn deep; apply three cones of moxibustion. *Jiǎ Yǐ* 《 甲乙 》 says: It is 5 cùn below the laryngeal prominence. The chapter on pediatric application of moxibustion in *Míng Xià* says: It is 3 cùn below the laryngeal prominence, in the depression between the two bones. (*Qiān* 《 千 》 named it Tiān Qú 天瞿 * Now I have corrected it by comparing all the other classics: The point is located 5 cùn below the laryngeal prominence.)

璇璣，在天突下一寸陷中，仰頭取之 。灸五壯，針入三分 。

Xuán Jī 璇璣 (Rèn 21): It is located in the depression 1 cùn below Tiān Tū 天突 (Rèn 22). Locate the point with the patient in a supine position. Apply five cones of moxibustion; needle 3 fēn deep.

華蓋，在璇璣下一寸陷中，仰頭取之 。針三分，灸五壯 。《 明下 》云：三壯 。一本云：五壯 。

Huá Gài 華蓋 (Rèn 20): It is located in the depression 1 cùn below Xuán Jī 璇璣 (Rèn 21). Locate the point with the patient in a supine position. Needle 3 fēn deep; apply five cones of moxibustion. *Míng Xià* 《 明下 》 says: Three cones. Another edition says: Five cones.

紫宮，在華蓋下一寸六分陷中，仰頭取之 。灸五壯，針三分 。《 明下 》云：在華蓋下一寸，灸七壯（ 小本亦同 ）。

Zǐ Gōng 紫宮 (Rèn 19): It is located in the depression 1.6 cùn below Huá Gài (Rèn 20). Locate the point with the patient in the supine position. Apply five cones of moxibustion; needle 3 fēn deep. *Míng Xià* says: It is 1 cùn below Huá Gài (Rèn 20). Burn seven cones of moxibustion (the small [edition of the] book says the same thing).

玉堂，一名玉英 。在紫宮下寸六分陷中 。灸五壯，針三分 。

Yù Táng 玉堂 (Rèn 18), another name is Yù Yīng 玉英: It is located in the depression 1.6 cùn below Zǐ Gōng (Rèn 19). Apply five cones of moxibustion; needle 3 fēn deep.

膻中，（ 一作亶 ），一名元兒 。在玉堂下一寸六分，橫直兩乳間陷中，仰臥取之 。灸七七壯，禁針，不幸令人夭 。《 明 》云：日灸七壯，止七七 。禁針，不幸令人死 。《 甲乙 》云：針三分 。《 下 》云：灸三壯 。《 千 》云：鳩尾上一寸 。

Dàn Zhōng 膻中 (Rèn 17), (also named *dǎn* 亶), another name is Yuán Ér 元兒: It is located in the depression 1.6 cùn below Yù Táng (Rèn 18), directly in line with the two nipples. Locate the point with the patient in a supine position. Burn seven times seven cones of moxibustion. Needling is contraindicated; it makes people die young. *Míng* 《明》 says: Burn seven cones daily, stop at seven time seven cones. Needling is contraindicated. It makes people die. *Jiǎ Yǐ* 《甲乙》 says: Needle 3 fēn deep. *Xià* 《下》 says: Burn three cones of moxibustion. *Qiān* 《千》 says: It is 1 cùn above Jiū Wěi 鳩尾 (Rèn 15).

《靈蘭秘典》云：膻中者，臣使之官，喜樂出焉。說者曰：膻中為氣之海，然心主為君，以敷宣教令。膻中主氣，以氣布陰陽，氣和志適，則喜樂由生，分布陰陽，故官為臣使也。然則膻中者，乃十二藏之一，臣使之官，為氣之海，分布陰陽，非其他穴比者。或患氣噎，鬲氣，肺氣上喘，不得下食，胸中如塞等疾，宜灸此。（◎《難疏》：氣會三焦，外筋直兩乳間。氣病治此）。

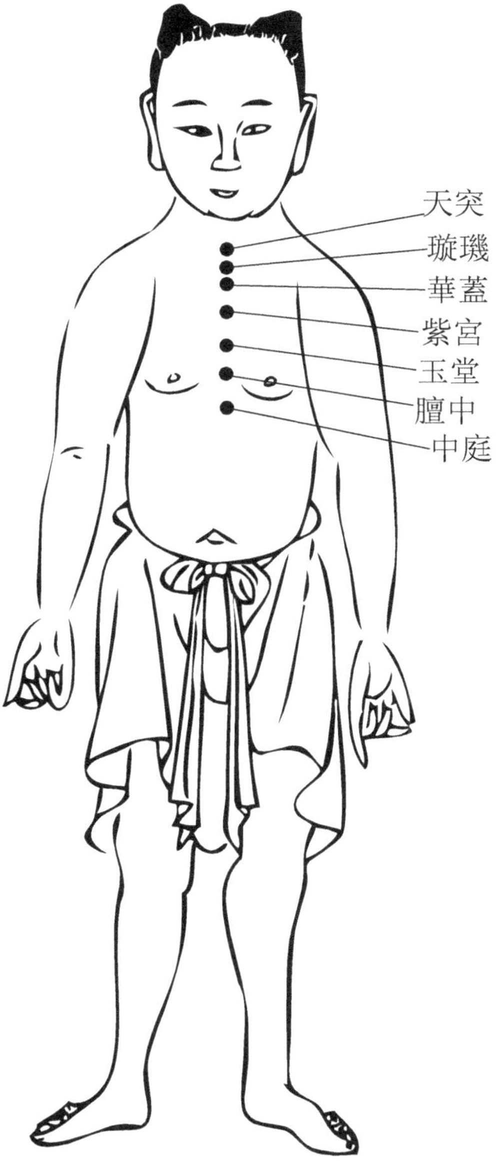

[Author's note:] *Líng Lán Mì Diǎn Lùn* 《靈蘭秘典》 (Treatise of the Arcane Book of the Orchid Chamber of the Spirit Tower)[67] says: Dàn Zhōng 膻中 is the officer who is the deputy and envoy, in order to make [the king] happy. It is said: Dàn Zhōng is the sea of qì. But the heart governs as the king, so [Dàn Zhōng] helps to propagate the regulations. Dàn Zhōng governs the qì. The qì spreads the yīn and yáng. When harmonious, the qì makes suitable aspirations, and happiness is engendered. [Dàn Zhōng] spreads the yīn and yáng, so it acts like the deputy and envoy. Dàn Zhōng [this term often refers to the pericardium itself] is one of the twelve viscera, the office of the deputy, the sea of qì, and it spreads the yīn and yáng. All these are incomparable. It is appropriate to apply moxibustion to it if the patient suffers from qì choking, qì occlusion, lung qì panting [shortness of breath], inability to get food down, and

天突
璇璣
華蓋
紫宮
玉堂
膻中
中庭

Fig. 1.20

67. This is referring to the *Sù Wèn* 《素問》 (Plain Questions), Chapter 8.

中庭，在膻中下寸六分陷中。灸五壯，針三分。《明》云：二分。《下》云：膻中下一寸，灸三壯。

Zhōng Tíng 中庭 (Rèn 16): It is located in the depression 1.6 cùn below Dàn Zhōng 膻中 (Rèn 17). Apply five cones of moxibustion; needle 3 fēn deep. *Míng*《明》says: 2 fēn deep. *Xià*《下》says: It is 1 cùn below Dǎn Zhōng (Rèn 17). Apply three cones of moxibustion.

1.16
Yīng Yú Dì Èr Háng Zuǒ Yòu Shí Èr Xué

膺俞第二行左右十二穴

The second line on the chest, 12 bilateral points [six on each side]

腧府（《素》作俞）二穴，在巨骨下，璇璣旁各二寸陷中，仰而取之。（《明》云：仰臥取之）。針三分，灸五壯。《明下》云：輸府，灸三壯。

Shù Fǔ 腧府 (KI 27) (*Sù*《素》writes *shù* 俞), bilateral point: It is located below the huge bone [clavicle], in the depression 2 cùn lateral to Xuán Jī 璇璣 (Rèn 21). Locate the point in the supine position. (*Míng*《明》says: Locate the point with the patient lying supine). Needle 3 fēn deep; burn five cones of moxibustion. *Míng Xià*《明下》says: Shū Fǔ 輸府 (KI 27): Burn three cones of moxibustion.

彧中二穴，在腧府下寸六分陷中，仰而取之（《明》云：仰臥取之）。針四分，灸五壯。《明下》云：輸府下一寸，灸三壯。

Yù Zhōng 彧中 (KI 26) bilateral point: It is located in the depression 1.6 cùn below Shù Fǔ (KI 27). Locate the point in the supine position. (*Míng* says: Locate the points with the patient lying supine.) Needle 4 fēn deep; burn five cones of moxibustion. *Míng Xià* says: 1 cùn below Shū Fǔ (KI 27); burn three cones of moxibustion.

神藏二穴，在彧中下寸六分陷中，仰而取之 。灸五壯，針三分 。

Shén Cáng 神藏 (KI 25), bilateral point: It is located in the depression 1.6 cùn below Yù Zhōng 彧中 (KI 26). Locate the point in the supine position. Burn five cones of moxibustion; needle 3 fēn deep.

靈墟二穴，在神藏下寸六分陷中，仰而取之 。針三分，灸五壯 。

Líng Xū 靈墟 (KI 24), bilateral point: It is located in the depression 1.6 cùn below Shén Cáng (KI 25). Locate the point in the supine position. Needle 3 fēn deep; burn five cones of moxibustion.

神封二穴，在靈墟下寸六分，仰而取之 。灸五壯，針三分 。

Shén Fēng 神封 (KI 23), bilateral point: It is located in the depression 1.6 cùn below Líng Xū (KI 24). Locate the point in the supine position. Burn five cones of moxibustion; needle 3 fēn deep.

步郎二穴，在神封下寸六分陷中，仰而取之 。針三分，灸五壯 。

Bù Láng 步郎 (KI 22), bilateral point: It is located in the depression 1.6 cùn below Shén Fēng (KI 23). Locate the point in the supine position. Needle 3 fēn deep; burn five cones of moxibustion.

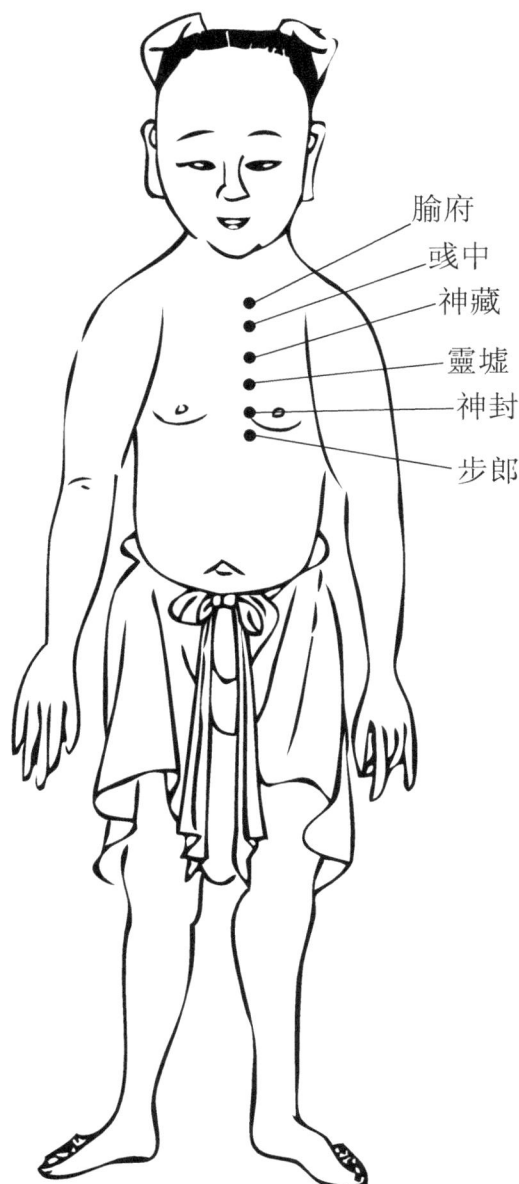

腧府
彧中
神藏
靈墟
神封
步郎

Fig. 1.21

1.17
Yīng Yú Dì Sān Háng Zuǒ Yòu Shí Èr Xué

膺俞第三行左右十二穴

The third line on the chest,
12 bilateral points [six on each side]

氣戶二穴，在巨骨下，俞府兩旁各二寸陷中，仰而取之。針三分，灸五壯。

Qì Hù 氣戶 (ST 13), bilateral point: It is located below the huge bone [clavicle]; in the depression 2 cùn lateral to Shù Fǔ 俞府 (KI 27). Locate the point in a supine position. Needle 3 fēn deep; burn five cones of moxibustion.

庫房二穴，在氣戶下寸六分陷中，仰而取之。灸五壯，針三分。

Kù Fáng 庫房 (ST 14), bilateral point: It is located in the depression 1.6 cùn below Qì Hù (ST 13). Locate the point in a supine position. Burn five cones of moxibustion; needle 3 fēn deep.

屋翳二穴，在庫房下寸六分陷中，仰而取之。灸五壯，針三分。

Wū Yì 屋翳 (ST 15), bilateral point: It is located in the depression 1.6 cùn below Kù Fáng (ST 14). Locate the point in a supine position. Burn five cones of moxibustion; needle 3 fēn deep.

膺窗二穴，在屋翳下寸六分。灸五壯，針四分。

Yīng Chuāng 膺窗 (ST 16), bilateral point: It is located in the depression 1.6 cùn below Wū Yì (ST 15). Burn five cones of moxibustion; needle 4 fēn deep.

乳中二穴，當乳是。足陽明脈氣所發。禁灸，灸不幸生蝕瘡。瘡中有清汁膿血，可治。瘡中有瘜肉，若蝕瘡者死。微刺三分。（亦相去寸六分。）

Rǔ Zhōng 乳中 (ST 17), bilateral point: It is located in [the center of] the nipple. It is where the qì of the foot yángmíng vessel is distributed. Moxibustion is contraindicated as it will cause eroding sores. It is treatable if there is clear fluid, pus, and blood in the sores; if there is a polyp and it looks like an eroding sore, the patient will die. Needle gently 3 fēn deep. (It is also 1.6 cùn away [from Yīng Chuāng 膺窗 (ST 16)]).

乳根二穴，在乳下寸六分陷中，
仰而取之。灸五壯，針三分。

Rǔ Gēn 乳根 (ST 18), bilateral point: It is located in the depression 1.6 cùn below the nipples. Locate the point in the supine position. Burn five cones of moxibustion; needle 3 fēn deep.

以上十二穴去膺中行各四寸，
遞相去寸六分。

The above 12 points are all located 4 cùn lateral to the midline of the chest, and 1.6 cùn from each other.

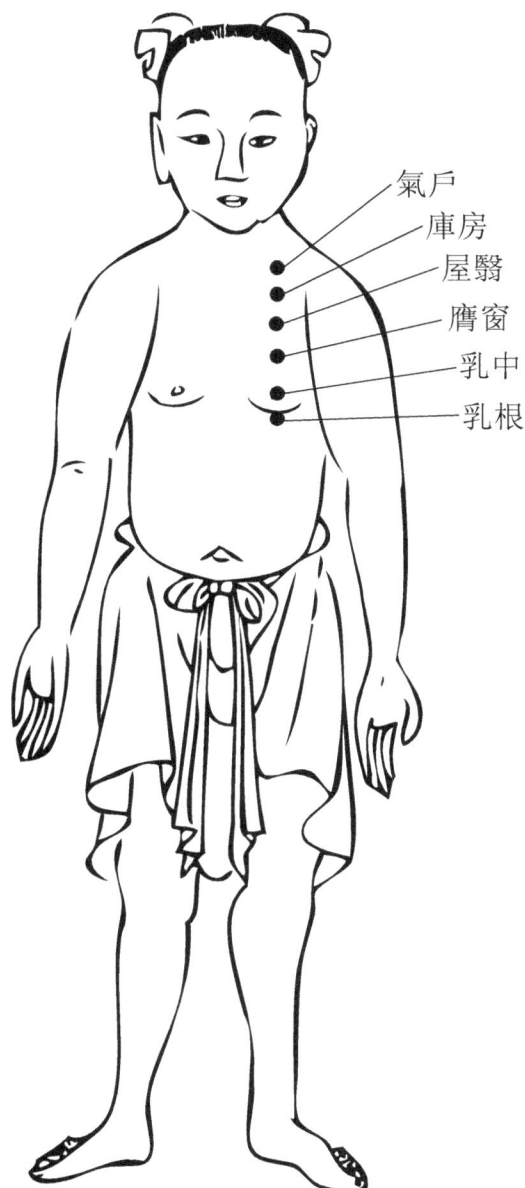

氣戶
庫房
屋翳
膺窗
乳中
乳根

Fig. 1.22

1.18

Yīng Yú Dì Sì Háng Zuǒ Yòu Shí Èr Xué

膺俞第四行左右十二穴

The fourth line on the chest, bilateral points [six on each side]

雲門二穴，在巨骨下，俠氣戶旁各二寸陷中。灸五壯，針三分，刺深使人氣逆，不宜深刺。《明》云：雲門在巨骨下，氣戶兩旁各二寸陷中，動脈應手，舉臂取之。《山眺經》云：在人迎下，第二骨間，相去二寸三分，通灸，禁針。《甲乙》云：灸五壯，針七分，若深令人氣逆。

Yún Mén 雲門 (LU 2), bilateral point: It is located below the huge bone [clavicle], in the depression 2 cùn lateral to Qì Hù 氣戶 (ST 13). Burn five cones of moxibustion; needle 3 fēn deep. Deep needling is not recommended, it causes the qì to counterflow. *Míng*《明》says: Yún Mén (LU 2) is located below the huge bone [clavicle], in the depression 2 cùn lateral to Qì Hù (ST 13). There is pulsating vessel that responds to the hand. Locate the point while raising [abducting] the arm. *Shān Tiào Jīng*《山眺經》[68] says: It is located below Rén Yíng 人迎 (ST 9), in the second bone depression [intercostal space], 2.3 cùn from [Rén Yíng (ST 9)]. Always apply moxibustion; needling is contraindicated. *Jiǎ Yǐ*《甲乙》says: Burn five cones of moxibustion; needle 7 fēn deep. Needling too deep causes the qì to counterflow.

中府二穴，一名膺中俞，肺之募。在雲門下一寸，乳上三肋間。針三分，留五呼，灸五壯。《素注》：在膺中行兩旁相去六寸，雲門下一寸，乳上三肋間，動脈應手陷中，仰而取之。

Zhōng Fǔ 中府 (LU 1), bilateral point, another name is Yīng Zhōng Shù 膺中俞; it is the alarm point of the lungs: It is located 1 cùn below Yún Mén (LU 2), in the depression three intercostal spaces above the nipples. Needle 3 fēn deep, retain the needle for five respirations; burn five cones of moxibustion. *Sù Zhù*《素注》says: It is located 6 cùn lateral to the midline of the chest, 1 cùn below Yún Mén (LU 2), in the depression three intercostal spaces above the nipples where there is pulsating vessel that responds to the hand. Locate the point in a supine position.

---

68. *Shān Tiào Jīng*《山眺經》: no information was found on this book.

周榮二穴，在中府下寸六分陷中，仰而取之 。針四分 。《 明下 》云：灸五壯 。

Zhōu Róng 周榮 (SP 20), bilateral point:
It is located in the depression 1.6 cùn below
Zhōng Fǔ 中府 (LU 1). Locate the point
in the supine position. Needle 4 fēn deep.
Míng Xià 《 明下 》 says: Burn five cones of
moxibustion.

胸鄉二穴，在周榮下寸六分陷中，
仰而取之 。針四分，灸五壯 。

Xiōng Xiāng 胸鄉 (SP 19), bilateral point:
It is located in the depression 1.6 cùn below
Zhōu Róng (SP 20). Locate the point in a
supine position. Needle 4 fēn deep; burn five
cones of moxibustion.

天溪二穴，在胸鄉下寸六分陷中，
仰而取之 。針四分，灸五壯 。

Tiān Xī 天溪 (SP 18), bilateral point: It is located in the depression 1.6 cùn below Xiōng
Xiāng (SP 19). Locate the point in the supine
position. Needle 4 fēn deep; burn five cones
of moxibustion.

食竇二穴，在天溪下寸六分陷中，
舉臂取之 。針四分，灸五壯 。

Shí Dòu 食竇 (SP 17), bilateral point: It is
located in the depression 1.6 cùn below Tiān
Xī (SP 18). Locate the point while raising
[abducting] the arm. Needle 4 fēn deep; burn
five cones of moxibustion.

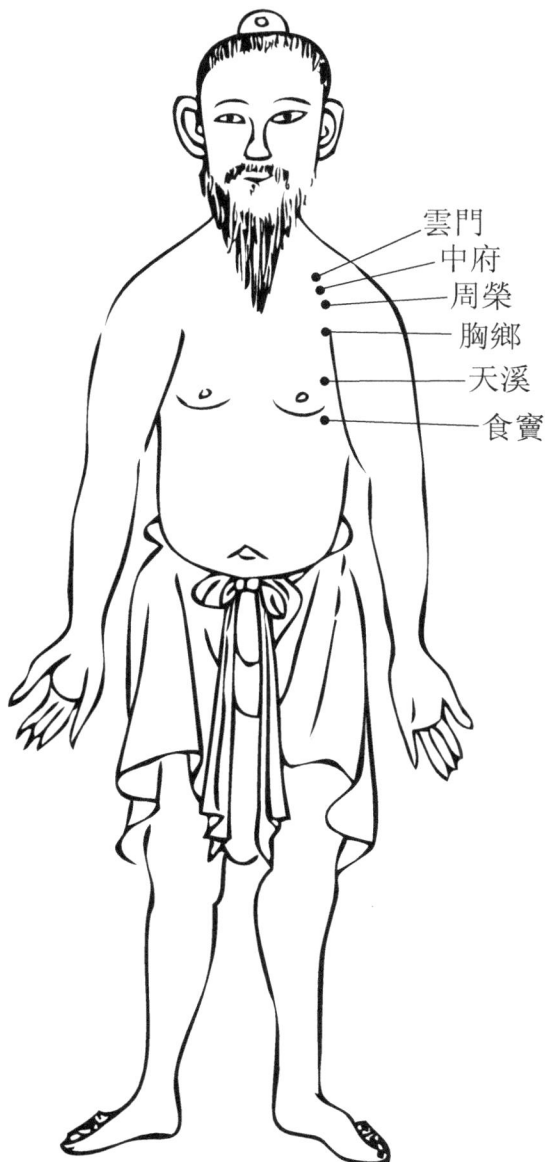

雲門
中府
周榮
胸鄉
天溪
食竇

Fig. 1.23

69

以上十二穴去膺中行各六寸六分。

以上十二穴去膺中行各六寸六分。

The above 12 points are all located 6.6 cùn[69] lateral to the midline of the chest.

1.19
Cè Yè Zuǒ Yòu Bā Xué

側腋左右八穴

Side of the axilla,
8 bilateral points [four on each side]

淵腋二穴，在腋下三寸宛宛中，舉臂得之。禁灸，灸之不幸令人生腫蝕馬瘍，內潰者死；寒熱生馬瘍可消。針三分。

Yuān Yè 淵腋 (GB 22), bilateral point: It is located in the depression, 3 cùn below the axilla. Locate the point while raising [abducting] the arm. Moxibustion is contraindicated. It causes swelling, erosion, and sores. [The patient] will die if the erosion ulcerates internally; or the erosion can be dispersed when the patient has cold and heat. Needle 3 fēn deep.

輒筋二穴，在腋下三寸，復前一寸著脅。灸三壯，針六分。

Zhé Jīn 輒筋 (GB 23), bilateral point: It is located 3 cùn below the axilla and runs 1 cùn anteriorly, adhering to the rib-sides. Burn three cones of moxibustion; needle 6 fēn deep.

天池二穴，一名天會。在乳後一寸，腋下三寸，著脅直腋橛肋間。灸三壯，針三分。

Tiān Chí 天池 (PC 1), bilateral point, another name is Tiān Huì 天會: It is located 1 cùn posterior to the nipples and 3 cùn below the axilla; it is on the line between the axilla and the intercostal

---

69. According to the text above, the statement here should read: 以上十二穴去膺中行各六寸，遞相去寸六分 (The above entries of 12 points are all located 6 cùn lateral to the midline of the chest, and 1.6 cùn from each other).

spaces of the peg ribs [free ribs], adhering to the rib-sides. Burn three cones of moxibustion; needle 3 fēn deep.

大包二穴，在淵腋下三寸。脾之大絡，布胸脅中，出九肋間。灸三壯，針三分。

Dà Bāo 大包 (SP 21), bilateral point: It is located 3 cùn below Yuān Yè 淵腋 (GB 22). It is the great network of spleen. It distributes [qì and blood] to the chest and rib-sides, exiting in the ninth intercostal space. Burn three cones of moxibustion; needle 3 fēn deep.

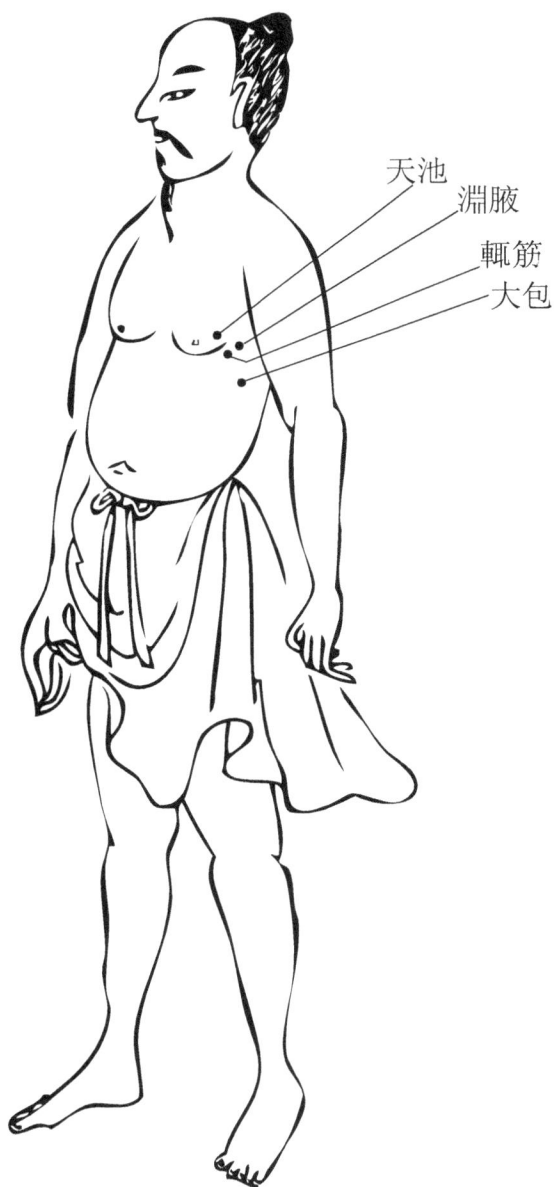

天池
淵腋
輒筋
大包

Fig. 1.24

1.20
Fù Bù Zhōng Háng Shí Wŭ Xué

腹部中行十五穴

Midline of the abdomen, 15 points

鳩尾，一名尾翳，一名𩩲骭。在臆前蔽骨下五分。不可灸，令人畢世少心力。此穴大難針，大好手方可下針，不然取氣多，令人夭。針三分，留三呼，瀉五吸，肥人倍之。忌同。《明下》云：灸三壯。《素注》：在臆前蔽骨下五分，不可灸刺。人無蔽骨者，從岐骨際下行一寸。

Jiū Wěi 鳩尾 (Rèn 15), another name is Wěi Yì 尾翳, also named Hé Gàn 𩩲骭: It is located 5 fēn below the covering bone [xiphoid process], anterior to the breast bone. Moxibustion is not recommended; it makes a person's heart lack strength for the rest of his life. It is very difficult to needle this point; only good hands [experienced people] can puncture it. Otherwise, it will consume too much qì and make people die young. Needle 3 fēn deep; retain the needle for three respirations and drain for five respirations; double the above for oversized patients. Follow the same contraindications [as Yì Xī 譩譆 (UB 45)]. *Míng Xià* 《明下》 says: Burn three cones of moxibustion. *Sù Zhù* 《素注》 says: It is 5 fēn below the covering bone, anterior to the breast bone. Moxibustion and needling are not recommended. If the patient has no [palpable] covering bone, locate the point 1 cùn below the border of the junction of the two bones [sternocostal angle].

巨闕，心之募。在鳩尾下一寸。鳩尾拒者，少令強一寸。中人有鳩尾拒之。針六分，留七呼，得氣即瀉，可灸七壯，止七七。忌同。

Jù Què 巨闕 (Rèn 14) is the alarm point of the heart. It is located 1 cùn below Jiū Wěi [turtledove tail-the xiphoid process]; if Jiū Wěi is square shaped, it is less than 1 cùn below. Some ordinary people have a square Jiū Wěi. Needle 6 fēn deep; retain the needle for seven respirations; drain [the point] as soon as qì arrives. Burn seven cones of moxibustion, stop at seven times seven cones. It has the same contraindications [as Yì Xī (UB 45)].

上脘（一作管），在巨闕下一寸（當寸五分），去蔽骨三寸（《明》云：去巨骨三寸）。針八分，先補後瀉，神驗。如風癇熱病，宜先瀉後補，立愈。

日灸二七壯至百壯，未愈倍之。忌同。《明下》云：三壯。（《千》：一名胃管。）

Shàng Wǎn 上脘 (Rèn 13) (also known as *guǎn* 管 [tube]): It is located 1 cùn (it should say 1.5 cùn) below Jù Què 巨闕 (Rèn 14), 3 cùn from [below] the covering bone [xiphoid process]. (*Míng* 《明》 says: It is 3 cùn from [below] the huge bone [clavicle]). Needle 8 fēn deep; drain first, then supplement. It will have magical results. For wind epilepsy and heat disease, drain first, then supplement. It will immediately cure the disease. Burn two times seven, up to a hundred cones of moxibustion daily. Double the dosage if the patient is not cured. Follow the same contraindications [as Yǐ Xī 譩譆 (UB 45)]. *Míng Xià* 《明下》 says: three cones. (*Qiān* 《千》 says: Another name is Wèi Guǎn 胃管)

中脘，一名太倉，胃之募。在上脘下一寸。上紀者，中脘也。針八分，留七呼，瀉五吸，疾出針，灸二七壯，止百壯。忌同。《明》云：日灸二七壯，止四百。（《千》一名胃募，在心下四寸，胃管下一寸。）

Zhōng Wǎn 中脘 (Rèn 12), another name is Tài Cāng 太倉: It is the alarm point of the stomach and is located 1 cùn below Shàng Wǎn (Rèn 13). Shàng Jì 上紀 (Upper Regulator) is [another name for] Zhōng Wǎn (Rèn 12). Needle 8 fēn deep; retain the needle for seven respirations; drain for five respirations; then remove the needle quickly. Burn two times seven cones of moxibustion, stop at a hundred [cones]. Follow the same contraindications [as Yǐ Xī (UB 45)]. *Míng* says: Burn two times seven cones of moxibustion daily, stop at four hundred [cones]. (*Qiān* says: Another name is Wèi Mù 胃募 and is located 4 cùn below the heart and 1 cùn below Wèi Guǎn).

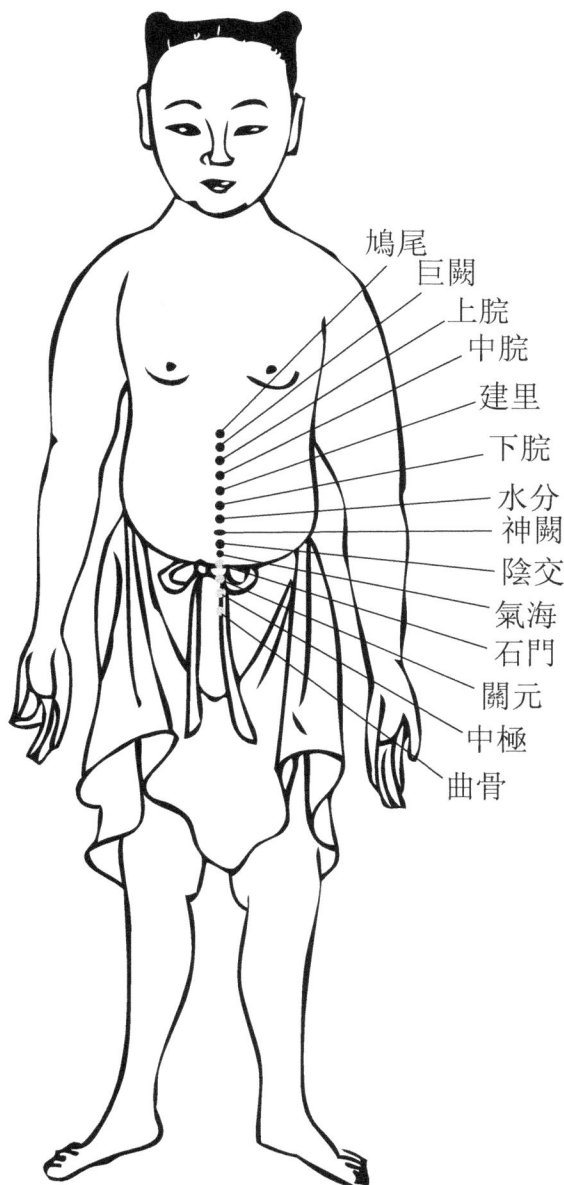

鳩尾
巨闕
上脘
中脘
建里
下脘
水分
神闕
陰交
氣海
石門
關元
中極
曲骨

Fig. 1.25

案《氣穴論》注云：中脘居心蔽骨與臍之中（上下各四寸），刺入寸二分，與《銅人》稍異，宜從《銅人》為穩。其日胃之募，蓋飲食蓄積於此也。予嘗苦脾疼，嘗灸此穴，覺冷氣從兩脅下而上至灸處即散，此灸之功也。自後頻灸之，亦每教人灸此。凡脾疼不可忍，飲食全不進者，皆宜灸。（《難疏》：腑會太倉，腑病治此。在心下四寸。）

[Author's note:] According to the Annotation to *Qì Xuè Lùn*《氣穴論》: Zhōng Wǎn 中脘 (Rèn 12) is located half way between the heart covering bone [xiphoid process] and the umbilicus (4 cùn from these upper and lower [landmarks]). Needle 1.2 cùn deep. This is a little bit different from *Tóng Rén*《銅人》. But following *Tóng Rén* is more appropriate. It is called the alarm point of the stomach because drink and food both accumulate here.

In the past, I suffered pain in my spleen. When I applied moxibustion on this point, I felt the cold qì flow upward from below my rib-sides, dissipating when it arrived at the site of moxibustion. This is the effect of moxibustion. I did it frequently from then on, and I also taught other people to burn moxibustion like this. It is appropriate to apply moxibustion on this point for unbearable pain in the spleen and inability to eat or drink. (*Nàn Shū*《難疏》says: It is the meeting [influential] point of the bowels; it treats diseases of the bowels. It is located 4 cùn below the heart.)

建里，在中脘下一寸。針五分，留十呼，灸五壯。《明》云：針寸二分。

Jiàn Lǐ 建里 (Rèn 11): It is located 1 cùn below Zhōng Wǎn (Rèn 12). Needle 5 fēn deep; retain the needle for ten respirations; burn 5 cones of moxibustion. *Míng*《明》says: Needle 1.2 cùn deep.

下脘，在建里下一寸。針八分，留三呼，瀉五吸。灸二七壯，止二百。

Xià Wǎn 下脘 (Rèn 10): It is located 1 cùn below Jiàn Lǐ (Rèn 11). Needle 8 fēn deep; retain the needle for three respirations; drain for five respirations. Burn two times seven cones of moxibustion, stop at two hundred.

水分，在下脘下一寸，臍上一寸。針八分，留三呼，瀉五吸。若水病，灸大良，可灸七壯，止百壯。禁針，針水盡即斃。《明》云：分水穴，若水病，灸大良，日灸七壯，止四百，針五分，留三呼。

Shuǐ Fēn 水分 (Rèn 9): It is located 1 cùn below Xià Wǎn (Rèn 10) and 1 cùn above the umbilicus. Needle 8 fēn deep; retain the needle for three respirations; drain for five respirations. It is very good to apply seven cones of moxibustion, stopping at a hundred cones for water disease [edema];

needling is contraindicated. The patient will die of water overflowing [if needled]. *Míng* 《 明 》 says: It is very good to apply seven cones of moxibustion on Fēn Shuǐ 水分 (Rèn 9), stopping at four hundred cones for water disease. Needle 5 fēn deep, retain the needle for three respirations.

（《明》云：水氣惟得針水溝，針餘穴，水盡即死。何於此卻云可針？◎今校勘不針為是。）

[Author's note:] (*Míng* says: Only needle Shuǐ Gōu 水溝 (Dū 26) for water qì [edema]. The patient will die of water overflowing if other points are needled. Why does it say to needle [Shuǐ Fēn (Rèn 9)] here? *Now corrected: It is better not to needle.)

《明堂》云：若是水病，灸之大良，針入五分。而《銅人》云：若是水病，灸之大良，禁不可針。針水盡即斃。是又不可針矣。恐人但知《明堂》之可針，不知《銅人》不可針也，於是書之，以示世醫云。（◎水分穴，校之不針為是）

[Author's note:] *Míng Táng* 《 明堂 》 says: It is very good to apply moxibustion on this point; needle 5 fēn deep. But *Tóng Rén* 《 銅人 》 says: It is very good to apply moxibustion, but needling is contraindicated. The patient will die of water overflowing if needled. That means it is not appropriate to needle it. I am afraid people just know that *Míng Táng* says acupuncture is acceptable, but do not know acupuncture is contraindicated in *Tóng Rén*. That is why I put it here – to show doctors nowadays. (*It is better not to needle Shuǐ Fēn (Rèn 9).)

神闕，一名氣合。當臍中。灸百壯，禁針。忌同。《素注》：禁刺，刺之使人臍中惡瘍潰，矢出者，死不可治。灸三壯。

Shén Què 神闕 (Rèn 8), another name is Qì Hé 氣合: It is located in the center of the umbilicus. Apply a hundred cones of moxibustion; needling is contraindicated. Follow the same contraindications [as Yì Xǐ 譩譆 (UB 45)]. *Sù Zhù* 《 素注 》 says: Needling is contraindicated. It causes malignity stroke and open ulcerated sores in the umbilicus. This is untreatable and the patient will die when there is a fecal incontinence. Burn three cones of moxibustion.

臍中，《千金》等經不言灸，只云禁針。《銅人》云：宜灸百壯。近世名醫遇人中風不省，急灸臍中，皆效。徐伾卒中不省，得桃源簿為灸臍中百壯始甦。更數月，乃不起。鄭糾云：有一親，卒中風，醫者為灸五百壯而甦，後年餘八十。向使徐伾灸使三五百壯，安知其不永年耶？（◎論神闕穴多灸極是。）

[Author's note:] *Qiān Jīn* 《千金》 and other classics do not discuss applying moxibustion in the center of the umbilicus; but they say acupuncture is contraindicated. *Tóng Rén* 《銅人》 says: It is appropriate to apply a hundred cones. Well-known doctors nowadays quickly apply moxibustion to the center of the umbilicus when the patient suffers wind stroke and unconsciousness. It is always effective. [A patient named] Xú Bēng suddenly suffered wind stroke and lost consciousness. He woke up after Táo Yuānbù[70] applied a hundred cones of moxibustion in the center of his umbilicus. But he still could not get up even after several months [of treatment]. Zhèng Jiū[71] said: I had a relative who suddenly suffered wind stroke. He woke up after the doctor applied five hundred cones of moxibustion and lived to be above the age of 80. If Xú Bēng had burned three or five hundred cones of moxibustion, the patient might have lived a long time, too. (*In discussing Shén Què 神闕 (Rèn 8), the maximum amount of moxibustion is often applied.)

陰交，一名橫戶。《素問》云：在臍下一寸。針八分，得氣即瀉，灸百壯止。《明》云：灸不及針，日三七壯，止百壯。

Yīn Jiāo 陰交 (Rèn 7), another name is Héng Hù 橫戶. *Sù Wèn* 《素問》 says: It is located 1 cùn below the umbilicus. Needle 8 fēn deep; drain [the point] as soon as qì arrives. Apply a hundred cones of moxibustion. *Míng* 《明》 says: Moxibustion is not as good as needling. Burn three times seven cones of moxibustion daily, stop at a hundred cones.

氣海，一名脖胦，一名下肓。在臍下寸半宛宛中。針八分，得氣即瀉，瀉後宜補之。灸百壯。今附：氣海者，是男子生氣之海也，治藏氣虛憊，真氣不足，一切氣疾久不差，皆灸之。忌同。《明下》云：灸七壯。

Qì Hǎi 氣海 (Rèn 6), another name is Bó Yāng 脖胦, also named Xià Huāng 下肓. It is located in the depression 1.5 cùn inferior to the umbilicus. Needle 8 fēn deep; drain [the point] as soon as qì arrives; supplement properly after [draining]. Burn a hundred cones of moxibustion. Appended here: Qì Hǎi (Rèn 6) is the sea of vital qì in males. It treats exhaustion of visceral qì, true qì insufficiency, and all long-lasting qì diseases. Apply moxibustion on it. Follow the same contraindications [as Yì Xī 譩譆 (UB 45)]. *Míng Xià* 《明下》 says: Burn seven cones.

此經以氣海為生氣之海，《難經疏》以為元氣之海。則氣海者，蓋人之元氣所生也。故柳公度曰：吾養生無它朮，但不使元氣佐喜怒，使氣海常溫爾。今人既不能不以元氣佐喜怒矣，若能時灸氣海使溫，亦其次也。予舊多病，常苦氣短。醫者教灸氣海，氣遂不促。自是每歲須一二次灸之，則以氣怯故也。

---

70. No information is available on Táo Yuānbù 桃源簿. He must have been an ancient doctor.
71. No information is available on Zhèng Jiū 鄭糾.

[Author's note:] This classic considered Qì Hǎi 氣海 (Rèn 6) the sea of vital qì. *Nàn Jīng Shū* 《難經疏》 thought it was the sea of original qì. So Qì Hǎi (Rèn 6 – the sea of qì) is generated from original qì. This is why Liǔ Gōngdù[72] said: I do not have any other method of life cultivation, except I do not allow joy and anger to accompany original qì; and I warm [apply moxibustion on] Qì Hǎi (Rèn 6) frequently. People living now cannot ensure that joy or anger do not accompany original qì, but if they can often warm Qì Hǎi (Rèn 6), this is the second [best choice].

I was easily sick in the past and suffered shortness of qì. The doctor told me to apply moxibustion on Qì Hǎi (Rèn 6), and I no longer have hasty breathing. So since then I have burned moxibustion on this point once or twice a year due to [my condition of] qì timidity.

石門，一名利機，一名精露。在臍下二寸。灸亦良，可灸二七壯，止百壯。婦人不可針，針之終身絕子。《明》云：《甲乙經》云：一名精露，一名丹田，一名命門。針八分，留三呼，得氣即瀉。《下》云：灸七壯。《千》云：灸絕孕，針五分。

Shí Mén 石門 (Rèn 5), another name is Lì Jī 利機, also named Jīng Lù 精露: It is located 2 cùn below the umbilicus. It is good to apply two times seven cones of moxibustion, stopping at a hundred cones. Needling is contraindicated in women, as it will cause infertility. *Míng* 《明》 says: *Jiǎ Yǐ Jīng* 《甲乙經》 says: Another name is Jīng Lù 精露, it is also named Dān Tián 丹田 and Mìng Mén 命門. Needle 8 fēn deep; retain the needle for three respirations; drain [the point] as soon as qì arrives. *Xià* 《下》 says: Burn seven cones of moxibustion. *Qiān* 《千》 says: Moxibustion can cause infertility. Needle 5 fēn deep.

臍下二寸名石門，《明堂》載《甲乙經》云：一名丹田。《千金》、《素問》注亦謂丹田在臍下二寸，世醫因是遂以石門為丹田，誤矣。丹田乃在臍下三寸，《難經疏》論之詳而有據，當以《難經疏》為正（詳見關元）。《銅人》云：針之絕子，《千金》云：灸之絕孕，要之，婦人不必針灸此。（◎論丹田穴，當以臍下二寸為是。）

[Author's note:] Shí Mén (Rèn 5) is located 2 cùn below the umbilicus. *Míng Táng* 《明堂》 recorded what was said in *Jiǎ Yǐ Jīng*: "It is also named Dān Tián (cinnabar field)." *Qiān Jīn* 《千金》 and the Annotation to *Sù Wèn* 《素問》 also say Dān Tián (cinnabar field) is located 2 cùn below the umbilicus. It is actually incorrect that doctors nowadays follow [the idea that] Shí Mén (Rèn 5) is Dān Tián (cinnabar field). Dān Tián (cinnabar field) is located 3 cùn below the umbilicus. *Nàn Jīng Shū* has a detailed discussion with proof which should be set as law. (For details see Guān Yuán 關元 (Rèn 4)). *Tóng Rén* 《銅人》 says: Needling will cause infertility. *Qiān Jīn*

72. Liǔ Gōngdù 柳公度 was the cousin of a famous calligrapher, Liǔ Gōngquán 柳公權 of the *Táng* Dynasty. He was an expert in life cultivation and lived a very long life.

says: Moxibustion will cause infertility. So do not use moxibustion or acupuncture on this point in women. (*Dān Tián 丹田 (cinnabar field) is actually located 2 cùn below the umbilicus.)

關元，在臍下三寸，小腸之募，足太陰、少陰、厥陰三陰、任脈之會。下紀者，關元也。針八分，留三呼，瀉五吸，灸百壯，止三百壯。忌同。《明》云：若懷胎，必不針。若針而落胎，胎多不出，而針外崑崙立出。灸不及針，日三十壯。《下》云：五壯。岐伯云：但是積冷虛乏，皆宜灸。

Guān Yuán 關元 (Rèn 4): It is located 3 cùn below the umbilicus. It is the alarm point of small intestine and the meeting point of the three foot yīn channels: foot tàiyīn, shàoyīn, and juéyīn with the rèn mài. Xià Jì 下紀 (Lower Regulator) is [another name for] Guān Yuán (Rèn 4). Needle 8 fēn deep; retain the needle for three respirations, and drain for five respirations. Burn a hundred cones of moxibustion, stop at three hundred cones. Follow the same contraindications [as Yǐ Xī 譩譆 (UB 45)]. *Míng* 《明》 says: Needling is contraindicated during pregnancy. If the patient has a miscarriage after needling this point, the fetus usually will not come out; but after puncturing external Kūn Lún 崑崙 (UB 60), it will come out immediately. Moxibustion is not as good as needling; burn thirty cones of moxibustion daily. *Xià* 《下》 says: five cones. Qí Bó said: It is appropriate to apply moxibustion for treating cold accumulations and vacuity fatigue.

關元乃丹田也。諸經不言，惟《難經疏》云：丹田在臍下三寸，方員四寸，著脊梁兩腎間中央赤是也。左青右白，上黃下黑，三寸法三光，四寸法四時，五色法五行。兩腎間名大海，而貯其血氣，亦名大中極。言取人身之上下四向最為中也。老醫與人灸，皆從此說。多者千餘壯，少亦三二百。不知全活者幾何人，然亦宜頻灸。故曰：若要安，丹田、三里不曾乾。

[Author's note:] Guān Yuán (Rèn 4) is the Dān Tián (cinnabar field). No other classics mentioned this except *Nàn Jīng Shū* 《難經疏》, which says: Dān Tián (cinnabar field) is located 3 cùn below the umbilicus and has a circumference of 4 cùn. It is attached to the spine and is located between the two kidneys. The color in the center is red, with green-blue on the left, white on the right, yellow on the top, and black on the bottom. **Three** cùn is modeled after the three luminaries [sun, moon and stars]; **four** cùn is modeled after the four seasons, and the **five** colors are modeled after the five elements. The space between the two kidneys is named Dà Hǎi 大海 (great sea), which stores blood and qì. It is also named Dà Zhōng Jí 大中極 (Rèn 4 – great central pole). It is said to be located in the exact center of the four directions [above, below, left and right] of the body. Old doctors all apply moxibustion on patients based on this theory, burning more than a thousand cones of moxibustion at the most, and two or three hundred cones at the least. Although we do not know how many people they have saved, they still do this moxibustion frequently. So it is said: If you want good health, do not let the Dān Tián (cinnabar field) and San Li 三里 (ST 36) become dry.

中極，一名玉泉，一名氣原 。在關元下一寸 。針八分，留十呼，得氣即瀉，
灸百壯，止三百 。《 明 》云：主婦人斷緒，四度針（ 《 銅人 》作以度針 ），
針即有子，故卻時任針也 。灸不及針，日三七壯 。《 下 》云：五壯 。

Zhōng Jí 中極 (Rèn 3), another name is Yù Quán 玉泉, also named Qì Yuán 氣原: It is located
1 cùn below Guān Yuán 關元 (Rèn 4). Needle 8 fēn deep; retain the needle for ten respirations;
drain [the point] as soon as qì arrives. Burn a hundred cones of moxibustion, up to three hundred.
Míng 《 明 》 says: It treats infertility[73] in women; they will become pregnant after four acupuncture treatments. (*Tóng Rén* 《 銅人 》 [mistakenly] writes *yǐ dù zhēn* 以度針 (consider using
acupuncture)[74]). So one should needle repeatedly. Moxibustion is not as good as needling; burn
three times seven cones of moxibustion. *Xià* 《 下 》 says: five cones.

曲骨，在橫骨上毛際陷中 。灸七壯，至七七，針二寸 。《 明下 》云：橫骨
上，中極下一寸毛際陷中 。《 千 》云：臍下五寸 。

Qū Gǔ 曲骨 (Rèn 2): It is located in a depression within the hairy region of the transverse bone
[pubic bone]. Burn seven cones of moxibustion, up to seven times seven cones; needle 2 cùn deep.
Míng Xià 《 明下 》 says: It is located on the transverse bone, in the depression within the hairy
region, 1 cùn below Zhong Ji 中極[75] (Rèn 3). *Qiān* 《 千 》 says: It is 5 cùn below the umbilicus.

會陰，一名屏翳 。在兩陰間，任脈別絡，俠督脈、衝脈之會 。灸三壯 。

Huì Yīn 會陰 (Rèn 1), another name is Píng Yì 屏翳: It is located between the two yīn [anus and
genitals]. It is the diverging network of the rèn mài. It also is a meeting point with the dū mài and
the chōng mài. Burn three cones of moxibustion.

---

73. *Duàn xù* 斷緒 (breaking pedigree) indicates infertility in women according to Volume 38
of *Zhū Bìng Yuán Hòu Lùn* 《 諸病源候論 》 (The Origin and Indicators of Disease) by Cháo
Yúanfāng 巢元方, published in 610 (*Suí* 隋).

74. The character *sì* 四 (four) is written as *yǐ* 以 (consider) in some editions of *Tóng Rén Tú Jīng*
《 銅人圖經 》.

75. *Jí* 極 was changed from *jí* 及 according to the chapter called "*Kǒng Xuè Xiàng Qù* 孔穴相去
(Distance between Points) in Volume 2 of this book. This change also matches Volume 100 of *Tài
Píng Shèng Huì Fāng* 《 太平聖惠方 》.

1.21
Fù Dì Èr Háng Zuǒ Yòu Èr Shí Èr Xué

腹第二行左右二十二穴

The second line on the abdomen, 22 bilateral points [eleven on each side]

幽門二穴，俠巨闕兩旁各五分。灸五壯，針五分。《明》云：在巨闕旁各寸半陷中。《千·腎藏》云：夾巨闕各一寸。

Yōu Mén 幽門 (KI 21), bilateral point: It is located 5 fēn lateral to Jù Què 巨闕 (Rèn 14). Burn five cones of moxibustion; needle 5 fēn deep. *Míng*《 明 》says: in the depression 1.5 cùn lateral to Jù Què (Rèn 14). *Qiān · Shèn Zàng*《 千·腎藏 》says: 1 cùn lateral Jù Què (Rèn 14).

《銅人》云：幽門夾巨闕，肓俞夾臍旁各五分（相去一寸）。《明堂》乃云：幽門在巨闕旁寸半，通谷夾上管旁相去三寸。按《千金》四滿（第二行穴）在丹田（◎今石門）兩邊各寸半，與《明堂》合。始知《銅人》誤云。

[Author's note:] *Tóng Rén*《 銅人 》says: Yōu Mén (KI 21) is located 5 fēn lateral to Jù Què (Rèn 14). Huāng Shù 肓俞 (KI 16) is located 5 fēn lateral to the umbilicus ([the left and right points are] 1 cùn from each other). *Míng Táng*《 明堂 》says: Yōu Mén (KI 21) is located 1.5 cùn lateral to Jù Què (Rèn 14) and Tōng Gǔ 通谷 (KI 20) is located lateral to Shàng Guǎn 上管[76] (Rèn 13), [with the right and left sides] 3 cùn from each other. According to *Qiān Jīn*《 千金 》, Sì Mǎn 四滿 (KI 14) (a point on the second line) is located 1.5 cùn lateral to Dān Tián 丹田 (cinnabar field) (*here referring to Shí Mén 石門 (Rèn 5)). This matches *Míng Táng*. So we know *Tóng Rén* was wrong.[77]

---

76. Shàng Guǎn 上管 is another name of Shàng Wǎn 上脘 (Rèn 13).

77. The location of Yōu Mén 幽門 (KI 21) in modern textbooks follows *Tóng Rén*《 銅人 》, which is 0.5 cùn lateral to the anterior midline.

通谷二穴，在幽門下一寸。針五分，灸五壯。《明》云：夾上管兩旁相去三寸。《下》云：灸三壯。

Tōng Gǔ 通谷 (KI 20), bilateral point: It is located 1 cùn below Yōu Mén 幽門 (KI 21). Needle 5 fēn deep; burn five cones of moxibustion. *Míng* 《明》 says: Lateral to Shàng Guǎn 上管 (Rèn 13). [The right and left sides are] 3 cùn from each other. *Xià* 《下》 says: Burn three cones of moxibustion.

陰都二穴，一名食宮。在通谷下一寸。灸三壯，針三分。

Yīn Dū 陰都 (KI 19), bilateral point, another name is Shí Gōng 食宮: It is located 1 cùn below Tōng Gǔ (KI 20). Burn three cones of moxibustion; needle 3 fēn deep.

石關二穴，在陰都下一寸。灸三壯，針一寸。

Shí Guān 石關 (KI 18), bilateral point: It is located 1 cùn below Yīn Dū (KI 19). Burn three cones of moxibustion; needle 1 cùn deep.

商曲二穴，在石關下一寸。灸五壯，針一寸。

Shāng Qū 商曲 (KI 17), bilateral point: It is located 1 cùn below Shí Guān (KI 18). Burn five cones of moxibustion; needle 1 cùn deep.

肓俞二穴，在商曲下一寸，臍旁各五分。灸五壯，針一寸。

Huāng Shù 肓俞 (KI 16), bilateral point: It is located 1 cùn below Shāng

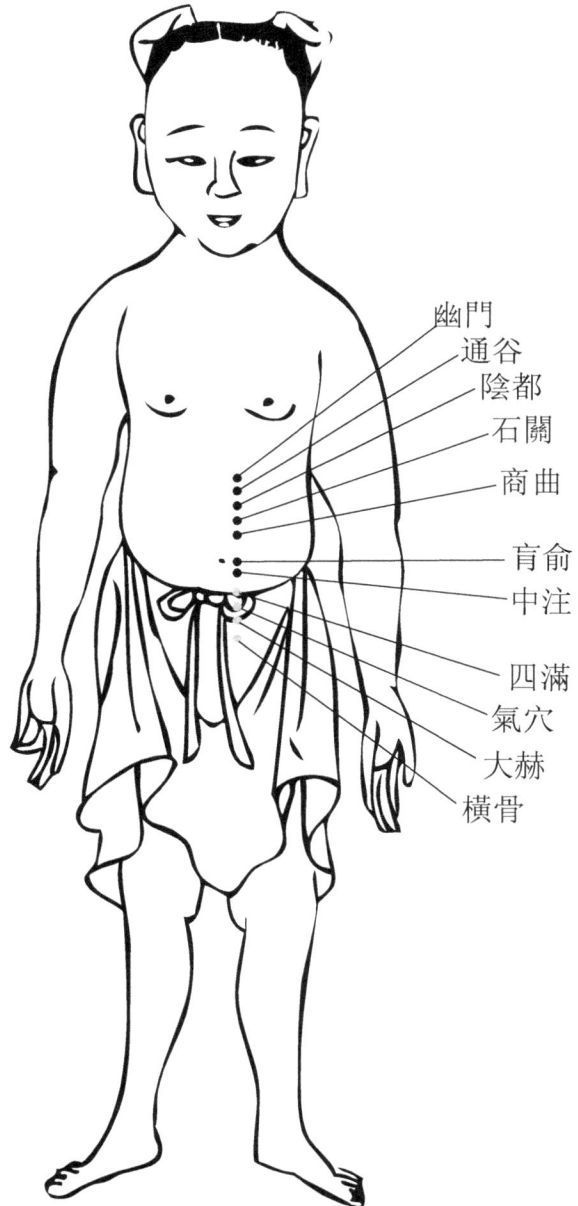

幽門
通谷
陰都
石關
商曲
肓俞
中注
四滿
氣穴
大赫
橫骨

Fig. 1.26

Qū (KI 17); 5 fēn lateral to the umbilicus. Burn five cones of moxibustion; needle 1 cùn deep.

中注二穴，在肓俞下一寸。灸五壯，針一寸。

Zhōng Zhù 中注 (KI 15), bilateral point: It is located 1 cùn below Huāng Shù 肓俞 (KI 16). Burn five cones of moxibustion; needle 1 cùn deep.

四滿二穴，一名髓府，在中注下一寸。針三分，灸三壯。

Sì Mǎn 四滿 (KI 14), bilateral point, another name is Suǐ Fǔ 髓府: It is located 1 cùn below Zhōng Zhù (KI 15). Needle 3 fēn deep; burn three cones of moxibustion.

（《千》：丹田旁各寸半，即心下八寸臍下横文是。◎今校勘，四滿二穴，《千金》云：在丹田旁各寸半，即心下八寸臍下横文是，尤証得丹田在二寸。）

([Author's note:] *Qiān*《千》says: [Sì Mǎn (KI 14) is located] 1.5 cùn lateral to the Dān Tián 丹田 (cinnabar field),[78] on the transverse crease below the umbilicus, 8 cùn below the heart. *Now corrected and revised: Sì Mǎn (KI 14), bilateral point: according to *Qiān Jīn*《千金》, it is located 1.5 cùn lateral to the Dān Tián, on the transverse crease below the umbilicus, 8 cùn below the heart. This proves that the Dān Tián (cinnabar field) is located 2 cùn [below the umbilicus].

氣穴二穴，一名胞門，一名子戶。在四滿下一寸。灸五壯，針三分。

Qì Xué 氣穴 (KI 13), bilateral point, another name is Bāo Mén 胞門; also named Zǐ Hù 子戶: It is located 1 cùn below Sì Mǎn (KI 14). Burn five cones of moxibustion; needle 3 fēn deep.

大赫二穴，一名陰維，一名陰關。在氣穴下一寸。灸五壯，針三分。

Dà Hè 大赫 (KI 12), bilateral point, another name is Yīn Wéi 陰維; also named Yīn Guān 陰關: It is located 1 cùn below Qì Xué 氣穴 (KI 13). Burn five cones of moxibustion; needle 3 fēn deep.

---

78. Traditionally, the Dān Tián 丹田 (cinnabar field) is considered to be a center of qì or life force energy. It is an important point of reference in qigong and other self-cultivation practices of exercise, breathing, and meditation, as well as in martial arts and in traditional Chinese Medicine. According to *Dōng Yī Bǎo Jiàn* 東醫寶鑒 (Exemplar of Korean Medicine) by Xǔ Jùn 許浚 (He Jun in Korean), the three main Dān Tiáns are typically emphasized: the upper Dān Tián is the brain, and is associated with consciousness and spirit (*shén*); the middle Dān Tián is the chest area, and is associated with storing life energy (qì); the lower Dān Tián is located three cùn below the umbilicus, and is associated with *jīng*-essence. The lower Dān Tián is particularly important as the focal point of breathing techniques, as well as the center of balance and gravity. This term usually indicates the area below the umbilicus. But there are different schools of thought on its exact location; it could be two cùn or three cùn below the umbilicus.

横骨二穴，在大赫下一寸。灸三壯。（《千》云：名屈骨端，在陰上橫骨中宛曲如卻月中央是。）

Héng Gǔ 橫骨 (KI 11), bilateral point: It is located 1 cùn below Dà Hè 大赫 (KI 12). Burn three cones of moxibustion. (*Qiān* 《 千 》 says: It is also named Qū Gǔ Dūan 屈骨端 (curved bone's end). It is located above the yīn (lower orifices), in the center of the transverse bone which is curved like a half moon.)

以上二十二穴去腹中行皆當為寸半，說見幽門。

[Author's note:] The above 22 points are all located 1.5 cùn lateral to the midline on the abdomen. Refer to the discussion under Yōu Mén 幽門 (KI 21).[79]

---

79. The vertical line of points in this section is considered to be 0.5 cùn lateral to the midline in modern texts.

1.22

Fù Dì Sān Háng Zuǒ Yòu Èr Shí Sì Xué

腹第三行左右二十四穴

The third line on the abdomen, 24 bilateral points [twelve on each side]

不容二穴，在幽門兩旁寸半。灸五壯，針五分。《明》云：在上管兩旁各一寸，灸三壯（《素注》：在第四肋端）。

Bù Róng 不容 (ST 19), bilateral point: It is located 1.5 cùn lateral to Yōu Mén 幽門 (KI 21). Burn five cones of moxibustion; needle 5 fēn deep. *Míng* 《明》 says: It is 1 cùn lateral to Shàng Guǎn 上管 (Rèn 13). Burn three cones of moxibustion. (*Sù Zhù* 《素注》 says: At the end of the fourth rib).

《素問》云：夾鳩尾外當乳下三寸，夾胃管各五，不容至太乙也；夾臍廣三寸各三，滑肉門、天樞、外陵也；下臍二寸夾之各三，大巨、水道、歸來也，皆腹第三行穴也。《新校正》云：《甲乙經》天樞在臍旁各二寸，與諸書同，特此經為異。信若是，則其穴不當乳下可也。必當乳下，則廣三寸之說為當。

[Author's note:] *Sù Wèn* 《素問》 says: There are five points [on the line] that is 3 cùn lateral to Jiū Wěi 鳩尾 (Rèn 15), below the nipples and lateral to Wèi Guǎn 胃管 (the stomach duct or Rèn 13): Bù Róng (ST 19) to Tài Yǐ 太乙 (ST 23). There are three points [on this same line] that is 3 cùn lateral to the umbilicus: Huá Ròu Mén 滑肉門 (ST 24), Tiān Shū 天樞 (ST 25), and Wài Líng 外陵 (ST 26). [Starting] 2 cùn below the umbilicus, there are three points [on this same line] that is lateral to the umbilicus: Dà Jù 大巨 (ST 27), Shuǐ Dào 水道 (ST 28), and Guī Lái 來 (ST 29). These are all points on the third line of the abdomen. *Xīn Jiào Zhèng* 《新校正》 says: According to *Jiǎ Yǐ Jīng* 《甲乙經》, Tiān Shū (ST 25) is located 2 cùn lateral to the umbilicus. All the other books agree except this Classic [*Jiǎ Yǐ Jīng*]. If we believe this, then the points must not be below the nipples; if the points are below the nipples, then they must be 3 cùn lateral.[80]

---

80. The distance of points from the midline is an area of disagreement in ancient texts. *Jiǎ Yǐ Jīng* 《甲乙經》 and *Líng Shū* 《靈樞》 place the distance between nipples as 9.5 cùn; in *Shén Yìng Jīng* 《神應經》, the distance between nipples is 8 cùn. Here, Wáng says it is 3 cùn from the mid-

承滿二穴，在不容下一寸。針三分，灸五壯。《明》云：三壯。（《千》：夾巨闕兩旁各一寸半。）

Chéng Mǎn 承滿 (ST 20), bilateral point: It is located 1 cùn below Bù Róng 不容 (ST 19). Needle 3 fēn deep; burn five cones of moxibustion. *Míng* 《明》 says: three cones. (*Qiān* 《千》 says: It is 1.5 cùn lateral to Jù Què 巨闕 (Rèn 14))

梁門二穴，在承滿下一寸。灸五壯，針三分。

Liáng Mén 梁門 (ST 21), bilateral point: It is located 1 cùn below Chéng Mǎn (ST 20). Burn five cones of moxibustion; needle 3 fēn deep.

關門二穴，在梁門下一寸。針八分，灸五壯。

Guān Mén 關門 (ST 22), bilateral point: It is located 1 cùn below Liáng Mén (ST 21). Needle 8 fēn deep; burn five cones of moxibustion.

太一二穴，在關門下一寸。灸五壯，針八分。

Tài Yī 太一[81] (ST 23), bilateral point: It is located 1 cùn below Guān Mén (ST 22). Burn five cones of moxibustion; needle 8 fēn deep.

滑肉門二穴，在太乙下一寸。灸五壯，針八分。（下一寸至天樞。）

Huá Ròu Mén 滑肉門 (ST 24), bilateral point: It is located 1 cùn below Tài Yī (ST 23). Burn five cones of moxibustion; needle 8 fēn deep. (1 cùn below it is Tiān Shū 天樞 (ST 25.)

天樞二穴，一名長溪，一名穀門，大腸之募。去肓俞寸半，夾臍旁各二寸陷中。灸五壯，針五分，留十呼。（《千》：魂魄之舍，不可針。合臍相去可三寸。）

---

line to the nipples, making the bilateral distance 6 cùn. Wáng states above that the kidney channel is 1.5 cùn lateral to the midline on the abdomen (although he acknowledges that others disagree); under the heading of Bù Róng 不容 (ST 19), above, he places the stomach channel 1.5 cùn lateral to the kidney channel. This accounts for his idea that the stomach channel is 3 cùn lateral to the midline of the abdomen and that these points are on the nipple line. In modern texts, the vertical line for points of the stomach channel on the abdomen is 2 cùn lateral to the midline, and halfway to the nipple line, which is 4 cùn lateral and belongs to the spleen.

81. Tài Yī 太一 is another name for Tài Yī 太乙 (ST 23).

Tiān Shū 天樞 (ST 25), bilateral point, another name is Cháng Xī 長溪; also named Gǔ Mén 榖門: It is the alarm point of the large intestine and is located 1.5 cùn lateral to Huāng Shù 肓俞 (KI 16), in the depression 2 cùn lateral to the umbilicus.[82] Burn five cones of moxibustion; needle 5 fēn deep; retain the needles for ten respirations. (*Qiān* 《千》 says: It is not appropriate to needle [because these right and left side points] are the house of the *hún* (Ethereal Soul) and *pò* (Corporeal Soul). They are 3 cùn away from the umbilicus.)[83]

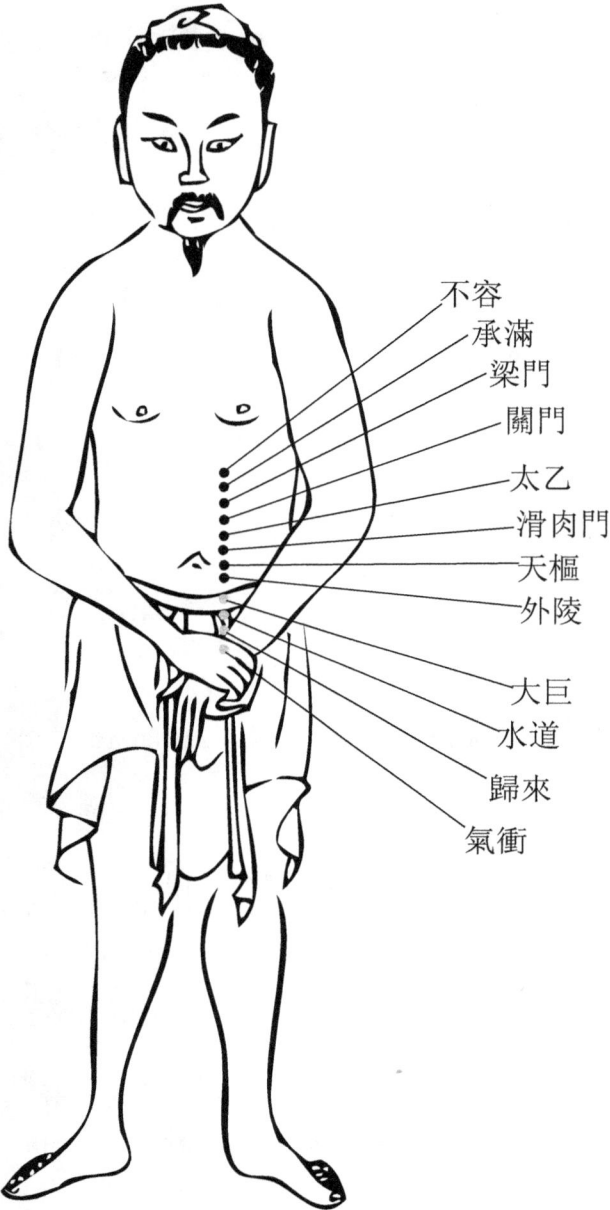

不容
承滿
梁門
關門
太乙
滑肉門
天樞
外陵
大巨
水道
歸來
氣衝

Fig. 1.27

外陵二穴，在天樞下一寸。灸五壯，針三分。

Wài Líng 外陵 (ST 26), bilateral point: It is located 1 cùn below Tiān Shū (ST 25). Burn five cones of moxibustion; needle 3 fēn deep.

大巨二穴，在長溪下二寸。灸五壯，針五分。（長溪，天樞也。《千》：在臍下一寸，兩旁各二寸。）

Dà Jù 大巨 (ST 27), bilateral point: It is located 2 cùn below Cháng Xī (ST 25). Burn five cones of moxibustion; needle 5 fēn deep. (Cháng Xī is [another name for] Tiān Shū (ST 25). *Qiān* says: It is 1 cùn below the umbilicus, 2 cùn lateral [to the midline].)

82. This puts the kidney channel back to 0.5 cùn lateral and the stomach channel 2 cùn lateral to the midline. But in the discussion above and in the conclusion of the sections on the second and third lines on the abdomen, they are stated to be 1.5 (also in *Míng* 《明》 and *Qiān* 《千》) and 3 cùn (also in *Sù Wèn* 《素問》) lateral. In modern texts, the vertical line of the kidney channel is 0.5 cùn and the stomach channel is 2 cùn lateral to the midline.

83. See footnote above.

水道二穴，在大巨下三寸。灸五壯，針三寸半。

Shuǐ Dào 水道 (ST 28), bilateral point: It is located 3 cùn[84] below Dà Jù 大巨 (ST 27). Burn five cones of moxibustion; needle 3.5 cùn deep.

歸來二穴，在水道下二寸。灸五壯，針八分。（《外臺》：水道下三寸。◎今校勘歸來二穴，在水道下二寸為是。）

Guī Lái 歸來 (ST 29), bilateral point: It is located 2 cùn below Shuǐ Dào (ST 28). Burn five cones of moxibustion; needle 8 fēn deep. (*Wài Tái* 《外臺》 says: It is 3 cùn below Shuǐ Dào (ST 28). *Now corrected [by comparing this with all the other classics], Guī Lái (ST 29) should be located 2 cùn below Shuǐ Dào (ST 28).)

氣衝二穴，一名氣街。在歸來下鼠鼷上一寸，動脈應手宛宛中。禁針，灸七壯立愈，炷如大麥。《明下》云：五壯。《素注》云：在腹臍下橫骨兩端鼠鼷上，針三分。《千》云：歸來下一寸。

Qì Chōng 氣衝 (ST 30), bilateral point, another name is Qì Jiē 氣街: It is located below Guī Lái 歸來 (ST 29), 1 cùn above the groin, in the depression where a pulsating vessel responds to the hand. Needling is contraindicated. Applying seven cones of moxibustion will cure [the disease] immediately. Use grain-of-wheat size cones. *Míng Xià* 《明下》 says: five cones. *Sù Zhù* 《素注》 says: In the groin region, at the end of the transverse bone [pubic bone], below the umbilicus. Needle 3 fēn deep. *Qiān* 《千》 says: It is 1 cùn below Guī Lái (ST 29).

以上二十六穴去腹中行當各三寸。

The above entries of 26 points are located 3 cùn lateral to the midline on the abdomen.

---

84. This seems to be a typo. Based on the point location we used now, *sān* 三 (three) is an error for *yī* 一 (one). In modern texts, the proportional measurement between the umbilicus and the upper boder of pubic symphysis is 5 cùn, which is different from *Líng Shū · Gǔ Dù* 《靈樞·骨度》 and *Zhēn Jiǔ Jiǎ Yǐ Jīng* 《針灸甲乙經》. In *Shén Yìng Jīng* 《神應經》 (Divinely Responding Classic) by Chén Huì 陳會 of the *Míng* Dynasty (1425), the distance is 5 cùn. The next point, Guī Lái 歸來 (ST 29), also has a similar discrepancy.

1.23
Fù Dì Sì Háng Zuǒ Yòu Shí Sì Xué

腹第四行左右十四穴

The fourth line on the abdomen,
14 bilateral points [seven on each side]

期門二穴，肝之募。在不容旁寸半，直兩乳第二肋端。針四分，灸五壯。
（《千》：直兩乳下第二肋端旁寸半，又云：乳直下寸半。）

Qī Mén 期門 (LV 14), bilateral point, the alarm point of the liver: It is located 1.5 cùn lateral to Bù Róng 不容 (ST 19),[85] at the end of the second rib that is directly below the nipples. Needle 4 fēn deep; burn five cones of moxibustion. (*Qiān*《千》 says: It is 1.5 cùn lateral to the end of the second rib that is directly below the nipples; it also says: 1.5 cùn directly below the nipples.)

日月二穴，膽之募。在期門下五分陷中。灸五壯，針五分。（《千》：名神光，一名膽募。）

Rì Yuè 日月 (GB 24), bilateral point, the alarm point of the gall bladder: It is located in the depression 5 fēn below Qī Mén (LV 14). Burn five cones of moxibustion; needle 5 fēn deep. (*Qiān* says: Another name is Shén Guāng 神光; it is also named Dǎn Mù 膽募.)

腹哀二穴，在日月下寸半。針三分。

Fù Āi 腹哀 (SP 16), bilateral point: It is located 1.5 cùn below Rì Yuè (GB 24). Needle 3 fēn deep.

大橫二穴，在腹哀下三寸半，直臍旁。灸三壯，針七分。

Dà Héng 大橫 (SP 15), bilateral point: It is located 3.5 cùn below Fù Āi (SP 16), lateral to the umbilicus. Burn three cones of moxibustion; needle 7 fēn deep.

---

85. The vertical line of Bù Róng 不容 (ST 19) here is 3 cùn lateral to the anterior midline.

肓俞，去臍旁當一寸半，天樞去臍當三寸，大橫去臍當四寸半，其去
章門合為六寸。《難經疏》乃云：章門在臍上二寸，兩旁九寸。為可
疑焉耳。

[Author's note:] Huāng Shù 肓俞 (KI 16) is located 1.5 cùn lateral to the umbilicus; Tiān Shù 天樞 (ST 25) is located 3 cùn lateral to the umbilicus; Dà Héng 大橫 (SP 15) is located 4.5 cùn lateral to the umbilicus; the total distance [from the umbilicus] to Zhāng Mén 章門 (LV 13) is 6 cùn. *Nàn Jīng Shū* 《 難經疏 》 says: Zhāng Mén (LV 13) is located 2 cùn above the umbilicus, [with the right and left sides] 9 cùn from each other. So it is doubtful.

腹結二穴，一名腸窟。在大
橫下三分。針七分，灸五
壯。

Fù Jié 腹結 (SP 14), bilateral point, another name is Cháng Kū 腸窟: It is located 3 fēn below Dà Héng (SP 15). Needle 7 fēn deep; burn five cones of moxibustion.

府舍二穴，在腹結下三寸，
足太陰、厥陰、陰維之交
會。此三脈，上下三入腹，
絡肝脾，結心肺，從脅上至
肩，此太陰郄，三陰、陽明
之別。針七分，灸五壯。

Fǔ Shè 府舍 (SP 13) bilateral point: It is located 3 cùn below Fù Jié (SP 14). It is the meeting point of foot tàiyīn, foot juéyīn and the yīnwéi [yīn linking vessel]. These three vessels enter the abdomen from the upper or lower [part of the abdomen], network with the liver and spleen, bind to the heart and lungs, and travel up

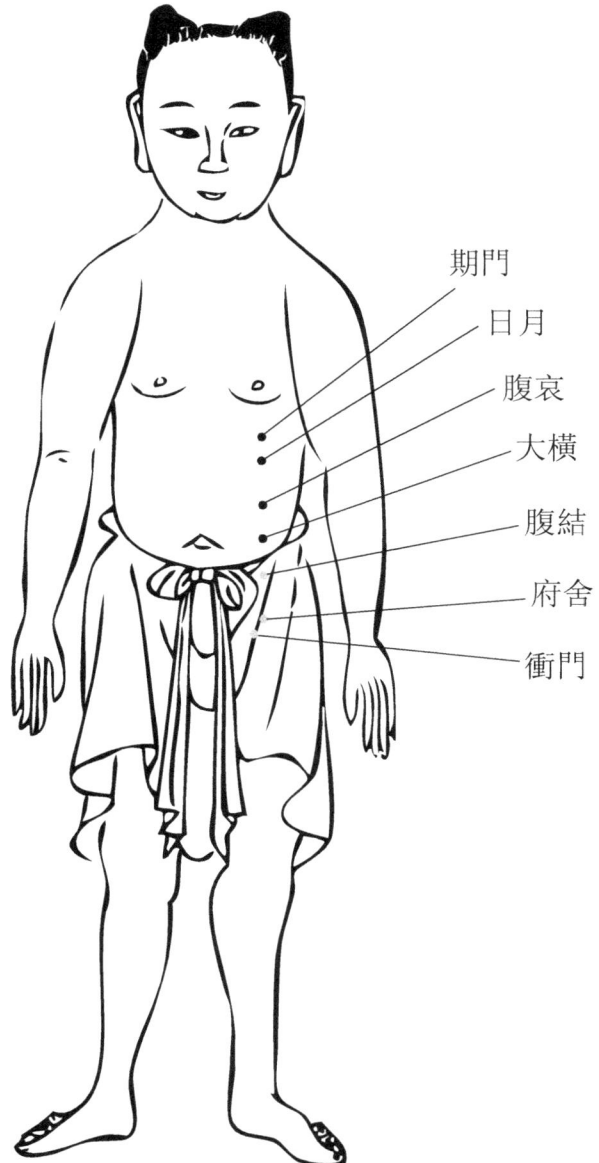

期門
日月
腹哀
大橫
腹結
府舍
衝門

Fig. 1.28

89

from the rib-sides to the shoulder. This point is the *xī*-cleft of the tàiyīn, and the divergence of the three yīn and yángmíng.[86] Needle 7 fēn deep; burn five cones of moxibustion.

衝門二穴，一名慈宮 。上去大橫五寸，府舍下橫骨兩端約中動脈 。針七分，灸五壯 。

Chōng Mén 衝門 (SP 12), bilateral point, another name is Cí Gōng 慈宮: It is located 5 cùn below Dà Héng 大橫 (SP 15). It is located below Fǔ Shè 府舍 (SP 13), on the pulsating vessel at the end of the transverse bone [pubic bone]. Needle 7 fēn deep; burn five cones of moxibustion.

以上十四穴去腹中行各當為四寸半。

The above 14 points are located 4.5 cùn[87] lateral to the midline on the abdomen.

---

86. The meaning of this passage is obscure.
87. In modern texts, they are 4 cùn lateral to the midline, on the abdomen.

1.24
Cè Xié Zuǒ Yòu Shí Èr Xué

側脅左右十二穴

Lateral rib-sides,
12 bilateral points [six on each side]

章門二穴，一名長平，一名脅髎，脾之募。在大橫外直臍季肋端，側臥屈上足伸下足，舉臂取之。針六分，灸百壯。《明》云：日七壯，止五百。忌同。（《難疏》：臟會季脅，章門也，臟病治此，是脅骨下短脅，在臍上二寸兩旁九寸。）

Zhāng Mén 章門 (LV 13), bilateral point, another name is Cháng Píng 長平, also named Xié Liáo 脅髎; it is the alarm point of the spleen: It is located at the end of the rib-sides, in line with the umbilicus, lateral to Dà Héng 大橫 (SP 15). Locate the point with [the patient] lying on their side, bending their upper leg, extending their lower leg, and raising their arms. Needle 6 fēn deep; burn a hundred cones of moxibustion. *Míng* 《明》 says: Burn seven cones of moxibustion daily, stop at five hundred cones. Follow the same contraindications [as Yì Xī 譩譆 (UB 45)]. *(Nàn Shū* 《難疏》 says: Zhāng Mén (LV 13) is the meeting [influential] point of the viscera and is located in the free rib region. It is used to treat diseases of the viscera and is located at the bottom of the rib-sides in the short ribs, 2 cùn above the umbilicus; [the right and left sides are] 9 cùn from each other.)

京門二穴，一名氣腧，一名氣府，腎之募。在監骨腰中季脅，本俠脊。灸三壯，針三分，留七呼。

Jīng Mén 京門 (GB 25), bilateral point, another name is Qì Shù 氣腧, also named Qì Fǔ 氣府; the alarm point of the kidneys: It is located on the lower back, on the haunch bone[88] in the free rib region, adjacent to the spine. Burn three cones of moxibustion; needle 3 fēn deep; retain the needle for seven respirations.

---

88. *Jiān gǔ* 監骨 (haunch bone) means *yāo jiān gǔ* 腰監骨 or *yāo kē* 腰髁. It indicates the pelvis. The text seems to be missing the word *shàng* 上 (above) after *jiān gǔ* 監骨 (haunch bone).

帶脈二穴，在季脅下寸八分陷中。針六分，灸五壯。《明下》云：三壯。（如帶繞身，管束諸經脈。《千》云：在季脅端。）

Dài Mài 帶脈 (GB 26), bilateral point: It is located in the depression 1.8 cùn below the free rib region. Needle 6 fēn deep; burn five cones of moxibustion. *Míng Xià*《明下》says: three cones. ([The Dài Mài 帶脈, which means both the dài vessel and this point,] is like a belt wrapped around the body and controls all the channel-vessels. *Qiān*《千》says: It is located at the end of the free rib region.)

五樞二穴，在帶脈下三寸。一云：在水道旁寸半陷中。針一寸，灸五壯。《明下》云：三壯。

Wŭ Shū 五樞 (GB 27), bilateral point: It is located 3 cùn below Dài Mài (GB 26). One source says: In the depression 1.5 cùn lateral to Shuĭ Dào 水道 (ST 28). Needle 1 cùn deep; burn five cones of moxibustion. *Míng Xià* says: three cones.

維道二穴，在章門下五寸三分。針八分，灸三壯。

Wéi Dào 維道 (GB 28), bilateral point: It is located 5.3 cùn below Zhāng Mén 章門 (LV 13). Needle 8 fēn deep; burn three cones of moxibustion.

居髎二穴，在章門下八寸三分監骨上陷中。灸三壯，針八分。

Jū Liáo 居髎 (GB 29), bilateral point: It is located 8.3 cùn below Zhāng Mén (LV 13), in the depression on the haunch bone. Burn three cones of moxibustion; needle 8 fēn deep.

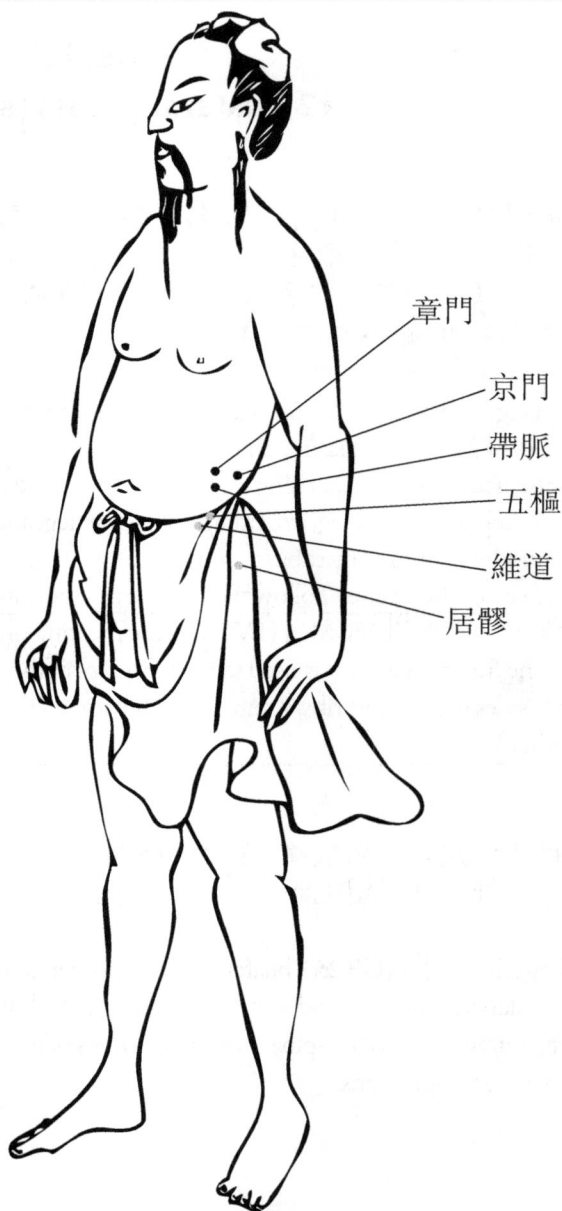

章門
京門
帶脈
五樞
維道
居髎

Fig. 1.29

脅堂二穴，在腋下二骨間陷中，舉腋取之 。灸五壯 。

Xié Táng 脅堂, bilateral point: It is located below the axilla in the depression between two bones. Locate the point with the patient raising the axilla [arms]. Burn five cones of moxibustion.

《明堂下經》有脅堂穴主胸脅、氣滿、噫饐、喘逆、目黃、遠視晎晎，而《銅人》無之，故附入於此。

[Author's note:] Xié Táng [is listed] in *Míng Táng Xià Jīng* 《 明堂下經 》. It controls the chest and rib-sides and treats qì fullness, belching and hiccups, panting counterflow, yellowing of the eyes, and seeing dimly afar [nearsightedness]. But [all this] is not in *Tóng Rén* 《 銅人 》, so I attached it here.

1.25
Shǒu Tài Yīn Fèi Jīng Zuǒ Yòu Shí Bā Xué

手太陰肺經左右十八穴

Hand Tàiyīn Lung Channel,
18 bilateral points [nine on each side]

少商二穴，木也 。在手大指端內側，去爪甲角如韭葉（《明》云：白肉際宛宛中 。）以三稜針刺之，微出血，洩諸藏熱湊，不宜灸。成君綽忽腮頷腫大如升，喉中閉塞，水粒不下 。甄權針之立愈。《明》云：針一分，留三呼，瀉五吸，宜針不宜灸，以三稜針刺之，令血出，勝氣針。所以勝氣針者，此脈脹腮之候，腮中有氣，人不能食，故刺出血以宣諸藏膜也 。忌冷熱食 。《下》云：灸三壯（《甲乙》作一壯 ）。

Shào Shāng 少商 (LU 11), bilateral point, wood[89]: It is located on the medial aspect of the thumb, a leek leaf's distance from the corner of the nail. (*Míng* 《 明 》 says: It is in the depression on the border of white flesh.) Prick it with a three-edged needle and bleed slightly to drain encroaching heat from all the viscera. Moxibustion is not recommended. [Provincial governor] Chéng Jūnzhuō 成君綽 suffered sudden swelling of his cheek and under his chin. [The swelling] was as big as a

---

89. In this section, wood point, fire point, earth point, metal point and water point, indicate the corresponding element (phase) of the point.

shēng.[90] He also had blockage of the throat and inability to get water and food down. Zhēn Quán needled this point and cured the disease immediately. *Míng* 《明》 says: Needle 1 fēn deep; retain the needle for three respirations; drain for five respirations. Needling is recommended, but not moxibustion. It is better to prick and bleed it with a three-edged needle. [This is called] needling to overcome [evil] qì. The reason [it is called] needling to overcome [evil] qì is: swollen cheeks are a symptom of this vessel [the lung channel]. There is [evil] qì within the cheeks and the sufferer cannot eat, so we drain the interstices and viscera by puncturing and bleeding. Cold and hot foods are both contraindicated. *Xià* 《下》 says: Burn three cones of moxibustion. (*Jiǎ Yǐ* 《甲乙》 says: one cone).

魚際二穴，火也。在手大指本節後內側散脈中。針一分，留二呼。《素注》：二分，灸三壯。

Yú Jì 魚際 (LU 10), bilateral point, fire: It is located posterior to the base joint of the thumb, on the scattered vessels medial [to the base joint]. Needle 1 fēn deep; retain the needle for two respirations. *Sù Zhù* 《素注》 says: Needle 2 fēn deep; burn three cones of moxibustion.

太淵二穴，在掌後陷中。灸三壯，針一分。《素注》：二分。《明下》云：太泉在手中掌後橫文頭陷中，灸五壯。（《難》：掌後魚際下。脈會太淵，脈病治此。）

Tài Yuān 太淵 (LU 9), bilateral point: It is located in the depression posterior

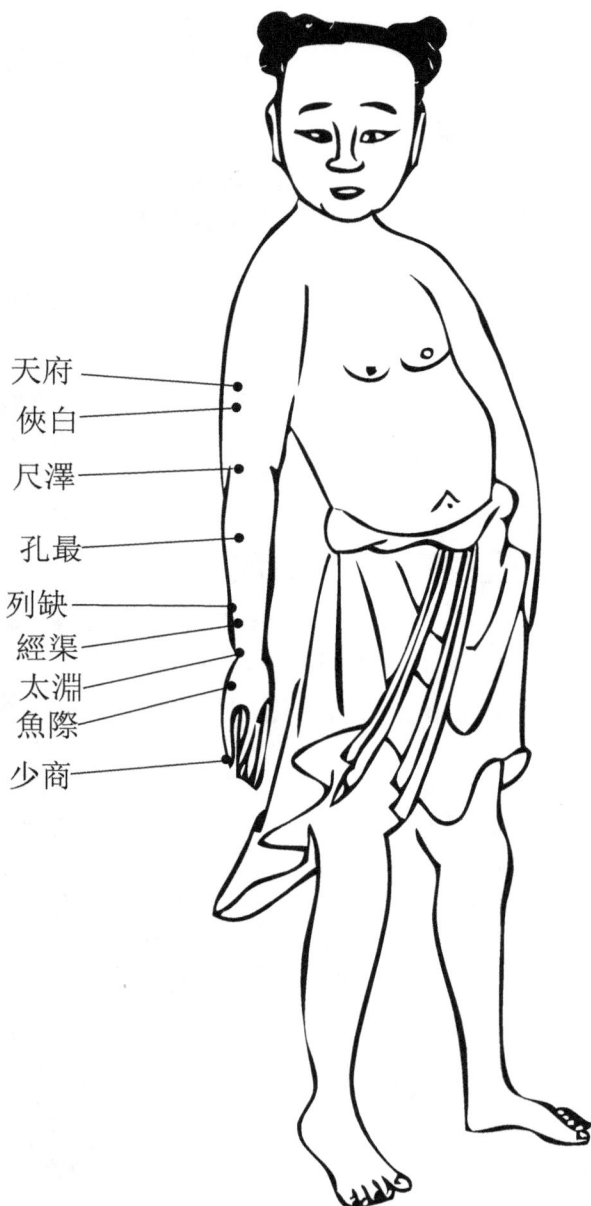

天府
俠白
尺澤
孔最
列缺
經渠
太淵
魚際
少商

Fig. 1.30

---

90. *Shēng* 升 is a unit of dry measurement for grain, equal to about 1 deciliter. Here it indicates the size of the swelling.

[proximal] to the palm. Burn three cones of moxibustion; needle 1 fēn deep. *Sù Zhù* 《素注》 says: 2 fēn deep. *Míng Xià* 《明下》 says: Tài Quán 太泉 (LU 9) is [located] at the end of the transverse crease posterior to the palm. Burn five cones of moxibustion. (*Nàn* 《難》 says: It is located below [proximal to] the fish's margin [thenar eminence, is also the name of LU 10]. Tài Yuān (LU 9) is the meeting [influential] point of the vessels. It treats diseases of the vessels.)

《銅人》曰：太淵，《明堂》曰：太泉，疑是二穴也。予按《千金方》注云：太泉即太淵也。避唐祖名改之，於是書之，以示世醫。（泉腋、清冷泉同。）

[Author's note:] *Tóng Rén* 《銅人》 calls it Tài Yuān (LU 9); while *Míng Táng* 《明堂》 calls it Tài Quán (LU 9); it sounds like two different points. I note based on *Qiān Jīn Fāng* 《千金方》: Tài Quán (LU 9) means Tài Yuān (LU 9). The name change was due to the [name] taboo for Emperor [Gāo] Zǔ of the *Táng* Dynasty.[91] I put it here to let doctors nowadays know. (The same thing occurred with Qúan Yè 泉腋 [Yuān Yè 淵腋] (GB 22) and Qīng Lěng Qúan 清冷泉 [Qīng Lěng Yuān 清冷淵] (SJ 11)).

經渠二穴，金也。在寸口陷中。針二分，留三呼。禁灸，灸傷人神。

Jīng Qú 經渠 (LU 8), bilateral point, metal [point]: It is located in the depression at the *cùn kǒu* [inch opening, the radial pulse]. Needle 2 fēn deep; retain the needle for three respirations. Moxibustion is contraindicated. It damages the human spirit.[92]

列缺二穴，在腕側上寸半。（《明堂下》云：腕上一寸）。以手交叉頭指末兩筋兩骨罅中。針二分，留二呼，瀉五吸，灸七壯，忌同。《明》云：針三分，日灸七壯。若患偏風灸至百，若患腕勞灸七七。《下》云：三壯。《素注》云：腕上寸半。

Liè Quē 列缺 (LU 7), bilateral point: It is located 1.5 cùn above the [radial] side of the wrist [crease]. (*Míng Táng Xià* 《明堂下》 says: It is 1 cùn above the wrist). When the two hands are

---

91. The personal name of the first emperor of the *Táng* Dynasty was Lǐ Yuān 李淵. This is the same character *yuān* as in Tài Yuān 太淵 (LU 9). In ancient China, it was forbidden to use the same Chinese character as the name of the emperor, so people used a similar character, with the same or similar pronunciation, to replace the original name.

92. *Rén shén* 人神 (human spirit): This is an ancient acupuncture prohibition for certain times and places in the body. The theory says there is a human spirit on duty in different part of the body at different times. The location changes based on the season, month, day and time. If this location is punctured, an accident will occur; people can even die in severe cases. For details, see Volume 2 of this book and *Zhēn Jiǔ Dà Chéng* 針灸大成 (The Great Compendium of Acupuncture and Moxibustion), Volume 4.

crossed, it is located at the end of the index finger, between the two sinews, in the cleft of the two bones. Needle 2 fēn deep; retain the needle for two respirations, drain for five respirations. Burn seven cones of moxibustion. Follow the same contraindications [as Shào Shāng 少商 (LU 11)]. *Míng*《明》says: Needle 3 fēn deep; burn seven cones of moxibustion daily. Apply up to a hundred cones for hemilateral wind and seven times seven cones for wrist taxation. *Xià*《下》says: three cones. *Sù Zhù*《素注》says: It is 1.5 cùn above the wrist.

孔最二穴，在腕上七寸（《明下》云：陷者宛宛中）。手太陰郄。治熱病汗不出，此穴可灸三壯，即汗出。咳逆臂厥痛。針三分，灸五壯。《明下》云：灸三壯。

Kǒng Zuì 孔最 (LU 6), bilateral point: It is located 7 cùn above the wrist (*Míng Xià*《明下》 says: in the depression [7 cùn above the wrist]). It is the xī-cleft point of hand tàiyīn. It treats heat disease with absence of sweating. Apply three cones of moxibustion on this point; it will induce sweating immediately. It also treats coughing counterflow and reversal pain of the arms. Needle 3 fēn deep; burn five cones of moxibustion. *Míng Xià* says: Burn three cones.

尺澤二穴，水也。在肘中約上動脈中。針三分，灸五壯。《明》云：肘中約上兩筋動脈中。甄權云：在臂屈伸橫文中筋骨罅陷中，不宜灸。主癲病，不可向手臂，不得上頭。《素·刺禁》云：刺肘中內陷，氣歸之，為不屈伸。注云：肘中謂肘屈折之中，尺澤穴中也。刺過陷脈，惡氣歸之，氣閉關節，故不屈伸。（《難疏》言：尺之一寸外為尺澤也，言尺脈入澤，如水入大澤。）

Chǐ Zé 尺澤 (LU 5), bilateral point, water: It is located on the pulsating vessel slightly above the center of the elbow. Needle 3 fēn deep; burn five cones of moxibustion. *Míng* says: On the pulsating vessel between the two sinews, slightly above the center of the elbow. Zhēn Quán says: It is in the depression between the bones and sinew, in the crease [that appears] when the patient bends and stretches the arm. Moxibustion is not recommended. It governs epilepsy, inability of the head to turn toward the arm, and the arm is unable to reach up to the head. *Sù · Cì Jìn*《素·刺禁》 says: When the inner depression in the center of the elbow is pricked, qì gathers there, so the arm becomes unable to bend and stretch. The Annotation says: The center of the elbow indicates the [area appearing] when the patient bends and stretches their arms; Chǐ Zé (LU 5) is located here. If one pricks through the vessel, evil qì gathers in it and blocks the joints. That is why the patient cannot bend and stretch their arms. (*Nàn Shū*《難疏》says: Chǐ Zé is 1 cùn lateral to the cubit. It indicates the place where the cubital pulse enters the marsh [Chǐ Zé 尺澤 means cubit marsh]; just like the water entering a large marsh.)

《銅人》云：灸五壯，《明堂下經》乃云：不宜灸。主癲病，不可向
手臂，不得上頭。既曰不宜灸矣，乃曰主癲病，是又可灸也。此必有
誤。且從《銅人》灸五壯，《明堂》亦云：禁穴許灸一壯至三壯故
也。

[Author's note:] *Tóng Rén* 《 銅人 》 says: Burn five cones of moxibustion. *Míng Táng Xià Jīng* 《 明堂下經 》 says: Moxibustion is not recommended. Chǐ Zé 尺澤 (LU 5) governs epilepsy, and inability of the head to turn toward the arm, and the arm is unable to reach the head. It says moxibustion is contraindicated, but also says moxibustion can be applied to treat epilepsy. So something must be wrong. [Perhaps we should] just follow the "five cones of moxibustion" of *Tóng Rén*, because *Míng Táng* 《 明堂 》 also says: One can apply one to three cones of moxibustion on points that are contraindicated for moxibustion.

俠白二穴，在天府下去肘五寸動脈中。針三分，灸五壯。

Xiá Bái 俠白 (LU 4), bilateral point: It is located below Tiān Fǔ 天府 (LU 3), 5 cùn from the elbow, on the pulsating vessel. Needle 3 fēn deep; burn five cones of moxibustion.

天府二穴，在腋下三寸動脈中，以鼻取之。禁灸，使人逆氣。今附：刺鼻衄
血不止，針四分，留三呼。《明》云：四分，留七呼，灸二七壯。不除，至
百壯。出《明堂經》，其《甲乙經》禁灸。

Tiān Fǔ (LU 3), bilateral point: It is located on the pulsating vessel 3 cùn below the axilla. Locate the point with the nose.[93] Moxibustion is contraindicated; it causes counterflow qì in patients. Now appended: This point treats incessant nosebleed. Needle 4 fēn deep, retain the needle for three respirations. *Míng* 《 明 》 says: Needle 4 fēn deep, retain the needle for seven respirations. Burn two times seven cones of moxibustion. Apply a hundred cones if the disease does not go away. This is from *Míng Táng Jīng* 《 明堂經 》. *Jiǎ Yǐ Jīng* 《 甲乙經 》 says: Moxibustion is contraindicated.

《甲乙》、《銅人》皆云禁灸，《明堂》乃云灸二七壯至百壯，亦甚
不同矣。要非大急不必灸。

[Author's note:] *Jiǎ Yǐ* 《 甲乙 》 and *Tóng Rén* both say moxibustion is contraindicated. But *Míng Táng* says: Burn two times seven cones, up to a hundred cones of moxibustion. That is a big difference. Do not apply moxibustion on Tiān Fǔ (LU 3) unless it is a very urgent condition.

---

93. Ask the patient to lift his arm to shoulder level, with the palm facing up. Then have the patient turn his head and bend toward the upper arm, letting his nose touch his arm. The point is located under the tip of his nose.

1.26
Shǒu Yáng Míng Dà Cháng Jīng Zuǒ Yòu Èr Shí Bā Xué

手陽明大腸經左右二十八穴

Hand Yángmíng Large Intestine Channel, 28 bilateral points [fourteen on each side]

商陽二穴，金也。一名絕陽。在手大指次指內側，去爪甲角如韭葉。灸三壯，針一分，留一呼。

Shāng Yáng 商陽 (LI 1), bilateral point, metal; another name is Jué Yáng 絕陽: It is located on the medial aspect of the index finger, a leek leaf's distance from the corner of the nail. Burn three cones of moxibustion. Needle 1 fēn deep; retain the needle for one respiration.

二間二穴，水也，一名間谷。在手大指次指本節前內側陷中。針三分，灸三壯。

Èr Jiān 二間 (LI 2), bilateral point, water; another name is Jiān Gǔ 間谷: It is located in the depression anterior [distal] to the base joint of the index finger, on the medial [radial] aspect. Needle 3 fēn deep; burn three cones of moxibustion.

三間二穴，木也，一名少谷。在手大指次指本節後內側陷中。針三分，留三呼，灸三壯。

Sān Jiān 三間 (LI 3), bilateral point, wood; another name is Shào Gǔ 少谷: It is located in the depression posterior [proximal] to the base joint of the index finger, on the medial [radial] aspect. Needle 3 fēn deep; retain the needle for three respirations. Burn three cones of moxibustion.

合谷二穴，一名虎口。在手大指次指岐骨間陷中（《明》云：手大指兩骨罅間宛宛中）。針三分，留三呼，灸三壯。今附：若婦人妊娠不可刺，刺損胎氣。（《千》云：手大指虎口兩骨間。）

Hé Gǔ 合谷 (LI 4), bilateral point, another name is Hǔ Kǒu 虎口: It is located in the depression within the junction of the bones between the thumb and index finger. (*Míng* 《明》 says: in the depression between the two bones [near] the thumb.) Needle 3 fēn deep; retain the needle for three respirations. Burn three cones of moxibustion. Now appended: Contraindicated during pregnancy. Needling damages the fetal qi. (*Qiān* 《千》 says: It is between the two bones in the Hǔ Kǒu (tiger mouth) [region] near the thumb.)

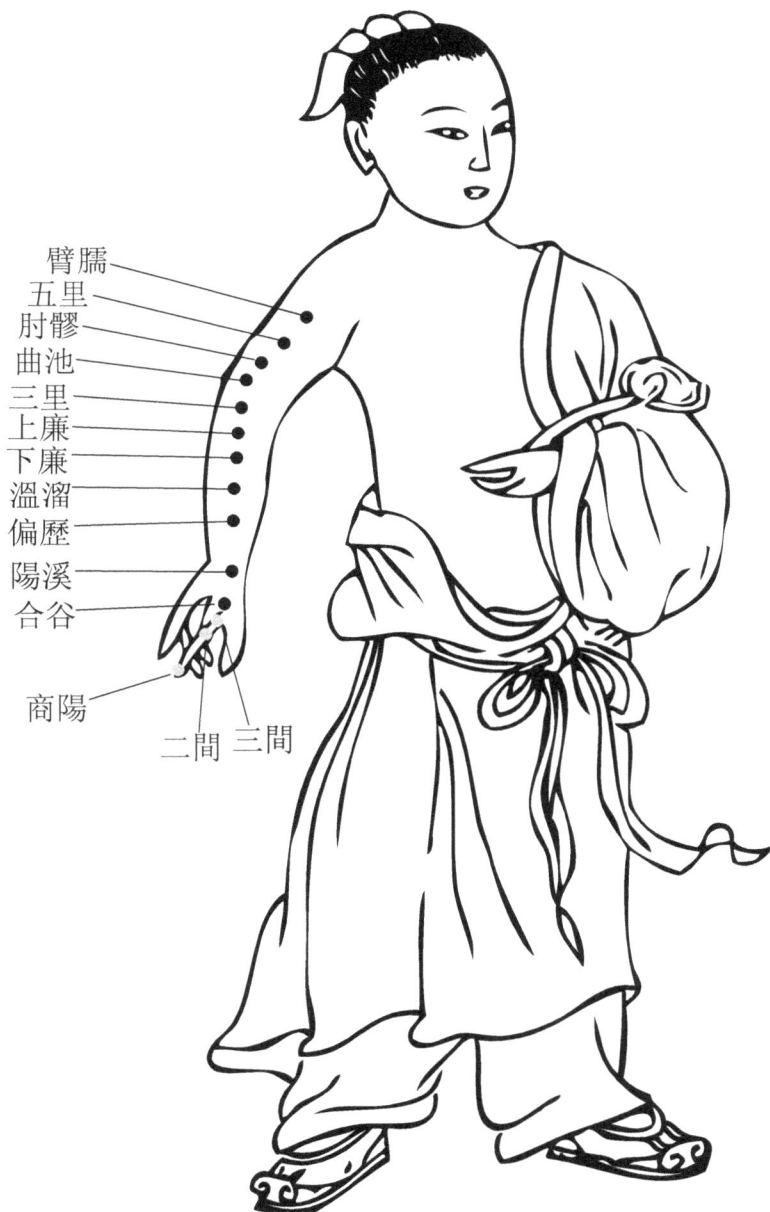

臂臑
五里
肘髎
曲池
三里
上廉
下廉
溫溜
偏歷
陽溪
合谷

商陽

二間 三間

Fig. 1.31

陽溪二穴，火也，一名中魁。在腕中上側兩筋間陷中。針三分，留七呼，灸二壯，忌同。

Yáng Xī 陽溪 (LI 5), bilateral point, fire; another name is Zhōng Kuí 中魁: It is located in the depression between the two sinews on the [radial] side of the wrist. Needle 3 fēn deep; retain the needle for seven respirations. Burn two cones of moxibustion. Follow the same contraindications [as Shào Shāng 少商 (LU 11)].

偏歷二穴，手陽明絡。在腕後三寸，別走太陰。針二分，留七呼，灸三壯。《明下》云：五壯。

Piān Lì 偏歷 (LI 6), bilateral point, the network [point] of the hand yángmíng: It is located 3 cùn posterior [proximal] to the wrist and diverges to the [hand] tàiyīn. Needle 2 fēn deep; retain the needle for seven respirations. Burn three cones of moxibustion. *Míng Xià*《明下》says: five cones.

溫溜二穴，一名逆注，一名池頭。在腕後，大士三寸，小士六寸。針三分，灸三壯。《明》云：在腕後五寸六寸間。

Wēn Liū 溫溜 (LI 7), bilateral point, another name is Nì Zhù 逆注, also named Chí Tóu 池頭: It is located posterior [proximal] to the wrist. [The distance from the wrist] is 3 cùn on a large person and 6 cùn on small person. Needle 3 fēn deep; burn three cones of moxibustion. *Míng*《明》says: It is 5 to 6 cùn posterior [proximal] to the wrist.

下廉二穴，在輔骨下，去上廉一寸，輔兌肉其分外斜。針五分，留二呼，灸三壯。

Xià Lián 下廉 (LI 8), bilateral point: It is located below the assisting bone [radius], 1 cùn from Shàng Lián 上廉 (LI 9). It is oblique to the lateral aspect of the tapered flesh [close to] the assisting bone. Needle 5 fēn deep; retain the needle for two respirations. Burn three cones of moxibustion.

此有下廉，足陽明亦有下廉，蓋在足者，乃下巨虛也。

[Author's note:] Here, there is Xià Lián 下廉 (LI 8); the foot yángmíng also has Xià Lián 下廉 (ST 39). That point is on the legs, so it is [also called] Xià Jù Xū 下巨虛 (ST 39).

上廉二穴，在三里下一寸，其分獨抵陽明之會外斜。針五分，灸五壯。

Shàng Lián 上廉 (LI 9), bilateral point: It is located 1 cùn below Sān Lǐ 三里 (LI 10). The muscle [under this point] runs obliquely and reaches the lateral aspect of yángmíng convergence.[94] Needle 5 fēn deep; burn five cones of moxibustion.

此有上廉，足陽明亦有上廉，蓋在足者，乃上巨虛也。

[Author's note:] Here, there is Shàng Lián 上廉 (LI 9); the foot yángmíng also has Shàng Lián 上廉 (ST 37). That point is on the legs, so it is [also called] Shàng Jù Xū 上巨虛 (ST 37).

三里二穴，在曲池下三寸。（手陽明穴云二寸），按之肉起，兌肉之端。灸三壯，針二分。《明》云：一名手三里，在曲池下二寸。

Sān Lǐ (LI 10), bilateral point: It is located 3 cùn inferior to Qū Chí 曲池 (LI 11) (the hand yángmíng points [section of *Tóng Rén* 《銅人》] says 2 cùn). The flesh rises up when pressed; it is at the end of the tapered flesh. Burn three cones of moxibustion; needle 2 fēn deep. *Míng* 《明》 says: Another name is Shǒu Sān Lǐ 手三里 (LI 10); it is located 2 cùn below Qū Chí (LI 11).

三里有二，有手三里，有足三里，此手三里。故《明堂》云：一名手三里是也。《銅人》云：三里在曲池下三寸，《明堂》乃云二寸。在手陽明穴亦云二寸。恐《銅人》本誤二字作三字也。

[Author's note:] There are two Sān Lǐ 三里: Shǒu [Hand] Sān Lǐ 手三里 (LI 10) and Zú [Foot] Sān Lǐ 足三里 (ST 36). [The point] here is the Hand Sān Lǐ (LI 10), so *Míng Táng* 《明堂》 says: Another name is Shǒu Sān Lǐ. *Tóng Rén* says: Sān Lǐ (LI 10) is located 3 cùn inferior to Qū Chí (LI 11) while *Míng Táng* says 2 cùn. The hand yángmíng point [section] also says 2 cùn. *Tóng Rén* may have accidentally written *sān* 三 (three) instead of *èr* 二 (two).

曲池二穴，土也。在肘外輔骨屈肘曲骨中，以手拱胸取之。針七分，得氣先瀉後補之，灸大良，可三壯。《明》云：曲池，木也。在肘外輔骨曲肘橫紋頭陷中。日灸七壯，至二百且停，十餘日更下火，止至二百罷。忌同。《下》云：在肘外輔屈肘曲骨中紋頭。《素注》：肘外輔屈肘兩骨中。《千》：肘外曲頭陷中。

---

94. This sentence is rather obscure.

Qū Chí 曲池 (LI 11), bilateral point, earth: It is located on the elbow, lateral to the assisting bone [radius], in the depression on the curved bone when the elbow is flexed. Locate the point with the arms encircling the chest [so as to flex the elbows]. Needle 7 fēn deep; drain first then supplement after the qì arrives. It is very good to burn moxibustion on the point; burn three cones of moxibustion. *Míng* 《明》 says: Qū Chí (LI 11) is wood. It is located on the elbow, lateral to the assisting bone of the elbow, in the depression at the end of the transverse crease when the elbow is flexed. Burn seven cones of moxibustion daily, stop temporarily at two hundred cones of moxibustion. Apply moxibustion again after ten days; stop at [another] two hundred cones. Follow the same contraindications [as Shào Shāng 少商 (LU 11)]. *Xià* 《下》 says: This point is located lateral to the assisting bone of the elbow, in the depression at the end of the crease of the curved bone when the elbow is flexed. *Sù Zhù* 《素注》 says: Lateral to the assisting bone of the elbow, between two bones. *Qiān* 《千》 says: On the lateral aspect of the elbow, in the depression at the end of the curved bone.

肘髎二穴，在肘大骨外廉陷中。灸三壯，針三分。

Zhŏu Liáo 肘髎 (LI 12), bilateral point: It is located on the elbow, in the depression on the lateral ridge of the big bone [humerus]. Burn three cones of moxibustion; needle 3 fēn deep.

五里二穴，在肘上三寸，行向裏大脈中央。灸十壯，禁針。《素問 · 氣穴論》云：大禁二十五，在天府下五寸。注云：謂五里穴也，謂之大禁者，禁不可刺也。又曰：五里者，尺澤之後五里，與此文同。

Wŭ Lĭ 五里 (LI 13), bilateral point: It is located 3 cùn above the elbow, running medially and in the center of the big vessel [the radial collateral artery]. Burn ten cones of moxibustion. Needling is contraindicated. *Sù Wèn* · *Qì Xuè Lùn* 《素問 · 氣穴論》 says: The Great Prohibition of 25[95] is located 5 cùn below Tiān Fŭ 天府 (LU 3). The Annotation says: It is named Wŭ Lĭ (LI 13); what is called "the great prohibition" means needling is contraindicated. Another source says: Wŭ Lĭ (LI 13) is located posterior [proximal] to Chĭ Zé 尺澤 (LU 5). This opinion is the same as the statement in this paragraph.

五里有二，其一在足厥陰肝經部，與此穴為二，此當為手五里也。《素問》所謂在天府下者，指此五里也。注云：尺澤之後五里，亦指此五里也。尺澤穴在手太陰。

---

95. *Dà jìn èr shí wŭ* 大禁二十五 (Great Prohibition of 25) indicates Wŭ Lĭ 五里 (LI 13). Chapter 60 of *Líng Shū* · *Yù Băn* 《靈樞 · 玉版》 (Magic Pivot · The Jade Slip) says: If Wŭ Lĭ (LI 13) is drained, visceral qì stops right in the middle while traveling. The true qì of one viscus lasts only about five respirations. If we drain the point five times, the visceral qì becomes exhausted. Five [viscera] times five [breaths of draining technique] is twenty-five, so this exhausts the points.

[Author's note:] There are two Wǔ Lǐ 五里: One is located on the foot juéyīn liver channel; that is different from the one here. This is Shǒu [Hand] Wǔ Lǐ 手五里 (LI 13). What is said in *Sù Wèn* 《素問》: "It is located below Tiān Fǔ 天府 (LU 3)," indicates this Wǔ Lǐ (LI 13). The Annotation says: 'Wǔ Lǐ (LI 13) is located posterior [proximal] to Chǐ Zé 尺澤 (LU 5).' This also indicates the Wǔ Lǐ (LI 13) here. Chǐ Zé (LU 5) is located on the hand tàiyīn.

臂臑二穴，在肘上七寸䐃肉端，手陽明絡。灸三壯，針三分。《明》云：在肩髃下一夫，兩筋兩骨罅陷宛中，平手取之，不得拿手令急，其穴即閉。宜灸不宜針，日七壯至百，若針，不得過三五，過多恐惡，忌同。《千》名頭衝。

Bì Nào 臂臑 (LI 14), bilateral point: It is located 7 cùn above the elbow, at the end of the muscle. It is a hand yángmíng network. Burn three cones of moxibustion; needle 3 fēn deep. *Míng* 《明》 says: It is located one hand [breadth] below Jiān Yú 肩髃 (LI 15), in the depression between the two bones and two sinews. Locate the point with the arm relaxed. If the patient lifts his arm and tightens [the muscle], the point will close up [disappear]. Moxibustion is recommended, but not acupuncture. Burn seven cones of moxibustion daily, up to a hundred cones. This point should not be pricked more than three or five times; with more there is the risk of a bad outcome. Follow the same contraindications [as Shào Shāng 少商 (LU 11)]. *Qiān* 《千》 called it Tóu Chōng 頭衝.

（ 肩髎在肩部 。 ）

(Jiān Liáo 肩髎 (SJ 14)[96] is located on the shoulder [so it is described elsewhere].)

---

96. This should say Jiān Yú 肩髃 (LI 15) instead of Jiān Liáo 肩髎 (SJ 14).

1.27

手少陰心經左右十八穴

Shǒu Shàoyīn Xīn Jīng Zuǒ Yòu Shí Bā Xué

Hand Shàoyīn Heart Channel,
18 bilateral points [nine on each side]

少衝二穴，木也，一名經始。在手小指內廉端（《明下》作側）去爪甲角如韭葉。針一分，灸三壯。《明》云：一壯。

Shào Chōng 少衝 (HT 9), bilateral point, wood; another name is Jīng Shǐ 經始: It is located at the tip of the medial ridge (*Míng Xià* 《明下》 says *cè* 側 (aspect)) of the little finger, a leek leaf's distance from the corner of the nail. Needle 1 fēn deep; burn three cones of moxibustion. *Míng* 《明》 says: one cone.

少府二穴，火也。在手小指本節後陷中。直勞宮（勞宮在手厥陰）。針二分，灸七壯。《明》云：三壯。

Shào Fǔ 少府 (HT 8), bilateral point, fire: It is located in the depression posterior [proximal] to the base joint of the little finger, directly in line with Láo Gōng 勞宮 (PC 8) (Láo Gōng (PC 8) is on the hand juéyīn). Needle 2 fēn deep; burn seven cones of moxibustion. *Míng* says: three cones.

神門二穴，土也，一名兌衝。在掌後兌骨端陷中。灸七壯，炷如小麥，針三分，留七呼。

Shén Mén 神門 (HT 7), bilateral point, earth; another name is Duì Chōng 兌衝: It is located in the depression at the end of the sharp bone [the styloid process of the ulna], posterior [proximal] to the palm. Burn seven cones of moxibustion. Use grain of wheat size cones. Needle 3 fēn deep; retain the needle for seven respirations.

陰郄二穴，在掌後脈中。去腕五分。針三分，灸七壯。

Yīn Xī 陰郄 (HT 6), bilateral point: It is located on the vessel posterior [proximal] to the palm; 5 fēn from the wrist. Needle 3 fēn deep; burn seven cones of moxibustion.

通里二穴，在腕後一寸陷中 。針三分，灸三壯 。《 明 》云：七壯 。

Tōng Lǐ 通里 (HT 5), bilateral point: It is located in the depression 1 cùn posterior [proximal] to the wrist. Needle 3 fēn deep; burn three cones of moxibustion. *Míng* 《 明 》 says: seven cones.

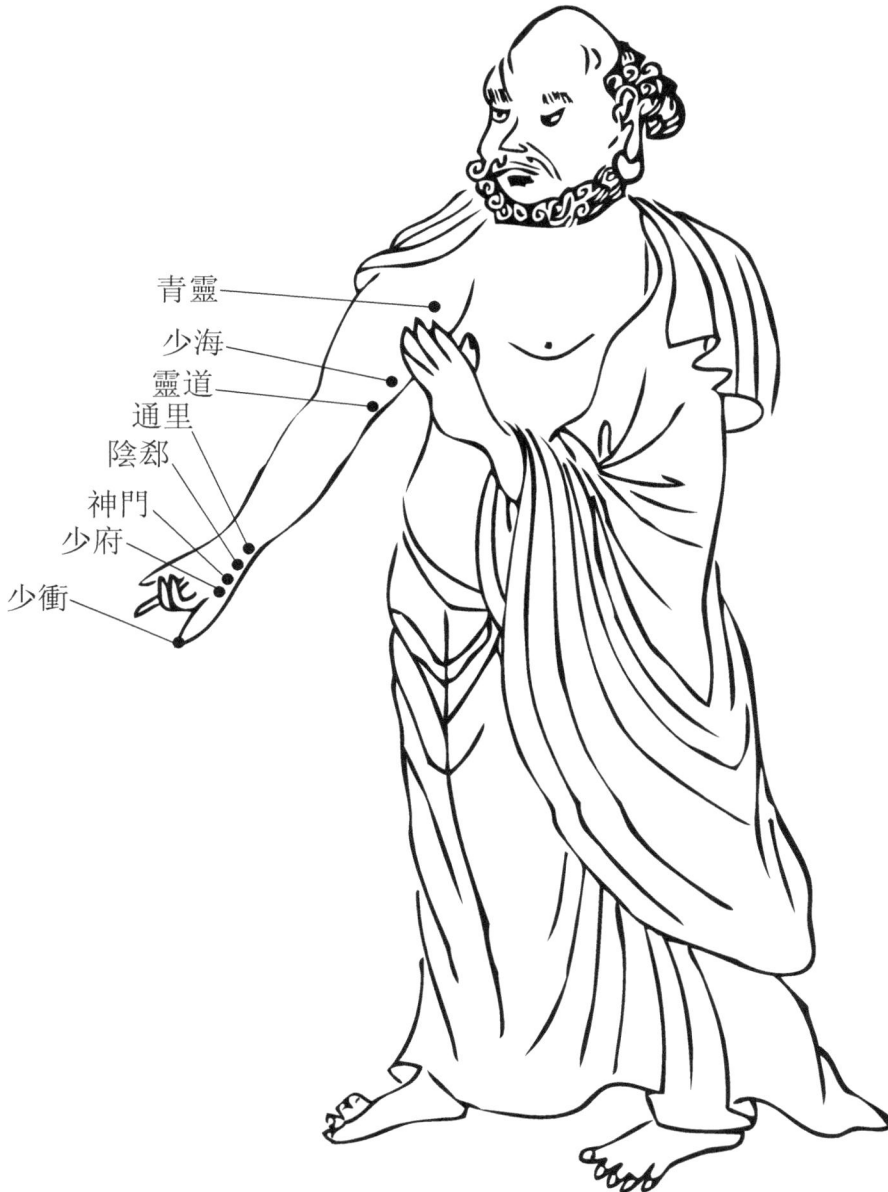

Fig. 1.32

靈道二穴，金也。去掌後寸半或一寸。灸三壯，針三分。

Líng Dào 靈道 (HT 4), bilateral point, metal: It is located 1.5 cùn or 1 cùn posterior [proximal] to the palm. Burn three cones of moxibustion; needle 3 fēn deep.

少海二穴，水也，一名曲節。在肘內廉節後。又云：肘內大骨外，去肘端五分，屈肘得之。針三分，灸三壯。甄權云：屈手向頭取之。治齒寒，腦風頭痛。不宜灸，針五分。《明》云：在肘內橫紋頭，屈手向頭取之陷宛中，《甲乙》云：穴在肘內廉即後陷中，動應手。針二分，留三呼，瀉五吸，不宜灸。《下》云：灸五壯。《素注》：五壯。

Shào Hǎi 少海 (HT 3), bilateral point, water; another name is Qū Jié 曲節: It is located on the medial aspect of the elbow, posterior [proximal] to the [elbow] joint. It also said: on the medial aspect the elbow, lateral to the big bone [medial epicondyle of the humerus], 5 fēn from the tip of the elbow. Locate the point while flexing the elbow. Needle 3 fēn deep; burn three cones of moxibustion. Zhēn Quán said: Locate the point with the patient flexing his hand toward his head. It treats cold teeth, brain wind, and headaches. Moxibustion is not recommended; needle 5 fēn deep. *Míng* 《明》 says: At the end of the transverse crease on the medial aspect of the elbow. Locate the point in the depression [that appears] when the patient flexes his hand toward his head. *Jiǎ Yǐ* 《甲乙》 says: The point is located in the depression posterior [proximal] to the medial aspect of the elbow. It responds to the hands when the patient moves [his arm]. Needle 2 fēn deep; retain the needle for three respirations; drain for five respirations. Moxibustion is not recommended. *Xià* 《下》 says: Burn five cones of moxibustion. *Sù Zhù* 《素注》 says: five cones.

《銅人》云：灸三壯，《明堂下經》、《素問》注皆云：灸五壯，《上經》、甄權皆云不宜灸，亦可疑矣。非大急，亦不必灸。

[Author's note:] *Tóng Rén* 《銅人》 says: Burn three cones of moxibustion. *Míng Táng Xià Jīng* 《明堂下經》 and the Annotation to *Sù Wèn* 《素問》 both say: Burn five cones of moxibustion. *Shàng Jīng* 《上經》 and Zhēn Quán both say: It is not appropriate to apply moxibustion. This is also doubtful. So do not apply moxibustion unless it is a very critical condition.

青靈二穴，在肘上三寸，伸肘舉臂取。灸七壯。《明下》云：三壯。

Qīng Líng 青靈 (HT 2), bilateral point: It is located 3 cùn above the elbow. Locate the point while the patient stretches his elbow and lifts his arm. Burn seven cones of moxibustion. *Míng Xià* 《明下》 says: three cones.

極泉二穴，在腋下筋間，動脈入胸。灸七壯，針三分。

Jí Quán 極泉 (HT 1), bilateral point: It is located below the axilla, [in the depression] between the sinews. There is a pulsating vessel that enters the chest. Burn seven cones of moxibustion; needle 3 fēn deep.

1.28
Shǒu Tàiyáng Xiǎo Cháng Jīng Zuǒ Yòu Shí Liù Xué

手太陽小腸經左右十六穴

Hand Tàiyáng Small Intestine Channel, 16 bilateral points [eight on each side]

少澤二穴，金也，一名小吉。在手小指端去爪甲下一分陷中。灸一壯，針一分。

Shào Zé 少澤 (SI 1), bilateral point, metal; another name is Xiǎo Jí 小吉: It is located at the tip of the little finger, in the depression 1 fēn from the corner of the nail. Burn one cone of moxibustion; needle 1 fēn deep.

前谷二穴，水也。在手小指外側本節前陷中。針一分，灸一壯。《明》云：三壯。

Qián Gǔ 前谷 (SI 2), bilateral point, water: It is located on the lateral aspect of the little finger, in the depression anterior [distal] to the base joint. Needle 1 fēn deep; burn one cone of moxibustion. *Míng* 《明》 says: three cones.

後溪二穴，木也。在手小指外側本節後陷中。灸一壯，針一分。《明》云：在手外側腕前起骨下陷中。灸三壯。

Hòu Xī 後溪 (SI 3), bilateral point, wood: It is located on the lateral aspect of the little finger, in the depression posterior [proximal] to the base joint. Burn one cone of moxibustion; needle 1 fēn deep. *Míng* says: It is located on the lateral aspect of the hand, in the depression below the bony protuberance anterior [distal] to the wrist. Burn three cones of moxibustion.

腕骨二穴，在手外側腕前起骨下陷中。灸三壯，針二分，留三呼。

Wàn Gǔ 腕骨 (SI 4), bilateral point: It is located on the lateral aspect of the hand, in the depression below the bony protuberance anterior [distal] to the wrist. Burn three cones of moxibustion; needle 2 fēn deep; retain the needle for three respirations.

陽谷二穴，火也。在手外側腕中兌（《素》作銳）骨下陷中。灸三壯，針二分，留二呼。

Yáng Gǔ 陽谷 (SI 5), bilateral point, fire: It is located in the depression inferior to the protuberant (*Sù*《素》says *ruì* 銳 sharp[97]) bone [styloid process of the ulna] on the lateral aspect of the hand. Burn three cones of moxibustion; needle 2 fēn deep; retain the needle for two respirations.

養老二穴，在手踝骨上空寸陷中。灸三壯，針三分。

Yǎng Lǎo 養老 (SI 6), bilateral point: It is located in the hollow 1 cùn above the wrist. Burn three cones of moxibustion; needle 3 fēn deep.

支正二穴，在腕後五寸。別走少陰。灸三壯，針三分。《明》云：在手太陽腕後五寸，去養老穴四寸陷中。灸五壯。

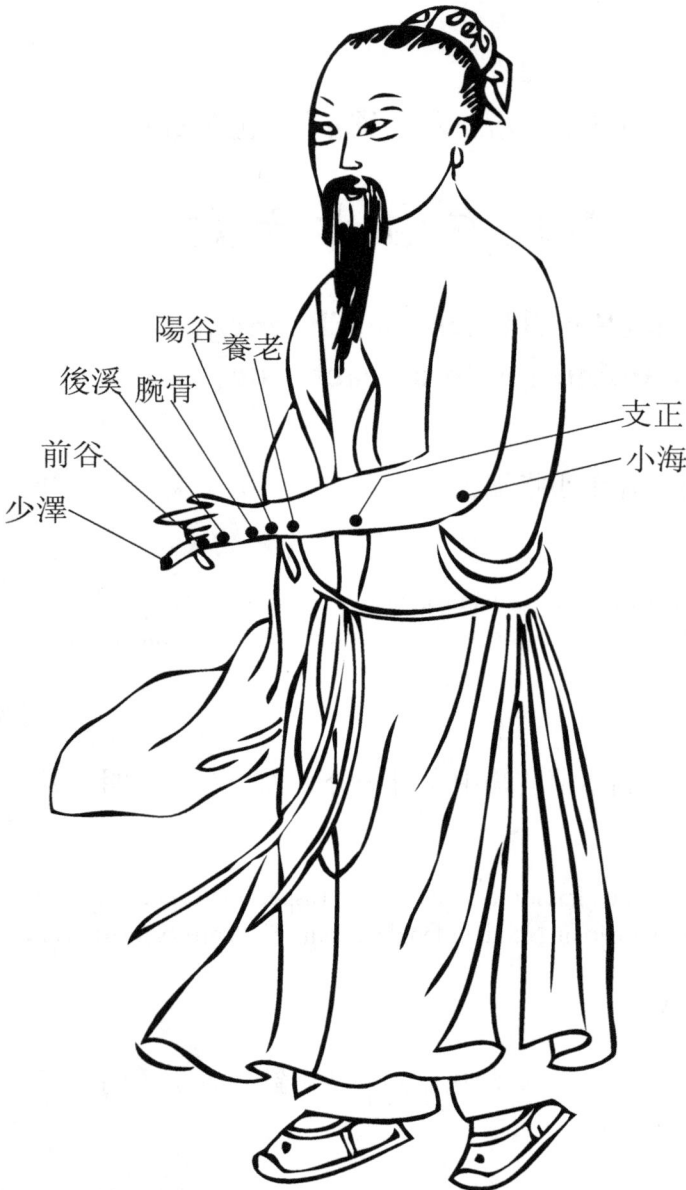

陽谷 養老
後溪 腕骨
前谷
少澤
支正
小海

Fig. 1.33

---

97. *Ruì* 兌 and *ruì* 銳 [sharp] were often read as the same character in ancient literature.

Zhī Zhèng 支正 (SI 7), bilateral point: It is located 5 cùn posterior [proximal] to the wrist. It diverges to the [hand] shàoyīn. Burn three cones of moxibustion; needle 3 fēn deep. *Míng* 《 明 》 says: It is located on the hand tàiyáng; 5 cùn posterior [proximal] to the wrist; in the depression 4 cùn from Yǎng Lǎo 養老 (SI 6). Burn five cones of moxibustion.

小海二穴，土也 。在肘內大骨外，去肘端五分陷中 。甄權云：屈手向頭取之 。灸三壯，針二分 。

Xiǎo Hǎi 小海 (SI 8), bilateral point, earth: It is located lateral to the big bone on the medial aspect of the elbow, in the depression 5 fēn from the tip of the elbow. Zhēn Quán said: Locate the point with the elbow flexed toward the head. Burn three cones of moxibustion; needle 2 fēn deep.

1.29

手厥陰心主脈左右十六穴

Shǒu Juéyīn Xīn Zhǔ Mài Zuǒ Yòu Shí Liù Xué

Hand Juéyīn Pericardium Channel, 16 bilateral points [eight on each side]

中衝二穴，木也，在手中指端，去爪甲如韭葉陷中 。針一分 。《 明 》云：灸一壯 。

Zhōng Chōng 中衝 (PC 9), bilateral point, wood: It is located on the tip of the middle finger, a leek leaf's distance from the nail. Needle 1 fēn deep. *Míng* 《 明 》 says: Burn one cone of moxibustion.

勞宮二穴，火也，一名五里 。在掌中央橫紋動脈中，屈無名指癢處是 。灸三壯 。《 明 》云：針二分，得氣即瀉 。祇一度針，過兩度，令人虛 。不可灸，灸令息肉日加 。忌同 。《 素注 》：灸三壯 。（ 一名掌中 。 ）

Láo Gōng 勞宮 (PC 8), bilateral point, fire; another name is Wǔ Lǐ 五里: It is located on the transverse crease in the center of the palm, on the pulsating vessel. Locate the point under the tip of the ring finger when it is bent and tickles [the palm]. Burn three cones of moxibustion. *Míng* says: Needle 2 fēn deep, drain [the point] as soon as qì arrives. Only needle once; needling twice can cause vacuity. Moxibustion is not recommended, as it makes polyps enlarge day by day. Follow the same contraindications [as Shào Shāng 少商 (LU 11)]. *Sù Zhù*《素注》says: Burn three cones of moxibustion. (Another name is Zhǎng Zhōng 掌中.)

趙岐釋《孟子》云：無名之指，手第四指也。今曰屈無名指著處是穴，蓋屈第四指也。（◎無名指當屈中指為是，今說屈第四指，非也。）

[Author's note:] Zhào Qǐ[98] explained Mèng Zǐ《孟子》[99] by saying: The ring finger is the fourth finger of the hand. Here it says: The point is located under the tip of the ring finger when it is bent. This must mean the fourth finger.[100] (* Here it should say the middle finger instead of the ring finger. What [the book] says, "to bend the fourth finger," is incorrect.)

大陵二穴，土也。在掌後兩筋間陷中。針五分，灸三壯。

Dà Líng 大陵 (PC 7), bilateral point, earth: It is located posterior [proximal] to the palm, in the depression between two sinews [palmaris longus tendon and flexor carpi radialis tendon]. Needle 5 fēn deep; burn three cones of moxibustion.

內關二穴，在掌後去腕二寸，別走少陽。針五分，灸三壯。

Nèi Guān 內關 (PC 6), bilateral point: It is located posterior [proximal] to the palm, 2 cùn above the wrist. It diverges to the [hand] shàoyáng. Needle 5 fēn deep; burn three cones of moxibustion.

間使二穴，金也。在掌後三寸兩筋間陷中。針三分，灸五壯。《明下》云：七壯。（《千》云：腕後三寸，或云：掌後陷中。）

Jiān Shǐ 間使 (PC 5), bilateral point, metal: It is located posterior [proximal] to the palm, 3 cùn above the wrist, in the depression between two sinews [palmaris longus tendon and flexor carpi

---

98. Zhào Qǐ 趙岐 (108-201) was a famous scholar who researched the classics. He was also a famous painter.

99. Mèng Zǐ《孟子》is the book that recorded the thoughts, speech, and stories of Mèng Zǐ 孟子. The author was Mèng Zǐ 孟子 and his students. The book contains seven chapters and was written during the middle and end of the Warring States period.

100. In Chinese, the fingers have different names than in English. The text here actually says "the nameless finger (無名指)," which we translate as "the ring finger." Both are idiomatic names for the fourth finger. The author is clarifying that the nameless (ring) finger is the same as the fourth finger. In the following sentence an editor states that this must be an error and the text should say the third or middle finger.

raidalis tendon]. Needle 3 fēn deep; burn five cones of moxibustion. *Míng Xià* 《 明下 》 says: Seven cones. (*Qiān* 《 千 》 says: It is 3 cùn posterior to the wrist; or it says: In the depression posterior to the palm.)

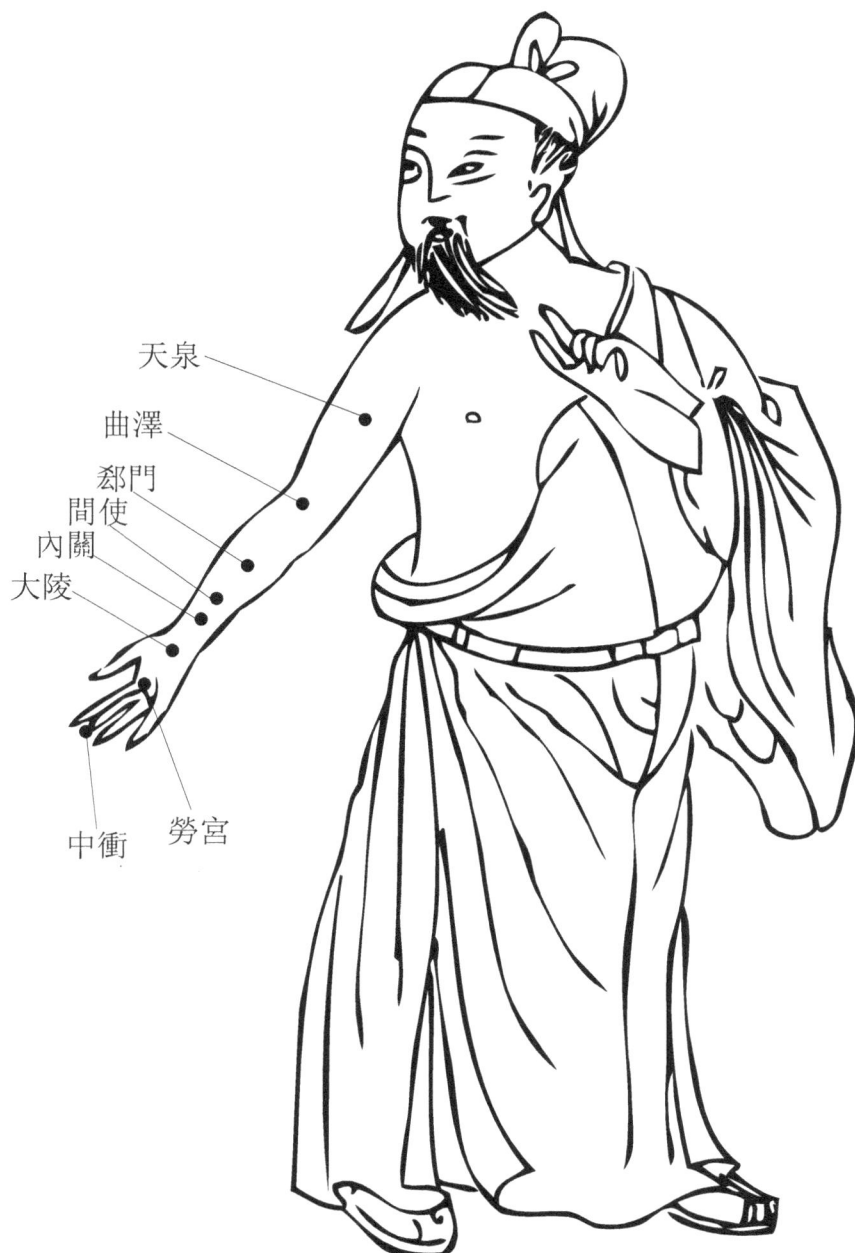

天泉
曲澤
郄門
間使
內關
大陵

中衝　勞宮

Fig. 1.34

111

郄門二穴，去腕五寸，手厥陰［郄］。針三分，灸五壯。

Xī Mén 郄門 (PC 4), bilateral point: It is located 5 cùn from the wrist. [It is the *xī*-cleft point[101] of] the hand juéyīn. Needle 3 fēn deep; burn five cones of moxibustion.

曲澤二穴，水也。在肘內廉陷中，屈肘取之。灸三壯，針三分，留七呼。《素注》：內廉下。

Qū Zé 曲澤 (PC 3), bilateral point, water: It is located in the depression on the inner aspect of the elbow. Locate the point with the elbow flexed. Burn three cones of moxibustion; needle 3 fēn deep; retain the needle for seven respirations. *Sù Zhù* 《素注》 says: It is below the inner aspect [of the elbow].

天泉二穴，一名天濕。在曲腋下二寸，舉臂取。針六分，灸三壯。

Tiān Quán 天泉 (PC 2), bilateral point, another name is Tiān Shī 天濕. It is located 2 cùn below the axillary fold. Locate the point while raising [abducting] the arm. Needle 6 fēn deep; burn three cones of moxibustion.

---

101. The character *xī* 郄 (*xī*-cleft point) is missing from original text. It is added here based on the standard passage for all the channels.

1.30
Shǒu Shàoyáng Sānjiāo Jīng Zuǒ Yòu Èr Shí Sì Xué

手少陽三焦經左右二十四穴

Hand Shàoyáng Sānjiāo Channel,
24 bilateral points [twelve on each side]

關衝二穴，金也。在手小指次指端，去爪甲角如韭葉。針一分，灸一壯。忌同。《素注》：三壯。（一云：握拳取之。）

Guān Chōng 關衝 (SJ 1), bilateral point, metal: It is located on the tip of the ring finger, a leek leaf's distance from the corner of the nail. Needle 1 fēn deep; burn one cone of moxibustion. Follow the same contraindications [as Shào Shāng 少商 (LU 11)]. *Sù Zhù* 《素注》 says: Burn three cones of moxibustion. (One source says: Locate the point while making a fist.)

液門二穴，水也。在手小指次指間陷中。針二分，灸三壯。（一云：握拳取之。）

Yè Mén 液門 (SJ 2), bilateral point, water: It is located in the depression between the little finger and the ring finger. Needle 2 fēn deep; burn three cones of moxibustion. (One source says: Locate the point while making a fist.)

中渚二穴，木也。在手小指次指本節後間陷中。針三分，灸三壯。《明》云：二壯。

Zhōng Zhǔ 中渚 (SJ 3), bilateral point, wood: It is located in the depression posterior [proximal] to the base joint of the ring finger. Needle 3 fēn deep; burn three cones of moxibustion. *Míng* 《明》 says: Two cones.

陽池二穴，一名別陽。在手表腕上陷中。針二分，留三呼，不可灸。忌同。《素注》：灸三壯。

Yáng Chí 陽池 (SJ 4), bilateral point, another name is Bié Yáng 別陽. It is located in the depression on the dorsum of wrist. Needle 2 fēn deep; retain the needle for three respirations. Moxibustion is contraindicated. Follow the same contraindications [as Shào Shāng 少商 (LU 11)]. *Sù Zhù* 《素注》 says: Burn three cones of moxibustion.

外關二穴，正少陽絡。在腕後二寸陷中。針三分，留七呼，灸二壯。《明》云：三壯。

Wài Guān 外關 (SJ 5) bilateral point, the network [vessel] of the [hand] shàoyáng: It is located in the depression 2 cùn posterior [proximal] to the wrist. Needle 3 fēn deep; retain the needle for seven respirations. Burn two cones of moxibustion. *Míng* 《明》 says: Three cones.

支溝二穴，火也。在腕後三寸兩骨間陷中。針二分，灸二七壯。忌同。《明》云：五壯。《素注》：三壯。（《千》云：腕後臂外三寸。）

Zhī Gōu 支溝 (SJ 6), bilateral point, fire: It is located 3 cùn posterior [proximal] to the wrist, in the depression between the two bones [radius and ulna]. Needle 2 fēn deep; burn two times seven cones of moxibustion. Follow the same contraindications [as Shào Shāng 少商 (LU 11)]. *Míng* says: Five cones. *Sù Zhù* says: Three cones. (*Qiān* 《千》 says: It is 3 cùn posterior to the wrist, on the lateral aspect of the arm.)

會宗二穴，在腕後三寸空中一寸。針三分，灸三壯。

Huì Zōng 會宗 (SJ 7), bilateral point: It is located in the 1-cùn-size hollow, 3 cùn posterior [proximal] to the wrist. Needle 3 fēn deep; burn three cones of moxibustion.

三陽絡二穴，在臂上大交脈（《明》云：肘前五寸外廉陷中），支溝上一寸。禁針，灸七壯。《明》云：五壯。

Sān Yáng Luò 三陽絡 (SJ 8), bilateral point: It is located on the arm, at the great intersection of the vessels [three yáng channels] (*Míng* says: It is in the depression 5 cùn anterior [distal] to the elbow, on the lateral aspect); 1 cùn above [proximal to] Zhī Gōu (SJ 6). Needling is contraindicated; burn seven cones of moxibustion. *Míng* says: Five cones.

四瀆二穴，在肘前一寸外廉陷中。灸三壯，針六分，留七呼。

Sì Dú 四瀆 (SJ 9), bilateral point: It is located in the depression 1 cùn anterior [distal] to the elbow, on the lateral aspect. Burn three cones of moxibustion; needle 6 fēn deep; retain the needle for seven respirations.

天井二穴，土也。在肘外大骨後，肘上（《明堂》作後。）一寸，兩筋間陷中，屈肘得之。甄權云：曲肘後一寸，又手按膝頭取之，兩筋骨罅。針三分，灸三壯，忌同。《明》云：五壯。《素注》：刺一寸。（《千》：肘後兩筋間。）

Tiān Jǐng 天井 (SJ 10), bilateral point, earth. It is located posterior [proximal] to the big bone, on the lateral aspect of the elbow, 1 cùn above (*Míng Táng*《明堂》 says: posterior to) [the tip of] the elbow, in the depression between two sinews. Locate the point while bending the elbow. Zhēn Quán said: It is 1 cùn posterior to the curve of the elbow. Locate the point while crossing the arms and pressing [the hands] on the knee caps; it is in the cleft of the bone between two sinews. Needle 3 fēn deep; burn three cones of moxibustion. Follow the same contraindications [as Shào Shāng 少商 (LU 11)]. *Míng*《明》 says: Five cones. *Sù Zhù*《素注》 says: Needle 1 cùn deep. (*Qiān*《千》 says: It is located posterior to the elbow, between two sinews.)

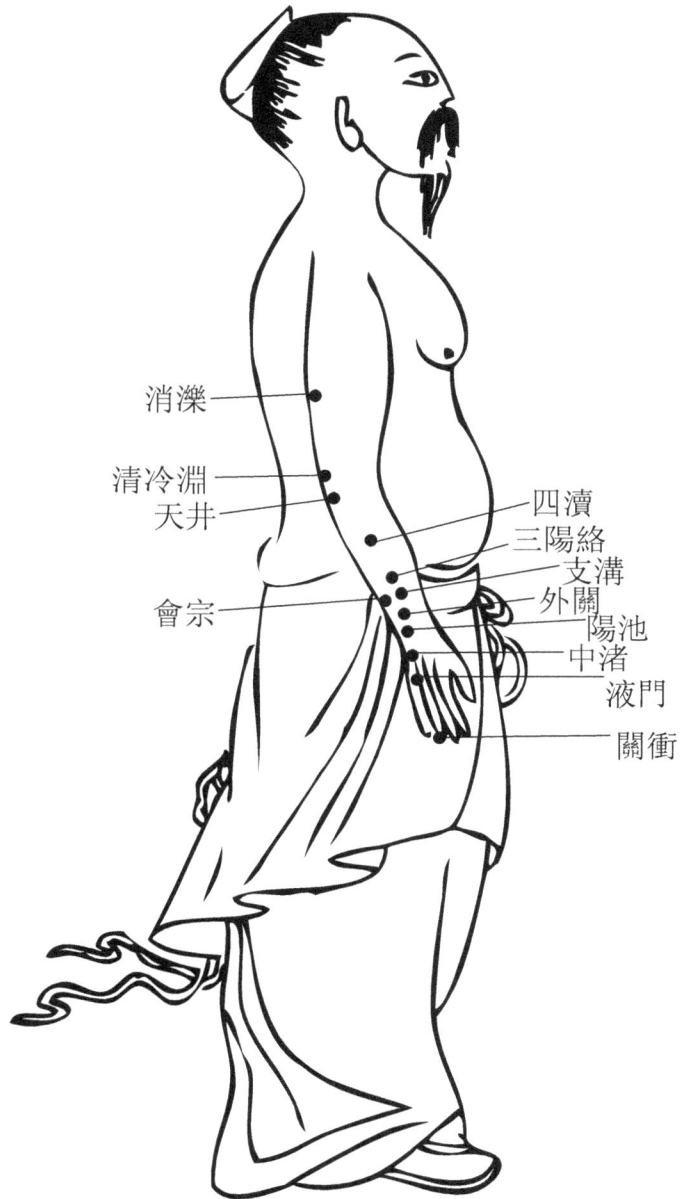

消濼

清冷淵
天井

會宗

四瀆
三陽絡
支溝
外關
陽池
中渚
液門

關衝

Fig. 1.35

清冷淵二穴，在肘上二寸，伸肘舉臂取。灸三壯，針三分。

Qīng Lěng Yuān 清冷淵 (SJ 11), bilateral point: It is located 2 cùn above the elbow. Locate the point while the patient stretches his elbow and lifts his arm. Burn three cones of moxibustion; needle 3 fēn deep.

消濼二穴，在肩下臂外腋斜肘分下行。針一分，灸二壯。《明》云：在肩下外關腋斜肘分下行。針六分，灸三壯。《素注》：肩下臂外關腋。

Xiāo Luò 消濼 (SJ 12), bilateral point: It is located below the shoulder, on the lateral aspect of the arm, oblique to the axilla, inferior to the muscles [near] the elbow. Needle 1 fēn deep; burn two cones of moxibustion. *Míng* 《明》 says: It is located below the shoulder, on the lateral gate[102] of the arm, oblique to the axilla, inferior to the muscles [near] the elbow. Needle 6 fēn deep; burn three cones of moxibustion. *Sù Zhù* 《素注》 says: It is below the shoulder, on the lateral aspect of the arm and axilla.

---

102. According to *Zhēn Jiŭ Jiǎ Yǐ Jīng* 《針灸甲乙經》, *guān* 關 (gate) should be *kāi* 開 (open). Then this phrase would read "*wài kāi* 外開," which means the lateral aspect. *Wài kāi* 外開 makes more sense than *wài guān* 外關 here.

1.31

足厥陰肝經左右二十二穴

Zú Juéyīn Gān Jīng Zuǒ Yòu Èr Shí Èr Xué

Foot Juéyīn Liver Channel,
22 bilateral points [eleven on each side]

大敦二穴，木也。在足大指端去爪甲如韭葉及三毛中。灸三壯，針三分，留六呼。《千》云：足大指聚毛中。

Dà Dūn 大敦 (LV 1), bilateral point, wood: It is located at the end of the big toe, a leek leaf's distance from the corner of the nail and in the three hairs[103] [region]. Burn three cones of moxibustion; needle 3 fēn deep; retain the needle for six respirations. *Qiān* 《千》 says: It is in the tuft of hair[104] on the big toe.

行間二穴，火也。在足大指間動脈應手陷中。灸三壯，針六分，留十呼。

Xíng Jiān 行間 (LV 2), bilateral point, fire: It is located in the depression [between] the big toe [and the second toe]. There is a pulsating vessel that responds to the hand. Burn three cones of moxibustion; needle 6 fēn deep; retain the needle for ten respirations.

太衝二穴，土也。在足大指本節後二寸或寸半陷中。今附：凡診太衝脈，可決男子病死生。針三分，留十呼，灸三壯。

Tài Chōng 太衝 (LV 3), bilateral point, earth. It is located in the depression 2 cùn or 1.5 cùn posterior [proximal] to the base joint of the big toe. Appended here: After diagnosing the Tài Chōng pulse, one can make a decision on the prognosis for diseases of male patients. Needle 3 fēn deep; retain the needle for ten respirations. Burn three cones of moxibustion.

---

103. *Sān máo* 三毛 (three hairs) indicates the region just proximal to the base of the nail of the big toe.

104. *Jù máo* 聚毛 (tuft of hair) indicates the region just proximal to the first metatarsophalangeal joint.

《明》云：在足大指本節後二寸，骨蹉間陷中。灸五壯。《素注》：在足大指間本節後二寸，動脈應手。《刺腰痛注》云：在大指本節後內間二寸。

[Author's note:] *Míng*《明》 says: It is located 2 cùn posterior [proximal] to the base joint of the big toe, in the cleft between the bones. Burn five cones of moxibustion. The *Sù Zhù*《素注》 says: It is located 2 cùn posterior to the base joint of the big toe. There is a pulsating vessel that responds to the hand. *Cì Yāo Tòng Zhù*《刺腰痛注》 (The Annotation to the Treatise on Needling Lower Back Pain)[105] says: It is 2 cùn posterior to the base joint of the big toe, on the inner aspect.

中封二穴，金也。在足內踝前一寸，仰足取之陷中，伸足乃得之。針四分，留七呼，灸三壯。《素注》：內踝前寸半。《甲乙》云：一寸。（《千》與《素》同。又云：內踝前一寸斜行小脈上。一名懸泉。）

Zhōng Fēng 中封 (LV 4), bilateral point, metal: It is located 1 cùn anterior to the medial malleolus, in the depression [that appears] when bending the foot [upward - dorsal flexion]. Locate the point while stretching the leg. Needle 4 fēn deep; retain the needle for seven respirations. Burn three cones of moxibustion. *Sù Zhù* says: It is 1.5 cùn anterior to the medial malleolus. *Jiǎ Yǐ*《甲乙》 says: 1 cùn. (*Qiān*《千》 and *Sù*《素》 agree. They also say: It is located 1 cùn anterior to the medial malleolus, on the small vessel that runs obliquely. Another name is Xuán Quán 懸泉.)

蠡溝二穴，在足內踝上五寸，別走少陽。針二分，留三呼，灸三壯。《明下》云：七壯。（又云：交儀在內踝上五寸，恐即蠡溝穴，但別出蠡溝，故不可曉。◎蠡溝二穴亦名交儀。）

Lǐ Gōu 蠡溝 (LV 5), bilateral point: It is located 5 cùn above the medial malleolus; it diverges to the [foot] shàoyáng. Needle 2 fēn deep; retain the needle for three respirations. Burn three cones of moxibustion. *Míng Xià*《明下》 says: Seven cones. (It also says: Jiāo Yí 交儀 is located 5 cùn above the medial malleolus; this might mean Lǐ Gōu (LV 5). But the divergence is from Lǐ Gōu (LV 5), so it is unknown [whether these two names are for the same point]. * Lǐ Gōu (LV 5), a bilateral point, is also named Jiāo Yí.)

中都二穴，一名中郄。在內踝上七寸胻骨中，與少陰相直。針三分，灸五壯。

---

105. This refers to Wáng Bīng's 王冰 annotation of *Sù Wèn* 素問 (Plain Questions), Chapter 41.

Zhōng Dū 中都 (LV 6), bilateral point, another name is Zhōng Xī 中郄: It is located on the tibia, 7 cùn above the medial malleolus, in line with the shàoyīn.[106] Needle 3 fēn deep; burn five cones of moxibustion.

膝關二穴，在犢鼻下二寸陷中 。針四分，灸五壯 。（ 犢鼻在足陽明 。 ）

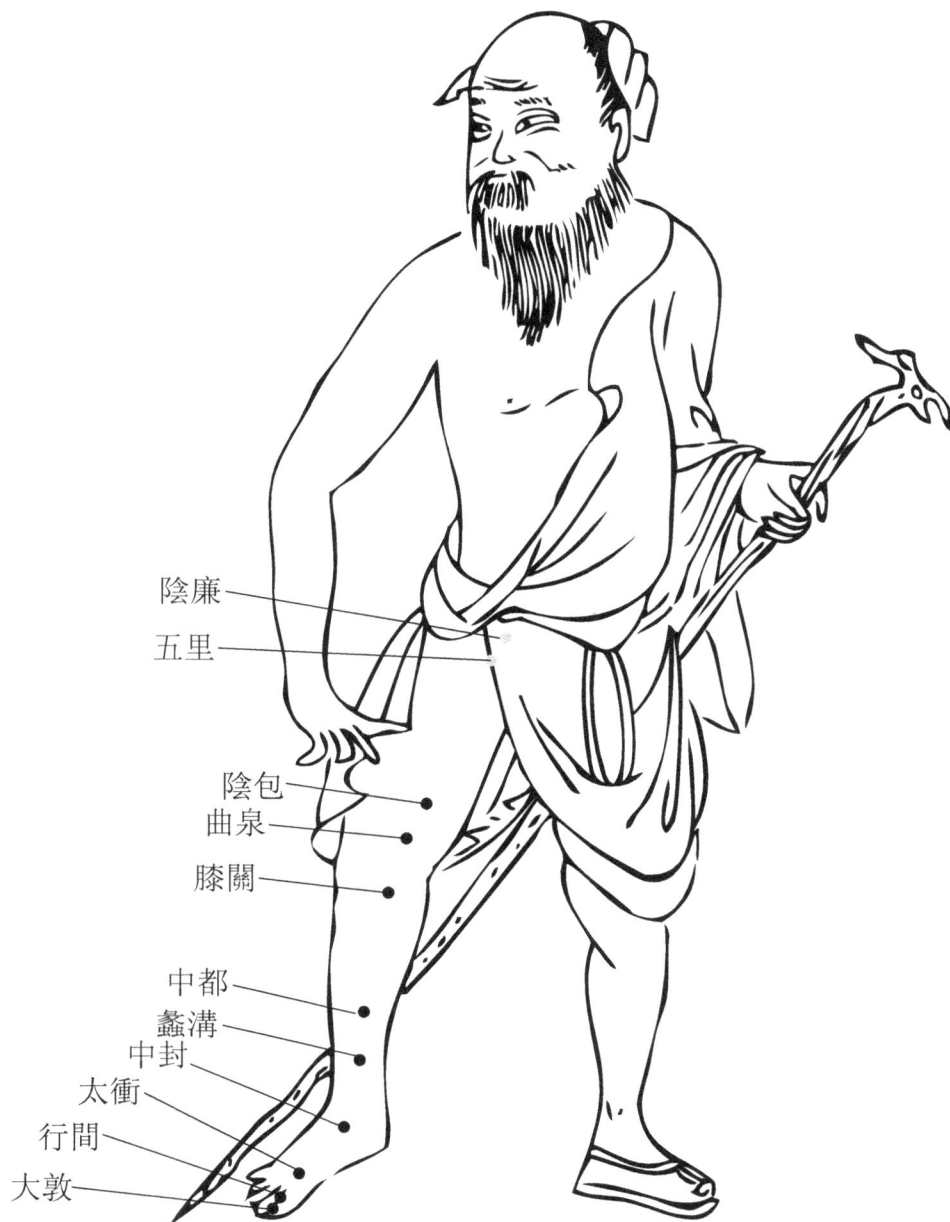

陰廉
五里
陰包
曲泉
膝關
中都
蠡溝
中封
太衝
行間
大敦

Fig. 1.36

---

106. The meaning of this phrase is obscure.

Xī Guān 膝關 (LV 7), bilateral point: It is located in the depression 2 cùn below Dú Bí 犢鼻 (ST 35).[107] Needle 4 fēn deep; burn five cones of moxibustion. (Dú Bí (ST 35) is on the foot yáng-míng.)

曲泉二穴，水也。在膝內輔骨下，大筋上小筋下陷中，屈膝取之。又云：正膝屈內外兩筋間宛宛中，又在膝曲橫紋頭。針六分，灸三壯。

Qū Quán 曲泉 (LV 8), bilateral point, water: It is located inferior to the medial aspect of the assisting bone of the knee [the region formed by medial epicondyle of the femur and medial condyle of the tibia], in the depression above the big sinew [semitendinosus tendon] and below the small sinew [the sartorius tendon]. Locate the point while flexing the knee. It also says: The point is located at the end of the transverse crease in the depression between the medial and lateral sinews while flexing the knee. Needle 6 fēn deep; burn three cones of moxibustion.

陰包（《明堂》作胞）二穴，在膝上四寸，股內廉兩筋間。針六分，灸三壯。《明》云：七壯。

Yīn Bāo 陰包 (LV 9) (Míng Táng 《明堂》 writes Bāo 胞), bilateral point: It is located 4 cùn above the knee, in the depression between two sinews on the medial aspect of the thigh. Needle 6 fēn deep; burn three cones of moxibustion. Míng 《明》 says: Seven cones.

五里二穴，在氣衝下三寸，陰股中動脈。灸五壯，針六分。治腸中滿，熱閉不得溺。氣衝在腹部第三行（陰廉穴，氣衝同。）

Wǔ Lǐ 五里 (LV 10), bilateral point: It is located 3 cùn below Qì Chōng 氣衝 (ST 30), on the pulsating vessel in the groin. Burn five cones of moxibustion; needle 6 fēn deep. It treats fullness in the intestines, heat blockage, and inability to urinate. Qì Chōng (ST 30) is located on the third line of the abdomen. (Yīn Lián 陰廉 (LV 11) and Qì Chōng (ST 30) are on the same [line].)

五里有二，其一在手陽明肘上三寸。其一在此，當為足五里也。

[Author's note:] There are two Wǔ Lǐ 五里: One is located on the hand yángmíng, 3 cùn above the elbow. Another is here, Zú [Foot] Wǔ Lǐ 足五里 (LV 10).

---

107. The stomach channel is on the lateral side of the leg, while the liver channel is on the medial side. So this must be an error.

陰廉二穴，在羊矢下，去氣衝二寸動脈中 。灸三壯，即有子，針八分，留七
呼 。

Yīn Lián 陰廉 (LV 11), bilateral point: It is located on the pulsating vessel, below Yáng Shǐ 羊矢
(LV 12); 2 cùn from Qì Chōng 氣衝 (ST 30). Someone can have children after applying three
cones of moxibustion. Needle 8 fēn deep; retain the needle for seven respirations.

1.32
Zú Shàoyáng Dǎn Jīng Zuǒ Yòu Èr Shí Bā Xué

足少陽膽經左右二十八穴

Foot Shàoyáng Gallbladder Channel,
28 bilateral points [fourteen on each side]

竅陰二穴，金也 。在足小指次指端，去爪甲如韭葉 。灸三壯，針一分 。

Qiào Yīn 竅陰 (GB 44), bilateral point, metal: It is located on the tip of the fourth toe, a leek leaf's
distance from the corner of the nail. Burn three cones of moxibustion; needle 1 fēn deep.

竅陰有二，其一在此，其一在側頭部。 此當為足竅陰也。

[Author's note:] There are two Qiào Yīn 竅陰: One is here; another is on the side of the head. This
is Zú [Foot] Qiào Yīn 足竅陰 (GB 44).

俠溪二穴，水也 。在足小指次指岐骨間，本節前陷中 。灸三壯，針三分 。《
明 》云：臨泣去俠溪寸半 。

Xiá Xī 俠溪 (GB 43), bilateral point, water: It is located between the junction of the bones of the
fourth toe [and little toe], in the depression anterior [distal] to the base joint. Burn three cones
of moxibustion; needle 3 fēn deep. *Míng* 《 明 》 says: Lín Qì 臨泣 (GB 41) is located 1.5 cùn
posterior [proximal] to Xiá Xī (GB 43).

地五會二穴，在足小指次指本節後陷中，去俠溪一寸。針一分，不可灸，灸使人羸瘦，不出三年卒。

Dì Wŭ Huì 地五會 (GB 42), bilateral point: It is located 1 cùn from Xiá Xī 俠溪 (GB 43), in the depression posterior [proximal] to the base joint of the fourth toe. Needle 1 fēn deep. Moxibustion is not recommended; it causes marked emaciation in a person and they will die in three years.

臨泣二穴，木也。在足小指次指本節後間陷中，去俠溪寸半。灸三壯，針二分。

Lín Qì 臨泣 (GB 41), bilateral point, wood: It is located in the depression posterior [proximal] to the base joint of the fourth toe, 1.5 cùn from Xiá Xī 俠溪 (GB 43). Burn three cones of moxibustion; needle 2 fēn deep.

偃伏第三行既有臨泣穴矣，此亦有臨泣穴。此當蓋足臨泣也。

[Author's note:] The chapter called Prone or Supine position; the third line [on the head] has Lín Qì 臨泣 (GB 15); it is also here, so this is Zú [Foot] Lín Qì 足臨泣 (GB 41).

丘墟二穴，在外踝下如前陷中，去臨泣三寸。灸三壯，針五分，留七呼。

Qiū Xū 丘墟 (GB 40), bilateral point: It is located inferior to the lateral malleolus, in the depression running anteriorly, 3 cùn from Lín Qì 臨泣 (GB 41). Burn three cones of moxibustion; needle 5 fēn deep; retain the needle for seven respirations.

懸鍾二穴，在足外踝上三寸動脈中。針六分，留七呼，灸五壯。《千》云：一名絕骨。（外踝上三寸，又云四寸。）

Xuán Zhōng 懸鍾 (GB 39), bilateral point: It is located 3 cùn above the lateral malleolus, on the pulsating vessel. Needle 6 fēn deep; retain the needle for seven respirations. Burn five cones of moxibustion. *Qiān*《千》 says: Another name is Jué Gŭ 絕骨 [meaning severed bone]. (It is 3 cùn above the lateral malleolus; it also says 4 cùn.)

陽輔二穴，火也。在外踝上四寸，輔骨前絕骨端如前三分，去丘墟七寸。灸三壯，針五分，留七呼。《千》云：外踝上輔骨前，餘同。

Yáng Fǔ 陽輔 (GB 38), bilateral point, fire: It is located 4 cùn above the lateral malleolus, running 3 fēn anterior to the assisting bone [fibula] and the tip of the severed bone [the region just superior to the lateral malleolus], 7 cùn from Qiū Xū 丘墟 (GB 40). Burn three cones of moxibustion; needle 5 fēn deep; retain the needle for seven respirations. *Qiān* 《千》 says: It is located above the lateral malleolus, anterior to the assisting bone [fibula]. The rest is the same.

光明二穴，在外踝上五寸。針六分，留七呼，灸五壯（《明下》云：七壯 ）。治腨疼不能久立，與陽輔療病同 。

Guāng Míng 光明 (GB 37), bilateral point: It is located 5 cùn above the lateral malleolus. Needle 6 fēn deep; retain the needle for seven respirations; burn five cones of moxibustion (*Míng Xià* 《明下》 says: seven cones). It treats pain of the lower leg and inability to stand for long. It treats the same diseases as Yáng Fǔ (GB 38).

外丘二穴，在外踝上七寸。針三分，灸三壯 。

Wài Qiū 外丘 (GB 36), bilateral point: It is located 7 cùn above the lateral malleolus. Needle 3 fēn deep; burn three cones of moxibustion.

陽交二穴，一名別陽 。在外踝上七寸，斜屬三陽分肉之間。灸三壯，針六分，留七呼 。《千》云：一名足髎，在外踝上七寸 。（一云：三寸。）

Yáng Jiāo 陽交 (GB 35), bilateral point, another name is Bié Yáng 別陽 (GB 35): It is located 7 cùn above the lateral malleolus on the muscle that runs obliquely

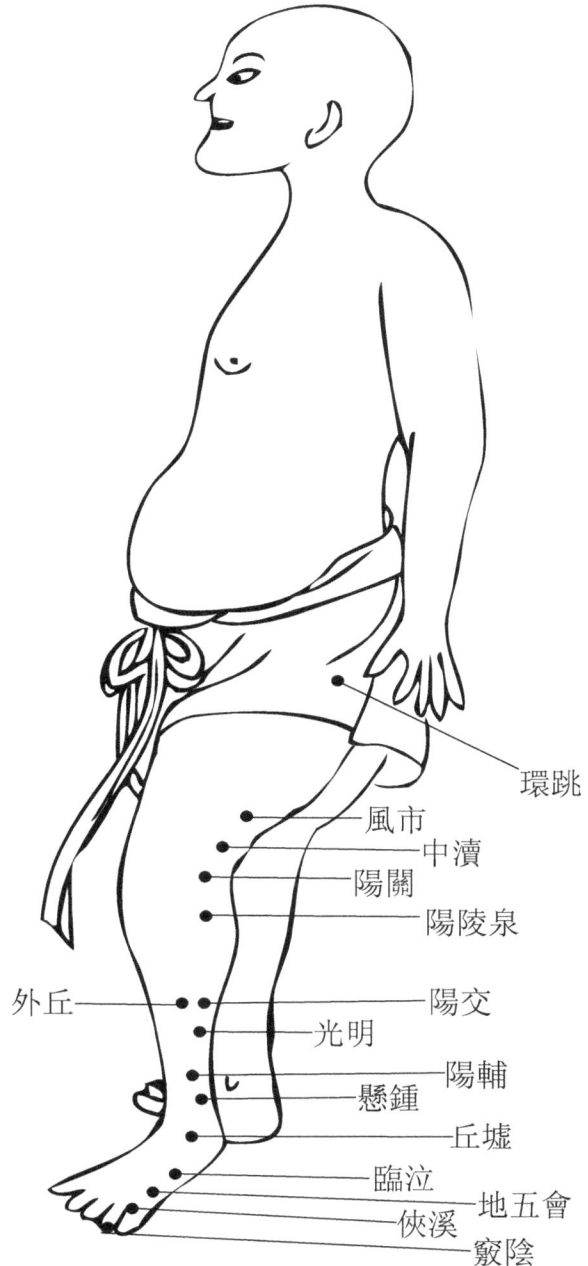

環跳
風市
中瀆
陽關
陽陵泉
外丘
陽交
光明
陽輔
懸鍾
丘墟
臨泣
地五會
俠溪
竅陰

Fig. 1.37

123

and homes to the three yáng [foot tàiyáng, shàoyáng and the yángmíng channels]. Burn three cones of moxibustion. Needle 6 fēn deep; retain the needle for seven respirations. *Qiān* 《千》 says: Another name is Zú Liáo 足窌; it is located 7 cùn above the lateral malleolus. (One source says: 3 cùn.)

陽陵泉二穴，土也。在膝下一寸外廉陷中。針六分，得氣即瀉，又宜久留針，灸七壯，至七七壯即止。《明下》云：一壯。《素注》：三壯。（《千》云：膝下外尖骨前。《難疏》：脛骨中微側少許。筋會陽陵泉，筋病治此。）

Yáng Líng Quán 陽陵泉 (GB 34), bilateral point, earth: It is located 1 cùn inferior to the knee, in the depression on the lateral aspect. Needle 6 fēn deep; drain [the point] as soon as qì arrives; retaining the needle for long time is also recommended. Burn seven cones of moxibustion, stop at seven times seven cones. *Míng Xià* 《明下》 says: One cone. *Sù Zhù* 《素注》 says: Three cones. (*Qiān* says: It is located below the knee, anterior to the lateral pointed bone [small head of fibula]. *Nàn Shū* 《難疏》 says: It is located slightly lateral to the tibia. It is the meeting [influential] point of the sinews. This point treats diseases of the sinews.

陽關二穴，在陽陵泉上二寸，犢鼻外陷中。針五分，不可灸。《千》云：關陽。（一云：關陵。）

Yáng Guān 陽關 (GB 33), bilateral point: It is located 2 cùn above Yáng Líng Quán (GB 34), in the depression lateral to Dú Bí 犢鼻 (ST 35). Needle 5 fēn deep. Moxibustion is contraindicated. *Qiān* calls it Guān Yáng 關陽. (One source says: Guān Líng 關陵.)

中瀆二穴，在髀骨外，膝上五寸分肉間陷中。灸五壯，針五分，留七呼。

Zhōng Dú 中瀆 (GB 32), bilateral point: It is located on the lateral aspect of the thigh bone [femur], 5 cùn above the knee, in the depression on the muscle. Burn five cones of moxibustion; needle 5 fēn deep, retain the needle for seven respirations.

環跳二穴，在髀樞中，側臥伸下足屈上足取之。灸五十壯，針一寸，留十呼，忌同。《明下》云：在硯子骨宛宛中，灸三壯。《甲乙》云：五壯。

Huán Tiào 環跳 (GB 30), bilateral point: It is located on the hip joint. Locate the point with the patient lying on his side, extending the lower leg and bending the upper leg. Burn fifty cones of moxibustion; needle 1 cùn deep, retain the needle for ten respirations. Follow the same contraindications [as Shào Shāng 少商 (LU 11)]. *Míng Xià* says: In the depression on the femur. Burn three cones of moxibustion. *Jiǎ Yǐ* 《甲乙》 says: Five cones.

風市二穴，在膝外兩筋間，立舒下兩手著腿，當中指頭陷中。療冷痹，腳脛麻，腿膝酸痛，腰重起坐難（《明下》）。

Fēng Shì 風市 (GB 31), bilateral point: It is located on the lateral aspect above the knee, between the two sinews. Ask the patient to relax his arms and touch his legs while standing. The point is in the depression under the tip of the middle finger. It treats cold *bì*-impediment, numbness of the feet and lower legs, aching pain of the legs and knees, and heaviness of the lower back with difficulty standing or sitting. (*Míng Xià* 《明下》).

予冬月當風市處多冷痹，急擦熱手溫之略止，日或兩三。痹偶謬刺以溫針遂愈，信乎能治冷痹也（亦屢灸此）。不特治冷痹，亦治風之要穴（見《明堂》）。《銅人》乃不載，豈名或不同將其本不全耶？

[Author's note:] I always had cold *bì*-impediment in the Fēng Shì (GB 31) area during the winter. It would get a little bit better after I rubbed my hands together to heat them up and quickly warmed this area. I did this two or three times a day. For *bì*-impediment, I applied the cross needling method[108] using warm needle on it and this cured the disease. You can believe that it will treat cold *bì*-impediment (also applying moxibustion on it frequently). This point is not only used to treat cold *bì*-impediment, but is also the main point to treat wind (see *Míng Táng* 《明堂》). *Tóng Rén* 《銅人》 has no record of this point. Could this be because the name is different or the edition [of the book] is not intact?

---

108. *Miu cì* 謬刺, also named as *mìu cì* 繆刺 (cross needling method), is one of nine needling methods in ancient times. It treats diseases on left side by puncturing the network vessels on the right side and vice versa.

1.33

Zú Tàiyīn Pí Jīng Zuǒ Yòu Èr Shí Èr Xué

足太陰脾經左右二十二穴

Foot Tàiyīn Spleen Channel, 22 bilateral points [eleven on each side]

隱白二穴，木也。在足大指端內側，去爪甲角如韭葉宛宛中。針三分。今附：婦人月事過時不止，刺立愈。《明》云：針一分，留三呼，灸三壯。

Yǐn Bái 隱白 (SP 1), bilateral point, wood: It is located on the medial aspect of the big toe, in the depression that is a leek leaf's distance from the corner of the nail. Needle 3 fēn deep. Appended here: For women with delayed menstruation and incessant bleeding, puncturing this point can cure the disease immediately. *Míng* 《明》says: Needle 1 fēn deep; retain the needle for three respirations. Burn three cones of moxibustion.

大都二穴，火也。在足大指本節後陷中。灸三壯，針三分。《千》注：本節內側白肉際。

Dà Dū 大都 (SP 2), bilateral point, fire: It is located in the depression posterior [proximal] to the base joint of the big toe. Burn three cones of moxibustion; needle 3 fēn deep. A note in *Qiān* 《千》says: On the border of the white flesh on the medial aspect of the base joint of the big toe.

太白二穴，土也。在足內側核骨下陷中。灸三壯，針三分。《千》云：足大指內側。

Tài Bái 太白 (SP 3), bilateral point, earth: It is located on the medial aspect of the big toe, in the depression inferior to the node bone [first metatarsophalangeal joint]. Burn three cones of moxibustion; needle 3 fēn deep. *Qiān* says: On the medial aspect of the big toe.

公孫二穴，在足大指本節後一寸。灸三壯，針四分。

Gōng Sūn 公孫 (SP 4), bilateral point: It is located 1 cùn posterior [proximal] to the base joint of the big toe, anterior to the medial malleolus. Burn three cones of moxibustion; needle 4 fēn deep.

商丘二穴，金也 。在內踝下微前陷中 。灸三壯，針三分 。

Shāng Qiū 商丘 (SP 5), bilateral point, metal: It is located in the depression inferior and slightly anterior to the medial malleolus. Burn three cones of moxibustion; needle 3 fēn deep.

三陰交二穴，在內踝上三寸，骨下陷中（《明》云：內踝上八寸陷中 ）。灸三壯，針三分 。昔宋太子善醫朮，出苑逢一妊婦，太子診曰女 。令徐文伯診，曰一男一女 。針之，瀉三陰交補合谷，應針而落，果如文伯言 。故妊娠不可刺 。《千》云：內踝上八寸骨下（ 又云：內踝上三寸 ）。

Sān Yīn Jiāo 三陰交 (SP 6), bilateral point: It is located 3 cùn above the medial malleolus, in the depression below the [shin] bone (*Míng*《明》 says: It is 8 cùn above the medial malleolus). Burn three cones of moxibustion; needle 3 fēn deep. In the past, a prince of the *Sòng* Dynasty was good at medicine. He encountered a pregnant woman on his way while hunting. He checked and predicted she would have a girl. He asked Xú Wénbó to confirm his diagnosis. Xú said she would have a girl and a boy [twins]. They needled the woman, draining Sān Yīn Jiāo (SP 6) and supplementing Hé Gǔ 合谷 (LI 4). She responded to the needles and miscarried. [The outcome] was just as Xú Wénbó said. So needling [Sān Yīn Jiāo (SP 6)] is contraindicated during pregnancy. *Qiān*《千》 says: It is 8 cùn above the medial malleolus, in the depression below the [shin] bone (It also said: 3 cùn above the medial malleolus).

漏谷二穴，亦名太陰絡 。在內踝上六寸骨下陷中 。針三分 。《明下》云：灸三壯 。

Lòu Gǔ 漏谷 (SP 7), bilateral point, also named Tài Yīn Luò 太陰絡: It is located 6 cùn above the medial malleolus, in the depression below the [shin] bone. Needle 3 fēn deep. *Míng Xià*《明下》 says: Burn three cones of moxibustion.

地機二穴，亦名脾舍，足太陰郄 。別走上一寸空，在膝下五寸 。灸三壯，針三分 。《明》云：膝內側轉骨下陷中，伸足取之 。

Dì Jī 地機 (SP 8), bilateral point, also named Pí Shè 脾舍; it is the *xī*-cleft point of foot tàiyīn: It is located in the 1 cùn-sized depression 5 cùn below the knee. Burn three cones of moxibustion; needle 3 fēn deep. *Míng* says: It is in the depression below the turning bone [medial condyle of the tibia][109] on the medial aspect of the knee. Locate the point while extending the leg.

---

109. *Zhuàn gǔ* 轉骨 (turning bone) may be a typographical error for *fǔ gǔ* 輔骨 (assisting bone), the region formed by the epicondyle of the femur and the condyle of the tibia.

陰陵泉二穴，水也 。在膝下內側輔骨下陷中，伸足取之 。針五分，當曲膝取
之 。

Yīn Líng Quán 陰陵泉 (SP 9), bilateral point, water. It is located below the knee, in the depression inferior to the medial assisting bone of the knee [the region formed by medial epicondyle of the femur and medial condyle of the tibia]. Locate the point while extending the leg. Needle 5 fēn deep. Locate the point right at the bend of the knee.

血海二穴，在膝臏上內廉白肉際
二寸中 。灸三壯，針五分 。《
千 》云：白肉際二寸半 。注云：
一作三寸 。

Xuè Hǎi 血海 (SP 10), bilateral point: It is located 2 cùn above the medial aspect of the patella, on the border of the white flesh. Burn three cones of moxibustion; needle 5 fēn deep. *Qiān* 《 千 》 says: It is 2.5 cùn [above the medial aspect of the patella], on the border of the white flesh. A note [to *Qiān*] says: 3 cùn.

箕門二穴，在魚腹上越筋間動脈
應手，在陰股內 。一云：上起筋
間 。灸三壯 。

Jī Mén 箕門 (SP 11), bilateral point: It is located in the groin, on the fish belly [muscle in the groin region], in [the depression] between the jumping sinews [sartorius tendon]. There is a pulsating vessel that responds to the hand. Another source says: In [the depression] between the rising sinews. Burn three cones of moxibustion.

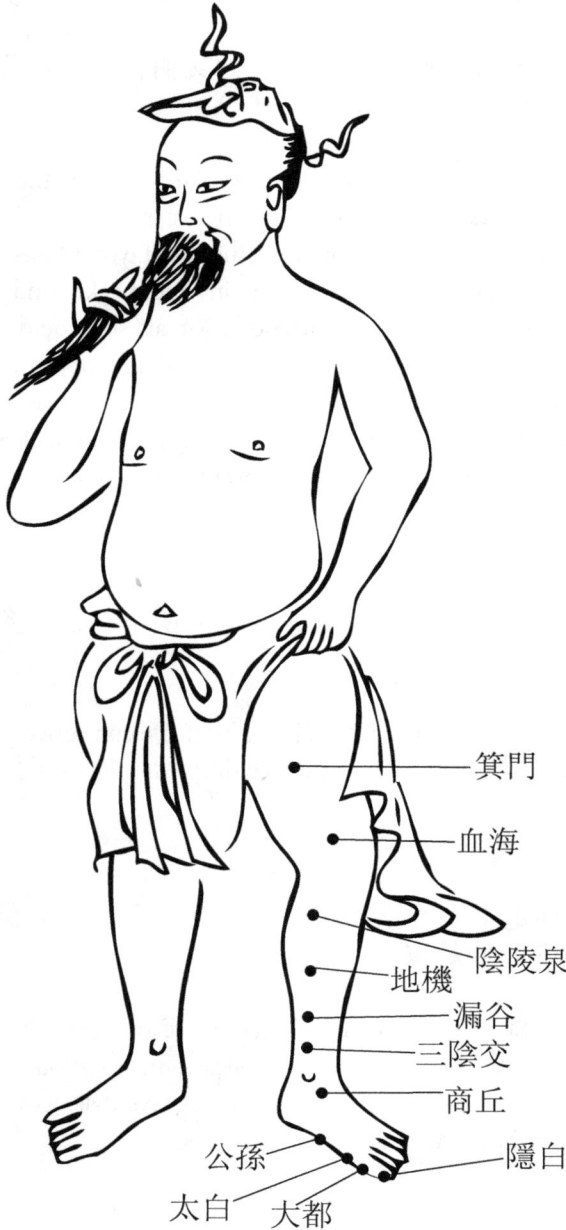

箕門
血海
陰陵泉
地機
漏谷
三陰交
商丘
公孫　　隱白
太白　大都

Fig. 1.38

128

1.34
Zú Yángmíng Wèi Jīng Zuǒ Yòu Sān Shí Xué

足陽明胃經左右三十穴

Foot Yángmíng Stomach Channel,
30 bilateral points [fifteen on each side]

厲兌二穴，金也。在足大指次指端去爪甲如韭葉。針一分，灸一壯。

Lì Duì 厲兌 (ST 45), bilateral point, metal: It is located at the tip of the second toe, a leek leaf's distance from the corner of the nail. Needle 1 fēn deep; burn one cone of moxibustion.

內庭二穴，水也。在足大指次指外間陷中。灸三壯，針三分。

Nèi Tíng 內庭 (ST 44), bilateral point, water: It is located in the depression lateral to the second toe. Burn three cones of moxibustion; needle 3 fēn deep.

陷谷二穴，木也。在足大指次指外間本節後陷中，去內庭二寸。針三分，留七呼，灸三壯。

Xiàn Gǔ 陷谷 (ST 43), bilateral point, wood: It is located on the lateral aspect of the second toe, in the depression posterior [proximal] to the base joint, 2 cùn from Nèi Tíng (ST 44). Needle 3 fēn deep; retain the needle for seven respirations. Burn three cones of moxibustion.

衝陽二穴，在足跗上去陷谷三寸。針五分，灸三壯。《素注》：跗上五寸骨間動脈，刺三分。《千》云：跗上五寸骨間，去陷谷三寸（一云：二寸）。

Chōng Yáng 衝陽 (ST 42), bilateral point: It is located on the dorsal aspect of the foot, 3 cùn from Xiàn Gǔ (ST 43). Needle 5 fēn deep; burn three cones of moxibustion. *Sù Zhù* 《素注》 says: On the dorsal aspect of the foot, 5 cùn [proximal to the toes], on the pulsating vessel between the bones. Needle 3 fēn deep. *Qiān* 《千》 says: On the dorsal aspect of the foot, 5 cùn [proximal to the toes], between the bones, 3 cùn from Xiàn Gǔ (ST 43). (One source says: 2 cùn)

解溪二穴，火也。在衝陽後寸半腕上陷中。《明下》云：在繫鞋處。針五分，灸三壯。《素注》：在衝陽後二寸半。《新校正》云：刺瘧注作三寸半，二注不同，當從《甲乙經》作寸半。

Jiě Xī 解溪 (ST 41), bilateral point, fire: It is located 1.5 cùn posterior [proximal] to Chōng Yáng 衝陽 (ST 42), in the depression on the ankle. *Míng Xià* 《明下》 says: [It is on the ankle] where the shoe laces are tied. Needle 5 fēn deep; burn three cones of moxibustion. *Sù Zhù* 《素注》 says: It is 2.5 cùn posterior to Chōng Yáng (ST 42). *Xīn Jiào Zhèng* 《新校正》 says: The Annotation to *Cì Nüè* 刺瘧 (Treatise on Needling Malaria)[110] says: 3.5 cùn. So the two annotations are different. We should follow the 1.5 cùn in *Jiǎ Yǐ Jīng* 《甲乙經》.

豐隆二穴，在外踝上八寸，下廉胻外廉陷中。針三分，灸三壯。《明下》云：七壯。

Fēng Lóng 豐隆 (ST 40), bilateral point: It is located 8 cùn above the lateral malleolus, in the depression lateral to the shin bone and lateral to Xià Lián 下廉 (ST 39). Needle 3 fēn deep; burn three cones of moxibustion. *Míng Xià* says: Seven cones.

下廉二穴，一名下巨虛，在上廉下三寸，當舉足取穴。針八分，灸三壯。《明》云：上廉下三寸，兩筋兩骨罅陷宛宛中，蹲地坐取之。針六分，得氣即瀉。《甲乙》云：針三分，灸三壯。主小腸氣不足，面無顏色，偏風熱風，冷痹不遂，風濕痹。灸亦良，日七七壯。《素注》：足陽明與小腸合，在上廉下三寸。針三分。

Xià Lián (ST 39), bilateral point, another name is Xià Jù Xū 下巨虛: It is located 3 cùn below Shàng Lián 上廉 (ST 37). The point is located while extending the foot upward [dorsal flexion]. Needle 8 fēn deep; burn three cones of moxibustion. *Míng* 《明》 says: It is 3 cùn below Shàng Lián (ST 37), in the depression in the cleft of the bone between two sinews. Locate the point in squatting position. Needle 6 fēn deep, drain [the point] as soon as qì arrives.

Jiǎ Yǐ says: Needle 3 fēn deep; burn three cones of moxibustion. It governs insufficient qì of the small intestine, pale facial complexion, hemilateral wind, hot wind, cold *bì*-impediment, paralysis, and wind-damp *bì*-impediment. Moxibustion also is good, burn seven times seven cones of moxibustion.

Sù Zhù 《素注》 says: It is the meeting point of the foot yángmíng and the small intestine [channels], and is located 3 cùn below Shàng Lián 上廉 (ST 37). Needle 3 fēn deep.

---

110. *Cì Nüè* 刺瘧 refers to *Sù Wèn* 《素問》 (Plain Questions), Chapter 36.

手陽明亦有下廉，此乃足下廉也。

[Author's note:] The hand yángmíng also has a Xià Lián 下廉 (LI 8); this is Zú [Foot] Xià Lián 足下廉 (ST 39).

條口二穴，在下廉上一寸，舉足取之。針五分。《明》云：在上廉下一寸，針八分，灸三壯。

Tiáo Kǒu 條口 (ST 38), bilateral point: It is located 1 cùn above Xià Lián (ST 39). Locate the point while lifting the foot upward [dorsal flexion]. Needle 5 fēn deep. *Míng* 《明》 says: It is 1 cùn below Shàng Lián (ST 37). Needle 8 fēn deep; burn three cones of moxibustion.

上廉二穴，一名上巨虛。在三里下三寸，當舉足取之。灸三壯，針三分。甄權云：治藏氣不足，偏風腰腿手足不仁。灸隨年為壯。《明》云：巨虛上廉在三里下三寸，兩筋兩骨罅陷宛宛中。針八分，得氣即瀉，灸大良，日七壯。《下》云：三壯。《素注》：在三里下三寸。又云：在膝犢鼻下胻外廉六寸。

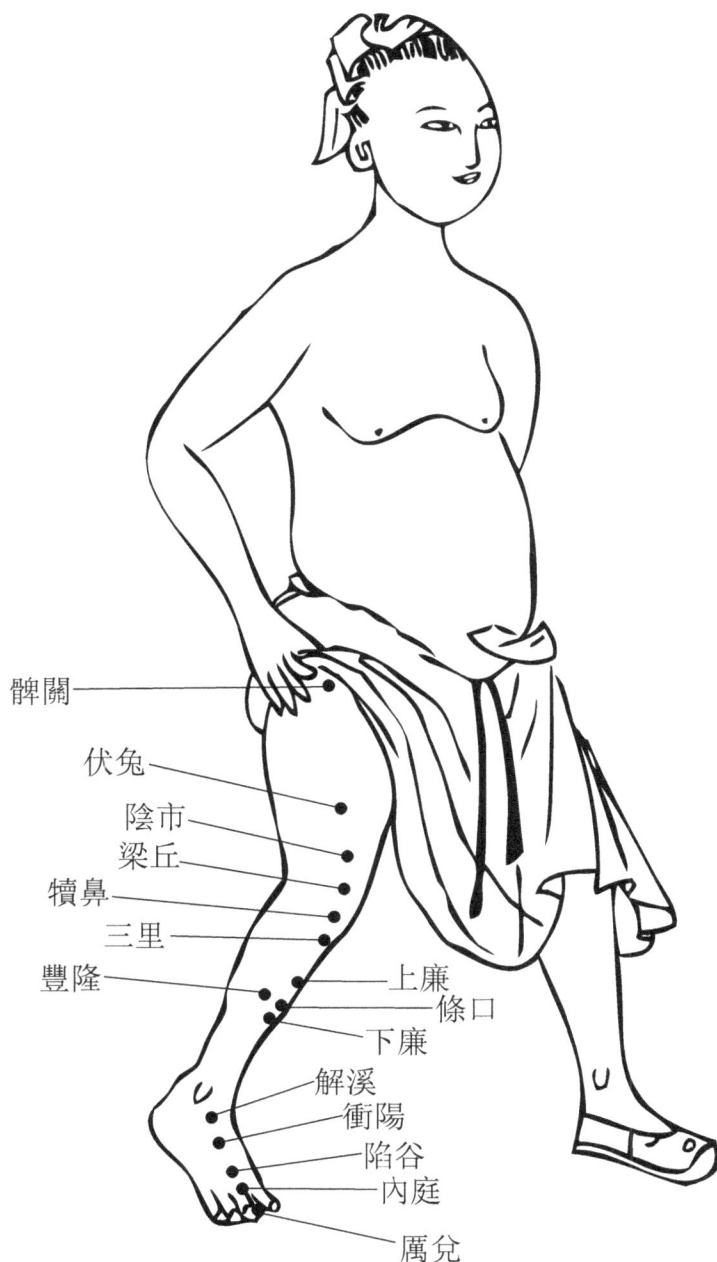

髀關

伏兔

陰市

梁丘

犢鼻

三里

豐隆

上廉

條口

下廉

解溪

衝陽

陷谷

內庭

厲兌

Fig. 1.39

131

Shàng Lián 上廉 (ST 37), bilateral point, another name is Shàng Jù Xū 上巨虛: It is located 3 cùn below Sān Lǐ 三里 (ST 36). Locate the point while extending the foot upward [dorsal flexion]. Burn three cones of moxibustion; needle 3 fēn deep. Zhēn Quán said: It treats insufficient visceral qì, hemilateral wind, and numbness of the lower back, hands and feet. Burn the same number of cones as the age of the patient. *Míng* says: Jù Xū Shàng Lián 巨虛上廉 (ST 37) is located 3 cùn below Sān Lǐ (ST 36), in the depression in the cleft of the two bones, between two sinews. Needle 8 fēn deep, drain [the point] as soon as qì arrives. Moxibustion also is good, burn seven cones of moxibustion daily. *Xià* 《下》 says: Three cones. *Sù Zhù* says: It is 3 cùn below Sān Lǐ (ST 36). It also says: On the lateral aspect of the shin bone, 6 cùn below Dú Bí 犢鼻 (ST 35), which is on the knee.

手陽明亦有上廉。　此乃足上廉也。

[Author's note:] The hand yángmíng also has a Shàng Lián 上廉 (LI 9); this is Zú [Foot] Shàng Lián 足上廉 (ST 37).

三里二穴，土也。在膝下三寸外廉兩筋間（一云：胻骨外大筋內），當舉足取之。秦承祖云：諸病皆治，食氣，水氣，蟲毒，痃癖，四肢腫滿，膝胻酸痛，目不明。華佗云：療五勞羸瘦，七傷虛乏，胸中瘀血，乳癰。

Sān Lǐ 三里 (ST 36), bilateral point, earth: It is located 3 cùn below the knee, in the depression between two sinews; on the lateral aspect [of the lower leg]. (One source says: medial to the big sinew and lateral to the shin bone.) Locate the point while extending the foot upward [dorsal flexion]. Qín Chéngzǔ[111] said: It can treat all diseases: consuming qì,[112] water qì, gǔ-toxins,[113] strings and aggregations (*xuán pì* 痃癖),[114] swelling of the limbs, aching pain of the knees and lower legs, and blurred vision. Huá Tuó said: It treats marked emaciation from the five taxations, vacuity from the seven damages, blood stasis in the chest, and mammary welling-abscess [acute mastitis].

---

111. Qín Chéngzǔ 秦承祖 was a famous doctor during the *Nán Běi Cháo* 南北朝 Southern and Northern Dynasties.

112. *Shì qì* 食氣 (consuming qì) is a Daoist ascetic practice. The practitioner chooses specific times of day to consume the clear qì of air through breathing techniques in order to reduce the consumption of food and get rid of turbid or evil qì inside the body. However, in the context of this sentence, it must be the name of a condition.

113. *Gǔ* 蠱 is a type of toxin that is said to be from various insects and reptiles (*chóng* 蟲). It affects the liver and spleen and can result in drum distention.

114. *Xuán pì* 痃癖 (strings and aggregations) are two kinds of abdominal masses, usually caused by cold phlegm accumulation with binding of qì and blood.

《外臺‧明堂》云：人年三十已上，若不灸三里，令氣上衝目，所以三里下氣也（《明》同）。灸三壯，針五分。《明》云：針腹背，每須去三里穴，針八分，留十呼，瀉七吸，日灸七壯，止百壯。《素注》：刺一寸。在膝下三寸胻骨外廉兩筋肉分間（《指》云：深則足趺陽脈不見。《集》云：按之太衝脈不動。）

Wài Tái ‧ *Míng Táng* 《外臺‧明堂》 says: When people are over the age of thirty, if they do not apply moxibustion on Sān Lǐ 三里 (ST 36), the qì surges upward into the eyes; Sān Lǐ (ST 36) can descend the qì (*Míng* 《明》 agrees). Burn three cones of moxibustion; needle 5 fēn deep. *Míng* says: When needling the abdomen and back, one should [also] go to [needle] Sān Lǐ (ST 36). Needle 8 fēn deep, retain the needle for ten respirations; drain for seven respirations. Burn seven cones moxibustion daily, stop at a hundred cones.

Sù Zhù 《素注》 says: Needle 1 cùn deep. It is located 3 cùn below the knee, on the lateral aspect of the shin bone, in the depression between two sinews and muscles. (*Zhǐ* 《指》 says: The *fū yáng* pulse[115] disappears [when Sān Lǐ (ST 36) is pressed] deeply. *Jí* 《集》 says: The *tài chōng* pulse stops when Sān Lǐ (ST 36) is pressed.)

手有三里，此亦曰三里，蓋足三里也。《銅人》云：在膝下三寸，《明堂》、《素問》注皆同。人多不能求其穴，每以大拇指次指圈其膝蓋，以中指住處為穴，或以最小指住處為穴。皆不得真穴所在也。予按《明堂》有膝眼四穴，蓋在膝頭骨下兩旁陷中也。又按《銅人》等經有犢鼻穴，蓋在膝髕下胻俠罅大筋中也。又按《銅人》有膝關二穴，蓋在犢鼻下二寸陷中也。而《新校正》、《素問》注巨虛上廉云：三里在犢鼻下三寸，則是犢鼻之下三寸方是三里，不可便從膝頭下去三寸為三里穴也。若如今人之取穴，恐失之太高矣。（《千》云：灸至五百壯，少亦一二百壯。）

[Author's note:] There is a Sān Lǐ 三里 (LI 10) on the hand which is also named Sān Lǐ. This is Zú [Foot] Sān Lǐ 足三里 (ST 36). *Tóng Rén* 《銅人》 says: It is located 3 cùn below the knee. This is the same as in *Míng Táng* 《明堂》 and the Annotation of *Sù Wèn* 《素問》. Most people cannot find the point. They all circle the knee cap with their thumb and index finger, and then locate the point under the tip of the middle finger or the little finger. But none of them can figure out exactly where the point is. I follow *Míng Táng*: Xī Yǎn 膝眼 [extra point] has four points [two on each side] which are located below the patella in the depressions on the sides [of the patellar ligament]. In *Tóng Rén*, there is also Dú Bí 犢鼻 (ST 35). It is located below the patella, on the big sinew, in the cleft between [the knee and] the shin bone. In *Tóng Rén*, there is also the bilateral point, Xī Guān 膝關 (LV 7), which is located in the depression 2 cùn below Dú Bí (ST

115. The *fū yáng* pulse refers to the pulsating vessel in the Chōng Yáng 衝陽 (ST 42) area. This point is located on the dorsum of the foot.

35). But in *Xīn Jiào Zhèng*《新校正》and the Annotation of *Sù Wèn*, it says [under the entry for] Jù Xū Shàng Lián 巨虛上廉 (ST 37): Sān Lǐ (ST 36) is located 3 cùn below Dú Bí (ST 35). That means the place 3 cùn below Dú Bí (ST 35) is Sān Lǐ (ST 36). So Sān Lǐ (ST 36) cannot be located at the place 3 cùn below the patella. The way people locate the point it today is too high. (*Qiān*《千》says: Burn up to five hundred cones of moxibustion, or a minimum of one to two hundred cones.)

犢鼻二穴，在膝臏下骱俠解（《明堂》作䐐）大筋中。治膝中痛不仁，難跪起。膝髕腫潰者不可治，不潰者可療。若犢鼻堅硬，勿便攻，先以洗熨，即微刺之愈。《明》云：針三分，灸三壯。

Dú Bí 犢鼻 (ST 35), bilateral point: It is located below the patella, on the big sinew in the depression between [the knee and] the shin bone. (*Míng Táng*《明堂》says: *xià* 䐐 (cleft).) It treats pain in the knee with numbness, and inability to kneel down and get up. It is not treatable if the patella is swollen and ulcerated; but it is treatable if there is no ulceration. If Dú Bí (ST 35) is very hard, do not attack [drain]. It can first be washed with the application of hot medicinal compresses, then needle gently. This will cure [the disease]. *Míng*《明》says: Needle 3 fēn deep; burn three cones of moxibustion.

按《素問·刺禁》云：刺膝髕出液為跛。犢鼻在膝髕下骱，用針者不可輕也。

[Author's note:] Note that *Sù Wèn · Cì Jìn*《素問·刺禁》says: The patient will become limp if the patella is punctured and fluid comes out. Dú Bí 犢鼻 (ST 35) is located below the patella, on the shin bone. The acupuncturist must not disparage this.

梁丘二穴，在膝上二寸（《明》云：三寸），兩筋間。灸三壯，針三分。《明》云：五分。

Liáng Qiū 梁丘 (ST 34), bilateral point: It is located 2 cùn above the knee (*Míng* says: 3 cùn), in the depression between two sinews. Burn three cones of moxibustion; needle 3 fēn deep. *Míng* says: 5 fēn.

《明堂》作三寸，《銅人》、《千金》皆作二寸，《千金》注謂或云三寸，姑兩存之。

[Author's note:] *Míng Táng*《明堂》says 3 cùn; *Tóng Rén*《銅人》and *Qiān Jīn*《千金》both say 2 cùn. A note to *Qiān Jīn* says: it might be 3 cùn. So I put both here.

陰市二穴，一名陰鼎，在膝上三寸，伏兔下陷中，拜而取之 。針三分，不可
灸 。《 明下 》云：灸三壯 。《 千 》注二十卷云：在膝上，當伏兔下行二寸，
臨膝取之 。（ 又云：膝內輔骨後，大筋下小筋上，屈膝得之 ）。

Yīn Shì 陰市 (ST 33), bilateral point, another name is Yīn Dǐng 陰鼎: It is located 3 cùn above
the knee, in the depression below Fú Tù 伏兔 (ST 32). Locate the point while kneeling. Needle 3
fēn deep; moxibustion is contraindicated. *Míng Xià* 《 明下 》 says: Burn three cones of moxibustion. The annotation of *Qiān* 《 千 》 in Volume 20[116] says: It is located above the knee, 2 cùn
below Fú Tù (ST 32). Locate the point close to the knee. (It also says: It is located posterior to the
medial assisting bone [the region formed by medial epicondyle of the femur and medial condyle of
the tibia], below the big sinew and above the small sinew. Locate the point with the knee flexed.)

《 銅人 》云：不可灸， 《 明堂 》乃云：灸三壯，豈以禁穴許灸一壯至
三壯耶？

[Author's notes:] *Tóng Rén* says: Moxibustion is not recommended. *Míng Táng* says: Burn three
cones of moxibustion. This might be [the theory of being able to] apply one to three cones of moxibustion on points that are contraindicated.

伏兔二穴，在膝上六寸，起肉正跪坐取之 。一云：膝蓋上七寸 。針五分，不
可灸 。《 明 》云：婦人八部諸病，通針三分 。

Fú Tù (ST 32), bilateral point: It is located 6 cùn above the knee, on the fleshy protuberance.
Locate the point when kneeling or sitting upright. One source says: 7 cùn above the knee. Needle 5
fēn deep; moxibustion is not appropriate. *Míng* 《 明 》 says: Needle 3 fēn deep in general for the
various female diseases.

髀關二穴，在膝上伏兔後交分中 。針六分 。《 明 》云：灸三壯 。

Bì Guān 髀關 (ST 31), bilateral point: It is located above the knee, in the convergence of muscles
posterior to Fú Tù (ST 32). Needle 6 fēn deep. *Míng* says: Burn three cones of moxibustion.

膝眼四穴，在膝頭骨下兩旁陷中 。主膝冷疼不已 。針五分，留三呼，瀉五
吸，禁灸 。（ 有人膝腫甚，人為灸此穴，遂致不救。蓋犯其所禁也。
）

---

116. The following quotation is actually from Volume 21.

Xī Yǎn 膝眼, four points [two on each side]: They are located below the patella, in the depression on the sides [of the patellar ligament]. They govern persistent cold pain in the knees. Needle 5 fēn deep, retain the needle for three respirations; drain for five respirations. Moxibustion is contraindicated. (Once when a patient suffered severe swelling of the knees, someone applied moxibustion on these points. The patient died. It might be because they offended the contraindication [for moxibustion of this point].)

《銅人》無此四穴，《明堂》有之，故附入於此。

[Author's note:] *Tóng Rén*《銅人》does not have these four points, but *Míng Táng*《明堂》 does, so it is appended here.

1.35
Zú Shàoyīn Shèn Jīng Zuǒ Yòu Èr Shí Xué

足少陰腎經左右二十穴

Foot Shàoyīn Kidney Channel,
20 bilateral points [ten on each side]

涌泉二穴，木也，一名地衝。在足心陷中，屈足捲指宛宛中。灸三壯，針五分，無令出血。淳於意云：漢北齊王阿母患足下熱，喘滿。謂曰熱厥也。當刺足心立愈。

Yǒng Quán 涌泉 (KI 1), bilateral point, wood; another name is Dì Chōng 地衝: It is located in the center of the sole. Locate the point in the depression while clenching the toes and bending the foot [plantar flexion]. Burn three cones of moxibustion; needle 5 fēn deep; it is not appropriate to bleed it. Chúnyú Yì[117] said: The wet nurse of King Běi Qí[118] of the *Hàn* Dynasty suffered a feeling of heat below her feet, with panting and fullness. It was called heat reversal and was cured right after puncturing the center of the sole.

---

117. Chúnyú Yì 淳於意 (205-150 B.C) was a famous doctor during the Western *Hàn* (西漢) Dynasty.
118. King Běi Qí 北齊王 of the *Hàn* Dynasty probably refers to King Jì Běi 濟北王.

《明》云：灸不及針，若灸廢人行動 。《下》云：在腳心底宛中白肉際 。灸三壯 。《素注》：刺三分 。《千》注：肝藏卷云在腳心大指下大筋 。（《史記》濟北王阿母足熱而懣，淳於意曰熱厥也 。刺足心各三所 。案之無出血，病巳 。病得之飲酒大醉 。）

Míng 《 明 》 says: Moxibustion is not as good as needling. Moxibustion will disable a person's movement [paralysis]. *Xià* 《 下 》 says: It is located in the center of the sole, in the depression on the border of the white flesh. Burn three cones of moxibustion. *Sù Zhù* 《 素注 》 says: Needle 3 fēn deep. A note to *Qián* 《 千 》 says: The volume on the liver says: It is located in the center of the sole, on the big sinew below the big toe. (*Shǐ Jì* 《 史記 》 (The Records of the Grand Historian) says: The wet nurse of King Jì Běi suffered hot feet and oppression. *Chúnyú Yì* said it was heat reversal. He pricked three places on the center of the sole. According to the record, there was no blood-letting, but the disease was cured. The disease was caused by severe drunkenness.)

然谷二穴，火也，一名龍淵 。在內踝前起大骨下陷中 。灸三壯，針三分，不宜見血 。《素注》：刺三分，刺此多見血，令人立飢飲食 。《千》注：《婦人方》云：在內踝前直下一寸 。

Rán Gǔ 然谷 (KI 2), bilateral point, fire; another name is *Lóng Yuān* 龍淵: It is located anterior to the medial malleolus, in the depression below the protuberance of the big bone [navicular bone]. Burn three cones of moxibustion; needle 3 fēn deep; it is not appropriate to bleed it. *Sù Zhù* 《 素注 》 says: Needle 3 fēn deep. If you prick it and let a lot of blood, it immediately makes people hungry for drink and food. A note to *Qián* 《 千 》 says: *Fù Rén Fāng* 《 婦人方 》 (Formulas for Women)[119] says: It is 1 cùn directly below the medial malleolus.

太溪二穴，土也 。在內踝後跟骨上動脈陷中 。灸三壯，針三分 。

Tài Xī 太溪 (KI 3), bilateral point, earth: It is located posterior to the medial malleolus, in the depression on the heel bone where there is a pulsating vessel. Burn three cones of moxibustion; needle 3 fēn deep.

大鍾二穴，在足跟後衝中 。灸三壯，針二分，留七呼 。

Dà Zhōng 大鍾 (KI 4), bilateral point: It is located on the posterior flat area of the heel. Burn three cones of moxibustion; needle 2 fēn deep; retain the needle for seven respirations.

---

119. *Fù Rén Fāng* 婦人方 (Formulas for Women) refers to Volume 2 of *Qīan Jīn Yào Fāng* 《 千金要方 》 (Prescriptions Worth a Thousand Pieces of Gold).

水泉二穴，去太溪下一寸，在內踝下 。灸五壯，針四分 。

Shuǐ Quán 水泉 (KI 5), bilateral point: It is located one cùn below Tài Xī (KI 3), inferior to the medial malleolus. Burn five cones of moxibustion; needle 4 fēn deep.

照海二穴，陰蹻脈所生 。在內踝下 。針三分，灸七壯 。（《千》云：在內踝下四分 。）《明上》云：陰蹻二穴，在內踝下陷宛中 。針三分，灸三壯 。《下》云：陰蹻二穴，在內踝下陷中 。灸三壯 。《千》云：內踝下容爪甲 。

Zhào Hǎi 照海 (KI 6), bilateral point; the origin of the yīnqiáo vessel 陰蹻脈: It is located below the medial malleolus. Needle 3 fēn deep; burn seven cones of moxibustion. (*Qiān* 《千》 says: It is 4 fēn below the medial malleolus.) *Míng Shàng* 《明上》 says: Yīn Qiáo, a bilateral point, is located in the depression below the medial malleolus. Needle 3 fēn deep; burn three cones of moxibustion. *Xià* 《下》 says: Yīn Qiáo, a bilateral point, is located in the depression below the medial malleolus. Burn three cones of moxibustion. *Qiān* 《千》 says: Below the medial malleolus, in the depression that can hold a fingernail.

《明堂》上下經有陰蹻穴，而《銅人》無之，惟有照海穴，亦在內踝下與陰蹻同，而未知其故。予按《素問·氣穴論》，陰陽蹻穴在內踝下，是謂照海，陰蹻所生，則與《銅人》照海穴合矣。則是陰蹻即照海也。故附陰蹻於照海之末。

[Author's notes:] In the Upper and Lower Canon of *Míng Táng* 《明堂》, there is a point [called] Yīn Qiáo 陰蹻, but it is not in *Tóng Rén* 《銅人》. [In *Tóng Rén*], there is only Zhào Hǎi (KI 6), which is also located below the medial malleolus just like Yīn Qiáo. I do not know the reason [for this discrepancy]. I follow *Sù Wèn · Qì Xuè Lùn* 《素問·氣穴論》: The Yīn Yáng[120] Qiáo 陰陽蹻 point is located below the medial malleolus. It called Zhào Hǎi (KI 6), and is where the yīnqiáo vessel starts. So this should be the same as Zhào Hǎi (KI 6) in *Tóng Rén*. The Yīn Qiáo [point] means Zhào Hǎi (KI 6). I have appended Yīn Qiáo at the end of the Zhào Hǎi (KI 6) [entry].

復溜二穴，金也，一名昌陽，一名伏白 。在內踝上二寸，動脈陷中 。針三分，留三呼，灸五壯 。《明》云：七壯 。

Fù Liū 復溜 (KI 7), bilateral point, metal; another name is Chāng Yáng 昌陽, also named Fú Bái 伏白: It is located 2 cùn above the medial malleolus, in the depression where there is a pulsating vessel. Needle 3 fēn deep, retain the needle for three respirations; burn five cones of moxibustion. *Míng* 《明》 says: Seven cones.

---

120. The character yáng 陽 should be removed, based on the meaning of the text.

交信二穴，在內踝上二寸，少陰前太陰後廉前筋骨間腨。灸三壯，針四分，
留五呼。《明下》云：內踝上二寸後廉筋骨陷中。《素問・氣穴論》：踝上
橫二穴。注云：內踝上者，交信穴也。

Jiāo Xìn 交信 (KI 8), bilateral point: It is located 2 cùn above the medial malleolus, anterior to the [foot] shàoyīn and posterior to the [foot] táiyīn; it is on the anterior ridge, in the depression between the sinews and bone on the calf. Burn three cones of moxibustion; needle 4 fēn deep; retain

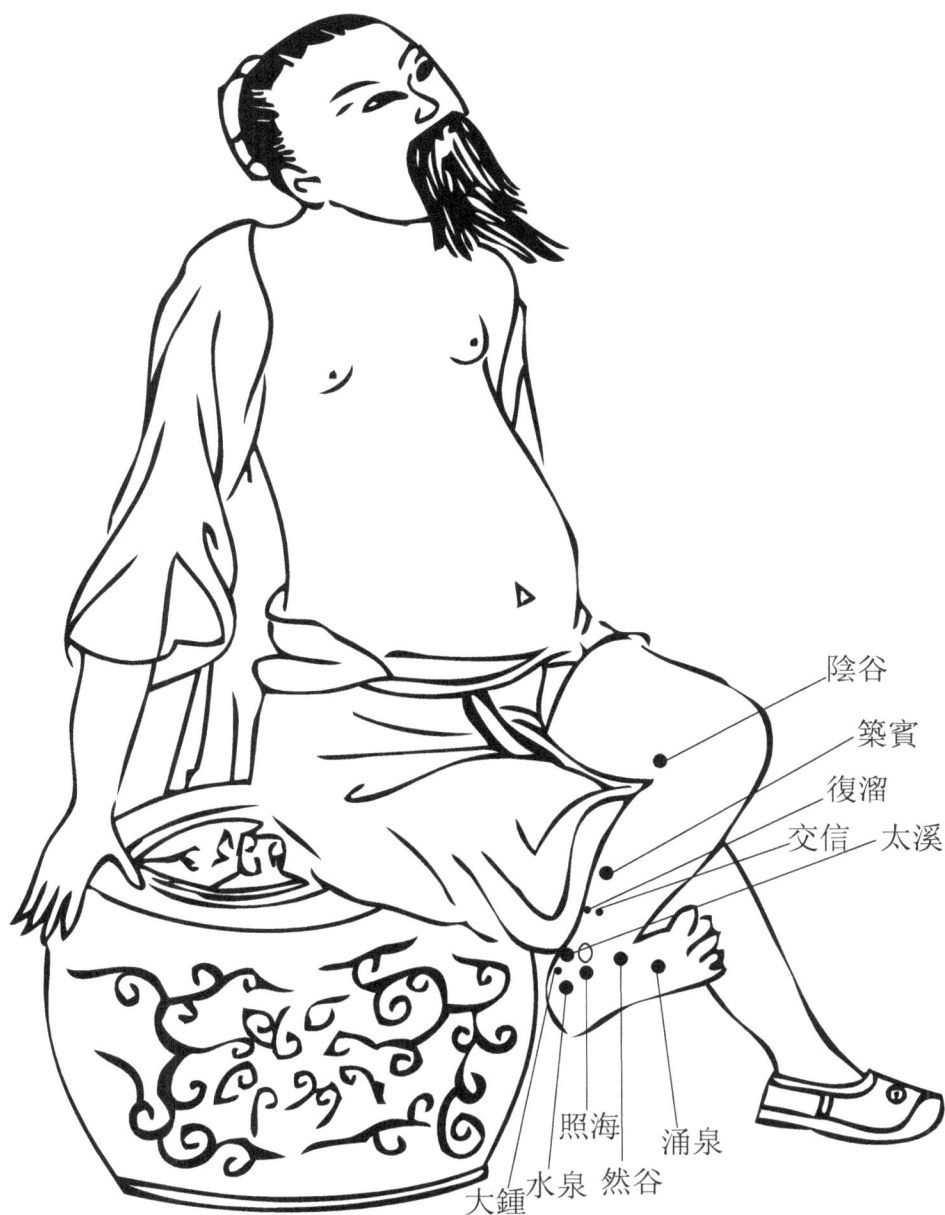

陰谷
築賓
復溜
交信　太溪
照海　涌泉
大鍾　水泉　然谷

Fig. 1.40

139

the needle for five respirations. *Míng Xià*《明下》says: It is 2 cùn above the medial malleolus, on the posterior aspect, in the depression between the sinews and bone. *Sù Wen • Qì Xuè Lùn* says: It is a bilateral point [located] transversely above the ankle. The Annotation says: [The point] above the medial malleolus is Jiāo Xìn (KI 8).

按《素問·氣府論》陰蹻穴注云：謂交信也，在內踝上二寸，少陰前太陰後筋骨間，陰蹻之郄。竊意陰蹻即交信也。至《氣穴論》陰陽蹻穴注乃云：陰蹻穴在內踝下，是謂照海，陰蹻所生，則是陰蹻乃照海，非交信矣。故《明堂下經》既有交信穴在內踝上，又出陰蹻穴在內踝下。上下不同，蓋二穴也。但不知《素問》之注何故前後自異，學者毋信其一注而不考其又有一注也。

> [Author's notes:] According to the Annotation to *Sù Wèn • Qì Fŭ Lùn*《素問·氣府論》on the Yīn Qiáo 陰蹻 point: Jiāo Xìn 交信 (KI 8) is located 2 cùn above the medial malleolus, anterior to the [foot] shàoyīn and posterior to the [foot] tàiyīn, in the depression between the sinews and bone. It is the *xī*-cleft point of the yīnqiáo [mài] 陰蹻[脈]. I personally thought the Yīn Qiáo point was Jiāo Xìn 交信 (KI 8). But the Annotation on the Yīn Yáng Qiáo 陰陽蹻 points in *Qì Xuè Lùn*《氣穴論》says: The Yīn Qiáo point is located below the medial malleolus; that is Zhào Hǎi 照海 (KI 6), where the yīnqiáo [mài] originates. So the Yīn Qiáo point is Zhào Hǎi (KI 6) and is not Jiāo Xìn (KI 8). *Míng Táng Xià Jīng*《明堂下經》has Jiāo Xìn (KI 8), which is located above the medial malleolus, and also has the Yīn Qiáo point which is located below the medial malleolus. "Above" and "below" differ from each other, so these must be two [different] points. I do not know why the Annotation to *Sù Wèn*《素問》has discrepancies in earlier and later [sections]. Scholars cannot simply trust one annotation without checking the others.

築賓二穴，在內踝上腨分中。灸五壯，針三分。《明》云：內踝上。灸三壯。

Zhù Bīn 築賓 (KI 9), bilateral point: It is located above the medial malleolus, in the muscle on the calf. Burn five cones of moxibustion; needle 3 fēn deep. *Míng*《明》says: It is above the medial malleolus. Burn three cones of moxibustion.

陰谷二穴，水也。在膝內輔骨後，大筋下小筋上，按之應手，屈膝乃取之。灸三壯，針四分，留七呼。

Yīn Gǔ 陰谷 (KI 10), bilateral point, water: It is located posterior to the medial assisting bone of the knee [the region formed by medial epicondyle of the femur and medial condyle of the tibia], below the big sinew and above the small sinew. It responds to the hand when it is pressed. Flex the knee to locate this point. Burn three cones of moxibustion; needle 4 fēn deep; retain the needle for seven respirations.

1.36

足太陽膀胱經左右三十六穴

Zú Tàiyáng Páng Guāng Jīng Zuǒ Yòu Sān Shí Liù Xué

Foot Tàiyáng Urinary Bladder Channel, 36 bilateral points [eighteen on each side]

至陰二穴，金也 。在足小指外側，去爪甲角如韭葉 。針二分，灸三壯 。

Zhì Yīn 至陰 (UB 67), bilateral point, metal: It is located on the lateral aspect of the little toe, a leek leaf's distance from the corner of the nail. Needle 2 fēn deep; burn three cones of moxibustion.

通谷二穴，水也 。在足小指外側，本節前陷中 。灸三壯，針二分 。

Tōng Gǔ 通谷 (UB 66), bilateral point, water: It is located on the lateral aspect of the little toe, in the depression anterior [distal] to the base joint. Burn three cones of moxibustion; needle 2 fēn deep.

束骨二穴，木也 。在足小指外側，本節後陷中 。灸三壯，針三分 。

Shù Gǔ 束骨 (UB 65), bilateral point, wood: It is located on the lateral aspect of the little toe, in the depression posterior [proximal] to the base joint. Burn three cones of moxibustion; needle 3 fēn deep.

京骨二穴，在足外側大骨下，赤白肉際陷中，按而得之 。針三分，灸七壯 。《明》云：五壯 。《素注》：三壯 。

Jīng Gǔ 京骨 (UB 64), bilateral point: It is located on the lateral aspect of the foot, inferior to the big bone, in the depression on the border of the red and white flesh. Press to find the point. Needle 3 fēn deep; burn seven cones of moxibustion. *Míng* 《明》 says: Five cones. *Sù Zhù* 《素注》 says: Three cones.

申脈二穴，陽蹻脈所出。在外踝下陷中，容爪甲白肉際。針三分。《千》
云：申脈在外踝下陷中。《明上》云：陽蹻二穴在外踝前一寸陷宛中。針三
分。《素問・氣穴》注：陽蹻穴是謂申脈，陽蹻所出，在外踝下陷中。《新
校正》云：按《刺腰痛篇》注：在外踝下五分。《繆刺論》注：外踝下半
寸，容爪甲。

Shēn Mài 申脈 (UB 62), bilateral point; the origin of the yángqiáo [mài] 陽蹻[脈]: It is located inferior to the lateral malleolus, in the depression that can hold a fingernail, on the border of the white flesh. Needle 3 fēn deep. *Qiān*《千》says: Shēn Mài (UB 62) is located in the depression inferior to the lateral malleolus. *Míng Shàng*《明上》says: The bilateral point Yáng Qiáo 陽蹻 is located in the depression 1 cùn anterior to the lateral malleolus. Needle 3 fēn deep. The Annotation to *Sù Wèn • Qì Xuè*《素問・氣穴》says: The Yáng Qiáo point means Shēn Mài (UB 62). It is the origin of the yángqiáo [mài] and is located in the depression below the lateral malleolus. *Xīn Jiào Zhèng*《新校正》says: According to the Annotation to *Cì Yāo Tòng Piān*《刺腰痛篇》: The point is located 5 fēn below the lateral malleolus. The Annotation to *Miù Cì Lùn*《繆刺論》(Treatise on Cross Needling)[121] says: It is 1.5 cùn below the lateral malleolus, in the depression that can hold a fingernail.

《明堂上經》有陽蹻穴，而《銅人》無此穴，惟有申脈二穴。陽蹻脈
所出在外踝下陷中，與陽蹻穴同，而未知其故。予按《素問・氣穴
論》陰陽蹻穴注云陽蹻穴是謂申脈。陽蹻所出，在外踝下陷中，以與
《銅人》申脈穴合，是則陽蹻即申脈也。故附《明堂》陽蹻於申脈之
後。

[Author's note:] In *Míng Táng Shàng Jīng*《明堂上經》, there is the Yáng Qiáo point, but *Tóng Rén*《銅人》does not have it; it only has the bilateral point of Shēn Mài (UB 62). The origin of the yángqiāo mài is in the depression below the lateral malleolus. This is the same [location] as the Yáng Qiáo point. But I do not know the reason [for the discrepancy in names]. I follow the Annotation on the Yīn Yáng Qiáo 陰陽蹻 points in *Sù Wèn • Qì Xuè Lùn*《素問・氣穴論》: The Yáng Qiáo point means Shēn Mài (UB 62). It is the origin of the yángqiāo mài and is located in the depression below the lateral malleolus. This matches Shēn Mài (UB 62) in *Tóng Rén*. So the Yáng Qiáo [point] is Shēn Mài (UB 62). I appended the Yáng Qiáo [point] from *Míng Táng*《明堂》at the end of the Shēn Mài (UB 62) [entry].

金門二穴，一名關梁。在外踝下。灸三壯，炷如小麥，針一分。

Jīn Mén 金門 (UB 63), bilateral point, another name is Guān Liáng 關梁: It is located below the lateral malleolus. Burn three grain-of-wheat size cones of moxibustion. Needle 1 fēn deep.

121. *Miù Cì Lùn*《繆刺論》(Treatise on Cross Needling) is Chapter 63 of *Sù Wèn*《素問》(Plain Questions).

僕參二穴，一名安耶 。在跟骨下陷中，拱足得之 。針二分，灸七壯 。《 明 》
云：三壯 。

Pú Cān 僕參 (UB 61), bilateral point, another name is Ān Yē 安耶: It is located in the lower depression on the heel bone [calcaneus]. Locate the point while arching the foot. Needle 2 fēn deep; burn seven cones of moxibustion. *Míng*《 明 》says: Three cones.

崑崙二穴，火也 。在外踝後，跟骨上陷中 。《 素注 》：細脈動應手 。灸三
壯，針三分 。《 明 》云：上崑崙，針五分 。下崑崙，外踝下一寸大筋下 。

Kūn Lún 崑崙 (UB 60), bilateral point, fire: It is located posterior to the lateral malleolus, in the depression on the heel bone [calcaneus]. *Sù Zhù*《 素注 》says: There is a thin pulsating vessel that responds to the hand. Burn three cones of moxibustion; needle 3 fēn deep. *Míng* says: Needle 5 fēn deep on upper Kūn Lún. Lower Kūn Lún is located 1 cùn below the lateral malleolus, inferior to the big sinew.

《明堂》有上崑崙， 又有下崑崙 。《 銅人 》祇云崑崙而不載下崑崙，
豈《 銅人 》不全耶， 抑名不同， 未可知也 。但《 上經 》云：內崑崙在
外踝下一寸， 《 下經 》云：內崑崙在內踝後五分 。未知其孰是， 予謂
既云內崑崙， 則當在內踝後矣 。《 下經 》之穴為通， 上崑崙在外踝故
也 。

In *Míng Táng*《 明堂 》, there is upper Kūn Lún and lower Kūn Lún, too. *Tóng Rén*《 銅人 》only discusses Kūn Lún and does not record lower Kūn Lún. I do not know if *Tóng Rén* is incomplete or if it uses a different name [for the point]. But *Shàng Jīng*《 上經 》says: Inner Kūn Lún is located 1 cùn below the **lateral** malleolus. *Xià Jīng*《 下經 》says: Inner Kūn Lún is located 5 fēn posterior to the **medial** malleolus. I do not know which one is correct, but I would say that if it is named **inner** Kūn Lún, it should be located posterior to the medial malleolus. The [explanation of the] point in *Xià Jīng* makes more sense, because upper Kūn Lún is located on the **lateral** malleolus.[122]

跗陽二穴，在外踝上三寸（ 足太陽穴同，《 千金 》亦同 。 ）陽蹻郄 。太陽
前，少陽後，筋骨間，陽蹻之郄 。灸三壯，針五分，留七呼 。《 明下 》云：
跗陽在外踝上二寸（恐二字當作三） 後，筋骨間宛宛中 。灸五壯 。《 素 ·
氣府論 》陰陽蹻各一注云：陽蹻謂跗陽穴也 。在外踝上三寸 。太陽前，少陽
後，筋骨間，陽蹻之郄 。

---

122. Inner Kūn Lún 崑崙 is Tài Xī 太溪 (KI 3); outer Kūn Lún and upper Kūn Lún both indicate Kūn Lún 崑崙 (UB 60); lower Kūn Lún is an extraodinary point which is located below Kūn Lún (UB 60).

Fū Yáng 跗陽 (UB 59), bilateral point: It is located 3 cùn above the lateral malleolus (the same as in the foot tàiyáng points [section in *Tóng Rén* 《銅人》] and *Qiān Jīn* 《千金》). It is the *xī*-cleft point of the yángqiáo [mài] 陽蹻[脈]. It is located anterior to the regular [foot] tàiyáng [pathway][123] and posterior to the [foot] shàoyáng, between sinews and bone. It is the *xī*-cleft point of yángqiáo [mài]. Burn three cones of moxibustion; needle 5 fēn deep, retain the needle for seven respirations. *Míng Xià* 《明下》 says: Fū Yáng (UB 59) is located 2 cùn (I suspect three (*sān* 三) may have accidentally been written as two (*èr* 二) here) above the lateral malleolus and runs posteriorly, in the depression between the sinews and bone. Burn five cones of moxibustion. The Annotation to the Yīn Yáng Qiáo 陰陽蹻 points in *Sù Wèn・Qì Fǔ Lùn* 《素・氣府論》 says: The Yáng Qiáo 陽蹻 [point] is Fū Yáng (UB 59) and is located 3 cùn above the lateral malleolus. It is located anterior to the [foot] tàiyáng and posterior to the [foot] shàoyáng, between the sinews and bone. It is the *xī*-cleft point of yángqiáo [mài].

按《素問・氣穴論》陽蹻穴注云謂跗陽穴也，在外踝上三寸。竊意陽蹻即跗陽也，及考《氣穴論》陰陽蹻四穴注云陽蹻穴是謂申脈，陽蹻所出。則是陽蹻乃申脈，非跗陽矣。故《明堂下經》既有跗陽在外踝上二寸，《上經》又有陽蹻在外踝前一寸。一寸二寸既異，是跗陽，陽蹻各是一穴也。但不知《素問》之注何故前後相背耶？

[Author's notes:] According to the Annotation to the Yáng Qiáo [point] in *Sù Wèn・Qì Xuè Lùn* 《素問・氣穴論》: The Yáng Qiáo point is called Fū Yáng (UB 59) and is located 3 cùn above the lateral malleolus. I personally thought Yáng Qiáo 陽蹻 meant Fū Yáng 跗陽 (UB 59). After I checked the Annotations for the four points of Yīn and Yáng Qiáo 陰陽蹻 in *Qì Xuè Lùn* 《氣穴論》: The Yáng Qiáo point is Shēn Mài 申脈 (UB 62), the origin of the yángqiáo mài 陽蹻[脈]. So the Yáng Qiáo [point] is Shēn Mài (UB 62) and is not Fū Yáng (UB 59). In *Míng Táng Xià Jīng* 《明堂下經》, there is Fū Yáng (UB 59), which is located 2 cùn above the lateral malleolus; *Shàng Jīng* 《上經》 has the Yáng Qiáo [point] which is located 1 cùn anterior to the lateral malleolus. 1 cùn and 2 cùn are different, so Fū Yáng (UB 59) and the Yáng Qiáo [point] are not the same. But I do not know why the annotations to *Sù Wèn* 《素問》 disagree with each other in earlier and later [sections].

飛揚二穴，一名厥陽。在外踝上九寸（《明堂》、《千金》並云：七寸）。針三分，灸三壯。《明》云：五壯。

Fēi Yáng 飛揚 (UB 58), bilateral point, another name is Jué Yáng 厥陽: It is located 9 cùn (*Míng Táng* 《明堂》 and *Qiān Jīn* 《千金》 say: 7 cùn) above the lateral malleolus. Needle 3 fēn deep; burn three cones of moxibustion. *Míng* 《明》 says: 5 cones.

---

123. "It is located anterior to the regular [foot] tàiyáng pathway" because the channel moves to the side of the leg on the lower leg.

承山二穴，一名魚腹，一名肉柱，一名傷山。在兌腨腸下分肉間陷中。灸一壯，針七分。《明》云：八分，得氣即瀉，速出針，灸不及針。止七七壯。《下》云：五壯。（**一云：在腿肚下分肉間。**）

Chéng Shān 承山 (UB 57), bilateral point, another name is Yú Fù 魚腹, also named Ròu Zhù 肉柱 and Shāng Shān 傷山: It is located below the tapered calf muscle [gastrocnemius], in the depression between the muscles. Burn one cone of moxibustion; needle 7 fēn deep. *Míng* says: 8 fēn deep; drain [the point] as soon as qì arrives. Remove the needle rapidly. Moxibustion is not as good as needling. Apply up to seven times seven cones of moxibustion. *Xià* 《下》 says: Five cones. (One source says: On the muscle below the calf.)

承筋二穴，一名腨腸，一名直腸。在腨腸中央陷中。灸三壯，禁針。《明》云：在脛後，從腳根後到上七寸，踹中央陷中。針三分。《千》云：從腳根上七寸踹中央。不刺。

Chéng Jīn 承筋 (UB 56), bilateral point, another name is Shuàn Cháng 腨腸, also named Zhí Cháng 直腸: It is located in the depression in the center of the calf muscle [gastrocnemius]. Burn three cones of moxibustion. Needling is contraindicated. *Míng* says: It is located on the posterior aspect of the lower leg, 7 cùn from the back of the heel, in the depression in the center of the calf muscle [gastrocnemius]. Needle 3 fēn deep. *Qiān* 《千》 says: 7 cùn above the heel, in the center of calf muscle. Needling is contraindicated.

《銅人》、《千金》皆云禁針，《明堂》乃云針三分，亦可擬矣，不針可也。

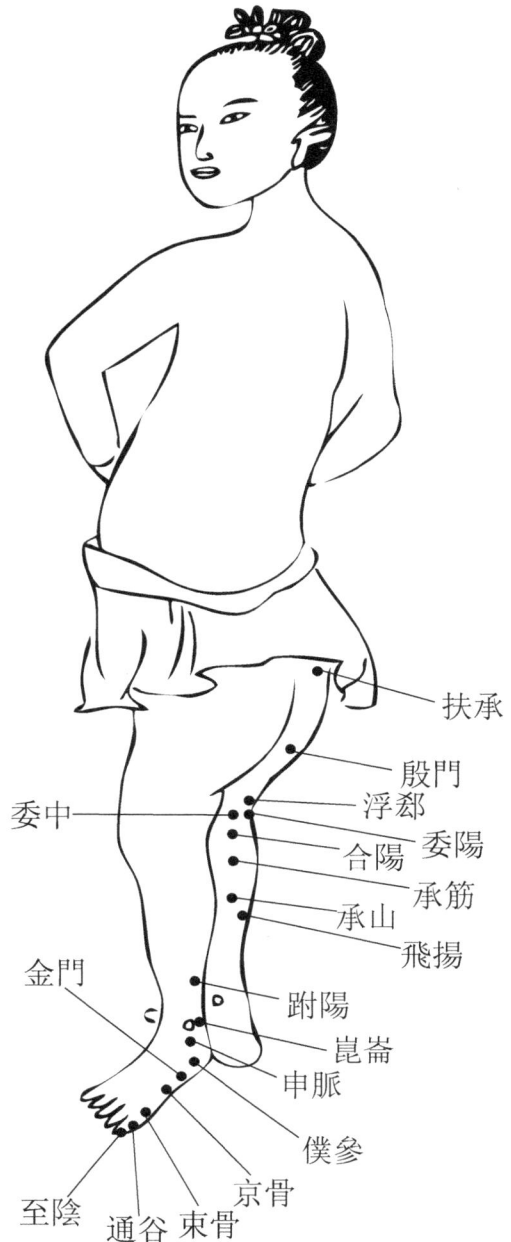

扶承
殷門
浮郄
委中
委陽
合陽
承筋
承山
飛揚
金門
跗陽
崑崙
申脈
僕參
至陰
通谷 束骨
京骨

Fig. 1.41

145

[Author's notes:] *Tóng Rén* 《銅人》 and *Qiān Jīn* 《千金》 all say: Needling is contraindicated. But *Míng Táng* 《明堂》 says: Needle 3 fēn deep. This is doubtful; it is appropriate not to needle.

合陽二穴，在膝約中央下二寸。（《千》作三寸）。針六分，灸五壯。

Hé Yáng 合陽 (UB 55), bilateral point: It is located 2 cùn below the center of the [posterior aspect of the] knee (*Qiān* 《千》 says: 3 cùn). Needle 6 fēn deep; burn five cones of moxibustion.

委中二穴，土也。在膕中央約紋中動脈。今附：委中者，血郄也。熱病汗不出，足熱厥逆滿，膝不得屈伸，取其經血立愈。《明》云：甄權云在曲跡髓內兩筋兩骨中宛宛是，令人面挺腹地而取之。針八分，留三呼，瀉五吸。《甲乙》云：針五分，留七呼，灸三壯。《素注》：在足膝後屈處，膕中央約紋中。又《骨空論》云：在膝解後，曲腳中背面取之。

Wěi Zhōng 委中 (UB 40), bilateral point, earth: It is located on the pulsating vessel in the center of popliteal fossa, on the crease. Appended here: Wěi Zhōng (UB 40) is the *xī*-cleft point of the blood. [If the patient suffers] heat disease with absence of sweating, heat reversal in the feet, counterflow fullness, and inability to flex the knees, bleed this point to cure the disease immediately.

Míng 《明》 says: Zhēn Quán said: It is located in the curved crease, in the depression between two sinews and two bones. Ask the patient to lie down with the abdomen against the ground and tilt the head; then locate the point. Needle 8 fēn deep, retain the needle for three respirations; drain for five respirations. *Jiǎ Yǐ* 《甲乙》 says: Needle 5 fēn deep, retain the needle for seven respirations. Burn three cones of moxibustion. *Sù Zhù* 《素注》 says: It is located in the curved area behind the knee, on the crease in the center of the popliteal fossa. *Gǔ Kōng Lùn* 《骨空論》 (Treatise on Bone Hollows)[124] says: It is at the back of the knee joint, in the curved crease. Locate the point with the patient turned around [in the prone position].

委陽二穴，三焦下輔腧也。在足太陽後，出於膕中外廉兩筋間，屈伸取之，扶承下六寸。灸三壯，針七分。《素注》：在足膕中外廉兩筋間。《千》云：足太陽前少陽後。

Wěi Yáng 委陽 (UB 39), bilateral point, the lower assisting point [lower sea point] of the sānjiāo: [Wěi Yáng] is located posterior to the foot tàiyáng channel. It emerges between two sinews at the lateral aspect of the popliteal fossa. Locate the point while bending and stretching [the leg]. It is

---

124. *Gǔ Kōng Lùn* 《骨空論》 (Treatise on Bone Hollows) from *Sù Wèn* 《素問》 (Plain Questions), Chapter 60.

located 6 cùn below Fú Chéng 扶承 (UB 36).[125] Burn three cones of moxibustion; needle 7 fēn deep. *Sù Zhù* 《 素注 》 says: It is located between two sinews at the lateral aspect of the popliteal fossa. *Qiān* 《 千 》 says: It is anterior to the foot tàiyáng channel and posterior to the foot shàoyáng channel.

浮郄二穴，在委陽上一寸，展膝得之 。灸三壯，針五分 。

Fú Xī 浮郄 (UB 38), bilateral point: It is located 1 cùn above Wěi Yáng (UB 39). Locate the point while extending the knee. Burn three cones of moxibustion; needle 5 fēn deep.

殷門二穴，在肉郄下六寸 。針七分 。

Yīn Mén 殷門 (UB 37), bilateral point: It is located 6 cùn below Ròu Xī 肉郄 (UB 36). Needle 7 fēn deep.

扶承二穴，一名肉郄，一名陰關，一名皮部 。在尻臀下，股陰衝上紋中 。針七分 。《 明下 》云：灸三壯 。《 千 》云：在尻臀下，股陰下紋中（**一云：尻臀下橫紋中**） 。

Fú Chéng 扶承 (UB 36), bilateral point, another name is Ròu Xī 肉郄; also named Yīn Guān 陰關 and Pí Bù 皮部: It is located below sacrum and gluteal region; on the crease above and facing the inner aspect of the thigh. Needle 7 fēn deep. *Míng Xià* 《 明下 》 says: Burn three cones of moxibustion. *Qiān* says: Below the sacrum and gluteal region; on the crease inferior to the inner aspect of the thigh (One source says: It is on the transverse crease below the sacrum and gluteal region).

以上諸穴皆依《銅人經》次第而編，《明堂》上下經有穴，而《銅人》不載亦或附入，惟有其穴而無其名者，無慮數十穴不編，當各依本經所說而針灸之，不可泥此經之無穴名而不針灸也。扁鵲灸鬼邪凡十三穴，與《銅人》、《明堂》同，而其名卻異，故不編入。許希《針經》之穴，既與諸經不同，其名又異，如興龍穴之類是已，亦不附入者，不欲以一人之私名，亂諸經之舊穴，以滋後學者惑也。

[Author's note:] The above entries of points are compiled following the order in *Tóng Rén Jīng* 《 銅人經 》. More than ten points were not included because, even though they are recorded in the Upper and Lower Canons of *Míng Táng* 《 明堂 》, *Tóng Rén* 《 銅人 》 does not record

---

125. 6 cùn seems incorrect here.

or append them, or it has the points, but without the [correct] name. We should use acupuncture and moxibustion on each point based on what is said in this classic [*Tóng Rén*]; but we cannot stop using acupuncture and moxibustion on a point simply because it is not [properly] named in this classic.

Biǎn Què[126] applied moxibustion on 13 points to treat ghost evils. These are the same [as points listed] in *Tóng Rén* and *Míng Táng*, but have different names, so I did not put them in my book. The points are in *Zhēn Jīng* 《針經》 (Acupuncture Classic) by Xǔ Xī 許希 are not the same as in other classics. Their names are also different, for example the Xīng Lóng 興龍 point, and so on. So I did not append them in my book either. I do not want to create disorder in the old [traditional] points from all the other classics just because of one person's own fame. That would confuse scholars later on.

---

126. Biǎn Què 扁鵲, also known as Qín Yüèrén 秦越人, is the name of a famous doctor during the Warring States (戰國) Period.

Zhēn Jiǔ Zī Shēng Jīng

《針灸資生經·第二》

2.01

Zhēn Jiǔ Xū Yào

針灸須藥

The necessity of acupuncture, moxibustion, and herbs

《千金》云：病有須針者，即針刺以補瀉之。不宜針者，直爾灸之。然灸之大法，其孔穴與針無忌，即下白針或溫針訖，乃灸之，此為良醫。

Qiān Jīn《千金》 says: For the diseases that require acupuncture treatment, needle and then apply supplementation and drainage [techniques]. For those that are not appropriate for needling, just apply moxibustion. Regarding the principles of moxibustion, if there is no taboo against acupuncture with a point, insert a plain needle or use warm needling first, then apply moxibustion afterward. That is a good doctor.

其腳氣一病，最宜針。若針而不灸，灸而不針，非良醫也。針灸而藥，藥不針灸，亦非良醫也。但恨下里間知針者鮮爾，所以學者須解用針。燔針、白針皆須妙解。

For the disease of leg qì, acupuncture is the best. If we needle without applying moxibustion; or apply moxibustion without needling – this is not a good doctor. Applying acupuncture and moxibustion [without]¹ using herbs, or using the herbs without applying acupuncture and moxibustion – this is not a good doctor either. But regretfully people in the countryside who know acupuncture are few, so someone who is studying it should understand how to use acupuncture. Red-hot needling and plain needling both need excellent explanations [by a competent doctor].

知針知藥，固是良醫，此言針灸與藥之相須也。今人或但知針而不灸，灸而不針，或惟用藥而不知針灸者，皆犯孫真人所戒也。而世所謂醫者，則但知有藥而已，針灸則未嘗過而問焉。人或誚之，則曰是外科也，業貴精不貴雜也。否則曰、富貴之家，未必肯針灸也，皆自文其過爾。吾故詳著《千金》之說以示人云。

---

1. Based on the text above and below, the word *bù* 不 (without) must be missing here.

Good doctors should know both acupuncture and herbal medicine, and [*Qiān Jīn* 《千金》] also mentions the necessity of using acupuncture, moxibustion, and herbs together. Currently, people only know acupuncture, but not moxibustion; or moxibustion, but not acupuncture; or only use herbs, but not acupuncture and moxibustion. They all violate the warnings of Sūn Zhēnrén.[2] And today's so-called doctors just know herbs, never trying acupuncture. When people tell them [they should], they say these are not within their scope of practice, and their profession values perfecting [one skill], rather than developing miscellaneous [skills]; or they say: The people from wealthy families will not accept acupuncture and moxibustion. These are all [excuses] to cover up their errors. So I wrote the theories from *Qiān Jīn* here in detail to show people.

2.02
Zhēn Jì

針忌

Contraindications of acupuncture

《千金》云：夫用針者，先明其孔穴，補虛瀉實，勿失其理。針毛皮腠理，勿傷肌肉。針肌肉，勿傷筋脈。針筋脈，勿傷骨髓。針骨髓，勿傷諸絡。

Qiān Jīn says: When performing acupuncture, [we must] clearly understand the points, as well as supplementing vacuity and draining repletion; we cannot miss this principle. When puncturing the body hair, skin, and interstices, we cannot damage the muscles. When puncturing the muscles, we cannot damage the sinews and vessels. When puncturing the sinews and vessels, we cannot damage the bones and marrow. When puncturing the bones and marrow, we cannot damage the network vessels.

傷筋膜者，愕視失魂。傷血脈者，煩亂失神。傷皮毛者，上氣失魄。傷骨髓者，呻吟失志。傷肌肉者，四肢不收，失智，此為五亂，因針所生，若更失度，有死之憂也。

Damage to the sinews and membranes results in a startled look and loss of the ethereal soul (*hún*). Damage to the blood vessels results in vexation, derangement, and loss of the spirit (*shén*). Damage to the skin and body hair results in qì ascent and loss of the corporeal soul (*pò*). Damage to the

---

2. Sūn Zhēnrén 孫真人 refers to Sūn Sīmiǎo 孫思邈, a famous doctor of the *Táng* (唐) Dynasty and the author of *Qiān Jīn* 《千金》.

bones and marrow results in groaning and loss of the will (*zhì*). Damage to the muscles results in loss of use of the limbs and loss of wisdom (*zhì*). These are the five derangements which develop from acupuncture. If they worsen, people may die.

《素問》亦云：刺骨無傷筋，刺筋無傷肉，刺肉無傷脈，刺脈無傷皮，刺皮無傷肉，刺肉無傷筋，刺筋無傷骨。刺中心，一日死。中肝，五日死。中腎，六日死。中肺，三日死。中脾，十日死。中膽，一日半死。刺跗上中大脈，血出不止死。刺頭中腦戶，入腦立死。

Sù Wèn 《素問》 also says: When puncturing the bones, do not damage the sinews. When puncturing the sinews, do not damage the muscles. When puncturing the muscles, do not damage the vessels. When puncturing the vessels, do not damage the skin. When puncturing the skin, do not damage the muscles. When puncturing the muscles, do not damage the sinews. When puncturing the sinews, do not damage the bones. A patient will die in one day if the heart is punctured; in five days if the liver is punctured; in six days if the kidneys are punctured; in three days if the lungs are punctured; in ten days if the spleen is punctured; in one and half days if the gallbladder is punctured. A patient will die if the big vessel on the dorsum of the foot is punctured, causing incessant bleeding; and a patient will die immediately if Nǎo Hù 腦戶 (Du 17) on the head is punctured and the needle enters the brain.

（又無刺大醉、大怒、大勞、大飢、大渴、大驚、新飽云云。詳見《素問》）

(It also says: Do not needle someone who is drunk, angry, suffers severe taxation, hunger, thirst, shock, or is just full from a meal. See *Sù Wèn* for details.[3])

---

3. This is in *Sù Wèn · Cì Jìn Lùn* 《素問 · 刺禁論》 (Treatise on Needling Contraindications), Chapter 52.

2.03
Kǒng Xué Xiāng Qù

孔穴相去

The distance between points

《甲乙經》云：自大椎下至尾骶骨二十一椎，長三尺，折量取俞穴。或云：第一椎上更有大椎在宛宛陷中，非有骨也。有骨處即是第一椎。若以大椎至尾骶二十一椎長三尺法校之，則上節云椎，每椎一寸四分，惟第七椎下至於膂骨多分之七，故上七節共九寸八分，分之七。下節十四椎，每椎一寸四分，分之五有奇，故下七節共二尺一分，分之三。此亦是一說也。但第一椎有骨，乃骨節之收。大椎雖無骨，實是穴名。既曰自大椎下至十一椎，豈可不量大椎以下。或者之說，於是不通矣。

Jiǎ Yǐ Jīng 《甲乙經》 says: It is 3 chǐ from the inferior aspect of Dà Zhuī 大椎[4] to the twenty-first vertebra [fourth sacral vertebra] at the [junction of] the sacrum and coccyx; use this measurement to locate points. Some say: Dà Zhuī (Du14) is in the depression above the first [thoracic] vertebra, not the bone; the bony site is the first vertebra.

If we check the 3 chǐ measurement from the [inferior aspect of] Dà Zhuī to the twenty-first vertebra [fourth sacral vertebra] at the [junction of] the sacrum and coccyx: each of the upper segments, called vertebra, is 1.4 cùn [tall], and there are seven-tenths of a fēn between the bottom of the seventh vertebra (C_7) and the [next] spine bone, so the total length of the upper seven vertebrae is 9.8 cùn plus seven-tenths of a fēn [9.87 cùn].[5]

There are fourteen vertebrae in the lower segment, and each vertebra is 1.4 cùn and five-tenths of a fēn [1.45 cùn tall]. So the length of the lower seven vertebrae[6] is 2 chǐ, one and three-tenths of a fēn

---

4. Dà Zhuī 大椎 is sometimes used to refer to the point, Du 14. Other times, Dà Zhuī 大椎 refers to the seventh cervical vertebra. Along with discussing the measurements, the author wants to clarify the use of this term in the passage that follows.

5. According to *Líng Shū · Gǔ Dù* 《靈樞·骨度》, Chapter 14, the upper seven vertebrae are each 1.41 cùn long, but the distance of seven-tenths of a fēn (0.01 cùn x 7 vertebrae = 0.07 cùn, which equals 0.7 fēn) is here counted together as below the seventh vertebra.

6. This must be in error for "the lower fourteen vertebrae," which would make more sense both in context and mathematically.

[2.013 chǐ].[7,8] This is another theory.

But the first vertebra is a bone, so it should be counted in the number of the vertebra.[9] Dà Zhuī 大椎 is not a bone; it is actually the name of the point [between the bones, Du 14]. But if we say the measurement is from the inferior aspect of Dà Zhuī to the twenty-first vertebra [fourth sacral vertebra],[10] then how can we not count what is below Dà Zhuī (Du 14)? So the theory mentioned above [from the words "Some say"] is incorrect.

自蔽骨下至臍八寸，而中管居其中（上下各四寸）。《氣穴論》注云：中管居心蔽骨與臍之中是也。按《明堂下經》云：鳩尾在臆前蔽骨下五分。人無蔽骨者從岐骨際下行一寸。則是欲定中管之中，又當詳有蔽骨無蔽骨也（當準人長短肥瘠量）。

It is 8 cùn from the covering bone [xiphoid process] to the umbilicus, and Zhōng Guǎn 中管 (Ren 12) is in the middle [4 cùn above and below]. The Annotation of *Qì Xùe Lùn*《氣穴論》says: Zhōng Guǎn (Ren 12) is located halfway between the heart covering bone [xiphoid process] and the umbilicus. According to *Míng Táng Xià Jīng*《明堂下經》: Jiū Wěi 鳩尾 (Ren 15) is located 5 fēn below the covering bone [xiphoid process] of the sternum. If the patient has no covering bone [xiphoid process], locate it 1 cùn below the ridge of bone junction [sternocostal angle]. So to ensure that Zhōng Guǎn (Ren 12) is located at the midpoint, [we should] clarify whether there is a covering bone [xiphoid process] or not [and measure according to a person's height and size].

自臍下寸半為氣海，三寸為丹田，至屈骨凡五寸。《千金》云：屈骨在臍下五寸。《明堂下經》亦云：屈骨在橫骨上、中極下一寸。當準人長短肥瘠量之。

Qì Hǎi 氣海 (Ren 6) is located 1.5 cùn below the umbilicus; Dān Tián 丹田 [cinnabar field] (Ren 4) is located 3 cùn below [the umbilicus]. There are 5 cùn from [the umbilicus] to Qū Gǔ 屈骨 (Ren 2). *Qiān Jīn*《千金》says: Qū Gǔ (Ren 2) is located 5 cùn below the umbilicus. *Míng Táng Xià Jīng*《明堂下經》also says: Qū Gǔ (Ren 2) is located on the transverse bone [pubic bone], 1 cùn below Zhōng Jí 中極 (Ren 3). Locate points according to a person's height and size.

7. If each vertebra is 1.45 cùn long, the length of 14 vertebrae would be 2.03 chǐ, so there must be some error in the description.

8. There are several discussions in different ancient literature regarding the height of the vertebrae, but these descriptions are confusing and disagree with each other. *Líng Shū·Gǔ Dù*《靈樞·骨度》and *Zhēn Jiǔ Jiǎ Yǐ Jīng*《針灸甲乙經》only talk about the upper seven vertebrae as described in the footnote above. *Shén Yìng Jīng*《神應經》says: Each of the upper seven vertebrae is 1.41 cùn, each of the middle seven vertebrae is 1.61 cùn, and each of lower seven vertebrae is 1.26 cun tall.

9. According to Volume 4 of *Pǔ Jì Fāng* 普濟方 (Universal Salvation Formulary), this should read 骨節之數 (the number of the vertebra), not 骨節之收 as is written here.

10. According to the text above, the Chinese should say the twenty-first (二十一) instead of eleventh (十一).

《銅人》云：幽門夾巨闕旁各五分，肓俞夾臍各五分（《明堂》云：在巨闕旁各寸半，通谷夾上管旁相去三寸），不容在幽門旁各寸半，天樞去肓俞寸半夾臍，期門在不容旁寸半，大橫直臍旁。（不容、天樞、期門既各寸半，則幽門、肓俞各五分誤矣。）

Tóng Rén 《銅人》says: Yōu Mén 幽門 (KI 21) is located 5 fēn lateral to Jù Qūe 巨闕 (Ren 14); Huāng Shù 肓俞 (KI 16) is located 5 fēn lateral to the umbilicus.

(*Míng Táng* 《明堂》says: [Yōu Mén (KI 21)] is located 1.5 cùn lateral to Jù Qūe (Ren 14); Tōng Gǔ 通谷 (KI 20) is located 3 cùn from each other, lateral to Shàng Guǎn 上管 (Ren 13)); Bù Róng 不容 (ST 19) is located 1.5 cùn lateral to Yōu Mén (KI 21); Tiān Shū 天樞 (ST 25) is located lateral to the umbilicus and 1.5 cùn lateral to Huāng Shù (KI 16); Qī Mén 期門 (LV 14) is located 1.5 cùn lateral to Bù Róng (ST 19); Dà Héng 大橫 (SP 15) is located in line with the umbilicus.

([The distance] for Bù Róng (ST 19), Tiān Shū (ST 25) and Qī Mén (LV 14) is 1.5 cùn, so [the distance] for Yōu Mén (KI 21) and Huāng Shù (KI 16) of 5 fēn might be wrong.)[11]

《銅人》云：腎俞在十四椎下兩旁各寸半，與臍平。肓門在十三椎下相去各三寸，與鳩尾相直。腎俞既與臍平，肓門乃與鳩尾相直亦可疑也。

Tóng Rén says: Shèn Shù 腎俞 (UB 23) is located 1.5 cùn lateral to the fourteenth vertebra [second lumbar vertebra] on both sides, level with the umbilicus; Huāng Mén 肓門 (UB 51) is located 3 cùn lateral to the thirteenth vertebra [first lumbar vertebra], in line with Jiū Wěi 鳩尾 (xiphoid process).

If Shèn Shù (UB 23) is level with the umbilicus, then it is doubtful that Huāng Mén (UB 51) is in line with Jiū Wěi (xiphoid process).

《甲乙經》云：人有長七尺五寸者，髮以下至頤一尺，結喉至𩪧骬（鳩尾也）一尺三寸，𩪧骬至天樞八寸，天樞至橫骨六寸半，橫骨至內輔上廉一尺八寸，內輔上廉至下廉三寸半，內輔下廉至內踝一尺三寸，內踝至地三寸。又膝膕至跗屬一尺六寸，跗屬至地三寸。又肩至肘一尺七寸，肘至腕一尺二寸半，腕至中指本節四寸，本節至末四寸半。

---

11. There is controversy in the old books regarding how far the channels are lateral to the midline on the abdomen. *Tóng Rén* says the kidney channel is 5 fēn (0.5 cùn) lateral to the midline, but *Míng Táng* says it is 1.5 cùn lateral (or three cùn between one side of the kidney channel and the other side). *Tóng Rén* says the stomach channel is 1.5 cùn lateral to the kidney channel, which would make it 2 cùn lateral to the midline, and Qī Mén 期門 (LV 14) is 1.5 cùn lateral to the stomach channel, which would make it 3.5 cùn lateral to the midline

Jiǎ Yǐ Jīng《甲乙經》says: If someone is 7 chǐ, 5 cùn tall:

- it is 1 chǐ from the hair[line] to the chin;
- 1 chǐ, 3 cùn from the laryngeal prominence [Adam's apple] to the breastbone (Jiu Wei 鳩尾 [the xiphoid]);
- 8 cùn from the breastbone to Tiān Shū 天樞 (ST 25);
- 6.5 cùn from Tiān Shū (ST 25) to the pubic bone;
- 1 chǐ, 8 cùn from the pubic bone to the superior medial aspect of the assisting bone [the region formed by medial epicondyle of the femur and medial condyle of the tibia];
- 3.5 cùn from the medial upper to the medial lower aspect of the assisting bone;
- 1 chǐ, 3 cùn from the lower medial aspect of the assisting bone to the medial malleolus;
- 3 cùn from the medial malleolus to the ground.
- It is also 1 chǐ, 6 cùn from the popliteal fossa to the dorsum of the foot;
- 3 cùn from the lateral aspect of the dorsum of the foot to the ground.
- It is 1 chǐ, 7 cùn from shoulder to the elbow;
- 1 chǐ, 2.5 cùn from the elbow to the wrist;
- 4 cùn from the wrist to the base joint of the middle finger;
- 4.5 cùn from the base joint [of the middle finger] to the tip.

2.04

Dìng Fà Jì

定髮際

Determining the hairline

《明堂下經》云：如後髮際亦有項腳長者，其毛直至骨頭；亦有無項腳者，毛齊至天牖穴。即無毛根，如何取穴？答曰：其毛不可輒定，大約如此，若的的定中府正相當即是，側相去各二寸。此為定穴。（《下》云：兩眉中直上三寸為髮際；後大椎直上三寸為髮際。）

Míng Táng Xià Jīng《明堂下經》says: If the posterior hairline runs a long way down the nape, the hair can reach the bone; if it does not run very far down, the hair can be level with Tiān Yǒu 天牖 (SJ 16).[12] How are the points located if there is no root to the hair? The answer is: Do not determine the hair[line] randomly; it is probably like this: if it is clear and distinct, the location of Zhōng

---

12. The Chinese cannot be translated literally in this sentence as the meaning is lost in English.

Fǔ 中府 (LU 1)[13] directly corresponds to it, or is 2 cùn to the sides. This is the determination of the points. (*Xià* 《下》 says: The [anterior] hairline is three cùn above the midpoint between the two eyebrows; the [posterior] hairline is three cùn directly above Dà Zhuī 大椎 (Du 14).)

2.05
Lùn Tóng Shēn Cùn

論同身寸

Discussion of proportional measurement [same-body cùn]

《下經》曰：岐伯以八分為一寸，緣人有長短肥瘠不同，取穴不準。扁鵲以手中指第一節為一寸，緣人有身長手短，身短手長，取穴亦不準。孫真人取大拇指節橫紋為一寸，亦有差互。今取男左女右手中指第二節內庭兩橫紋相去為一寸。（若屈指即旁取指則中節上下兩文角，角相去遠近為一寸，謂同身寸。）

Xià Jīng 《下經》 says: Qí Bó took 8 fēn as equivalent to 1 cùn, but people have different height and size, so this is not accurate for locating points. Biǎn Què took the first section of the middle finger as 1 cùn. But some people have a long body, but short hands; some people have a short body, but long hands. This [method] is not accurate for locating points either. Sūn Zhēnrén took the transverse crease of the thumb as 1 cùn, which is also different among people. Nowadays, we take the distance between the two transverse creases of the second section of the medial aspect of the middle finger as 1 cùn, using the left hand on males and the right hand on females. (We take the distance between the corners of the two transverse creases as 1 cùn when the finger is flexed. This is called proportional measurement [same-body cùn].)

自依此寸法與人著灸療病多愈。今以為準《銅人》亦曰取中指內文為一寸。《素問》云：同身寸是也。又多用繩度量，繩多出縮不準。今以薄竹片點量分寸，療病準的。亦有用蠟紙條量者。但薄篾易折，蠟紙亦黏手取。取稻稈心量卻易為，勝於用繩之信縮也。

People are often cured using this cùn-measurement to [locate points and] treat disease by applying moxibustion. Nowadays we use *Tóng Rén* 《銅人》 as the standard, which also says the distance

---

13. Zhōng Fǔ 中府 (LU 1) does not make sense here. It might be Fēng Fǔ 風府 (Dū 16).

between the medial creases of the middle finger is 1 cùn. *Sù Wèn*《素問》says: This is the proportional measurement [same-body cùn]. People also often use a string to measure, but it is not accurate because a string is elastic. Nowadays some people use thin bamboo strips to measure as the standard for treating disease. Others use wax paper strips to measure. But thin bamboo strips break easily and wax paper is sticky when grabbing it. It is easy to use the center of rice straw to measure and better than the string's elasticity.

2.06
Shěn Fāng Shū

審方書

Examining medical books

經云：爪甲與爪甲角、內間與外間、內側與外側、與夫陷中宛宛中，要精審。如某穴去某處幾寸，與其穴去處同者，自各有經絡。

The Classic says: We should check carefully [whether a book says] the nail or the corner of the nail; inner or outer; medial or lateral; in the sunken place or in the depression. For example, if a particular point is located a certain number of cùn away from some site, the point that is away from this same site must be on a different channel than a point located right at that site.

《灸膏肓》云：其間當有四肋三間，灸中間者，謂四肋必有三間，當中間灸，不灸邊兩間也。

Jiu Gāo Huāng《灸膏肓》says: [In locating Gāo Huāng 膏肓 (UB 43)] the space has four ribs with three intercostal spaces in between, apply moxibustion in the middle intercostal space. This means there should be three intercostal spaces between the four ribs. Apply moxibustion in the middle intercostal space means do not apply moxibustion to the intercostal space above or below.

《千金》曰：經云；橫三間寸者，則是三灸兩間，一寸有三灸，灸有三分，三壯之處，即為一寸也。

Qiān Jīn《千金》says: The Classic says: *Héng Sān Jiān Cùn* 橫三間寸 (The Transverse Three Cùn Method)[14] means to apply three moxibustion [cones] with two spaces between them. There are three [cones of] moxibustion within the length of one cùn; the [base of each cone] is three fēn, so the three cones equal [approximately] one cùn.

又曰：凡量一夫之法，覆手並舒四指，對度四指上下節橫過為一夫 。夫有兩種，有三指為一夫者，若灸腳弱，以四指為一夫也（ 見腳氣 ）。

It also says: When making a standard measurement with one hand, turn the hand over, relax the four fingers, and measure horizontally across the upper and lower joints of the four fingers. That is the standard for one hand. There are two types of hand standards. One type uses three fingers, but when applying moxibustion for weak legs use four fingers (See the section on leg qì).

---

14. *Héng Sān Jiān Cùn* 橫三間寸 (Transverse Three Cùn Method) is an ancient moxibustion technique, usually reserved for suppurating moxibustion. In plain English, three cones are placed in a line covering a total length of one cùn. The base of each is three fēn wide. Since one cùn equals ten fēn, there is only a half fēn space between the three cones. The name implies that these cones are applied perpendicular to the channel with the middle cone being on the channel itself; they are not placed above and below the point on top of the channel. This method will be mentioned a few times in the volumes on treatment.

2.07
Xué Míng Tóng Yì

穴名同異

Similarities and differences in the names of points

手有三里、五里，足亦有三里、五里。手有上廉、下廉，足亦有上廉、下廉。側頭部有竅陰，足少陽亦有竅陰。偃伏部有臨泣，足少陽亦有臨泣。既有五里矣，勞宮亦名五里。既有光明矣，攢竹亦名光明。肩有肩井，又有所謂中肩井。足有崑崙，又有所謂下崑崙。太淵、太泉之名或殊，天鼎、天頂之字有異。丹田初非石門，和髎（《明堂上經》誤作"和"字）亦非禾髎。陽蹻實為申脈本非跗陽，陰蹻實為照海本非交信。肩髃之名扁骨見於《外臺》，懸鐘之名絕骨，瞳子髎之名前關見於《千金》注。如此者眾，可不審處而針灸耶？苟不審處，則差之毫厘，有尋丈之謬矣。於是舉其略以示世醫，俾之謹於求穴云。

- There are Sān Lǐ 三里 (LI 10) and Wǔ Lǐ 五里 (LI 13) on the arm; there are also Sān Lǐ (ST 36) and Wǔ Lǐ (LV 10) on the leg.
- There are Shàng Lián 上廉 (LI 9) and Xià Lián 下廉 (LI 8) on the arm; there are also Shàng Lián (ST 37) and Xià Lián (ST 39) on the leg.
- There is Qiào Yīn 竅陰 (GB 11) on the side of the head; the foot shàoyáng also has Qiào Yīn (GB 44).
- There is Lín Qì 臨泣 (GB 15) in prone position section; there also is Lín Qì (GB 41) in foot shàoyáng.
- Although there is Wǔ Lǐ 五里 (LI 13), Láo Gōng 勞宮 (PC 8) is also called Wǔ Lǐ.
- Although there is Guāng Míng 光明 (GB 37), Zǎn Zhú 攢竹 (BL 2) is also named Guāng Míng.
- There is Jiān Jǐng 肩井 (GB 21) on the shoulder; there also is a point called Middle Jiān Jǐng (Jiān Yú 肩髃 (LI 15)).
- There is Kūn Lún 崑崙 (UB 60) on the foot; there also is a point named lower Kūn Lún.
- There might be a difference between the name of Tài Yuān 太淵 (LU 9) and Tài Quán 太泉; and the characters of Tiān Dǐng 天鼎 (LI 17) and Tiān Dǐng 天頂 are not the same.
- Dān Tián 丹田 (cinnabar field) was not Shí Mén 石門 (Ren 5) in the beginning.
- Hé Liáo 和髎 (SJ 22) (*Míng Táng Shàng Jīng* 《明堂上經》 accidentally wrote Hé 和) is not Hé Liáo 禾髎 (LI 19).
- Yáng Qiáo 陽蹻 is actually Shēn Mài 申脈 (BL 60) and is not Fū Yáng 跗陽 (BL 59);

- Yīn Qiáo 陰蹻 is actually Zhào Hǎi 照海 (KI 6) and is not Jiāo Xìn 交信 (KI 8).
- Biǎn Gǔ 扁骨 (flat bone) is another name for Jiān Yú (LI 15) found in *Wài Tái* 《外臺》;
- Jué Gǔ 絕骨 (severed bone) is another name for Xuán Zhōng 懸鐘 (GB 39) and Qián Guān 前關 (anterior gate) is another name for Tǒng Zǐ Liáo 瞳子髎 (GB 1) found in the Annotation of the *Qiān Jīn* 《千金》.

There are a lot points like this, so how can we perform acupuncture without checking the location? If we do not check the location, a small error may lead to a large discrepancy later on. So I give some examples here to show doctors, and help them to be serious when locating points.

2.08
Diǎn Xué

點穴

Locating points

《千金》云：人有老少，體有長短，膚有肥瘦，皆須精思商量，準而折之。又以肌肉紋理，節解縫會，宛陷之中，及以手按之，病者快然。如此仔細安詳用心者，乃能得之耳。許希亦云：或身短而手長，或手短而身短，或胸腹短，或胸腹長，或瘠或肥，又不可以一概論也。

Qiān Jīn says: There are old and young people, with tall and short bodies, fat and thin skin. So we need to consider this thoroughly and discuss it, and be precise when locating points. [Points are located] in the muscles, in the cleft of the joints, or in depressions. Patients feel happy when we press these points. If we locate the points carefully, peacefully, and serenely, we can find them [accurately]. Xú Xī also said: People may have a short body, but long arms; or a long body, but short arms; or a short chest and abdomen; or a long chest and abdomen. They may be fat or thin. So we cannot treat different matters as the same.

《千金》云：凡點灸法皆須平直四體，無使傾側，灸時恐穴不正，徒破好肉爾（《明堂》云：須得身體平直，四肢無令拳縮，坐點無令俯仰，立點無令傾側）。若坐點則坐灸，臥點則臥灸，立點則立灸，反此則不得其穴。

Qiān Jīn says: When applying moxibustion, [the patient's] four limbs must be straight and cannot lean to the side. [Otherwise,] the points may not be correct and we just damage the flesh in vain (*Míng Táng* 《 明堂 》 says: The patient should lie flat and straight, they cannot curl up their four limbs. If we locate points while the patient is sitting, then they cannot lie face down or face up [during treatment]; if we locate points while the patient is standing, then they cannot lean to the side). We need to apply moxibustion with the patient sitting if we located the points while the patient was sitting; we need to apply moxibustion with the patient lying down if we located the points while the patient was lying down; we need to apply moxibustion with the patient standing if we located the points while the patient was standing. We cannot reach the points if we violate this.

《 千金 》云：凡灸當先陽後陰 。言從頭向左而漸下，次後從頭向右而漸下，先上後下 。

Qiān Jīn 《 千金 》 says: When applying moxibustion, we should apply it on the yáng aspects first, and then on the yīn aspects. For example, start from the head and go down the left side first; then start from the head and go down the right side. Do the upper aspect first, then the lower aspect.

《 明堂下 》云：先灸於上，後灸於下，先灸於少，後灸於多，皆宜審之 。

Míng Táng Xià 《 明堂下 》 says: We should apply moxibustion on the upper part first, then the lower part; apply fewer cones of moxibustion first, then more cones. Everyone should examine this.

2.09
Lùn Zhuàng Shù Duō Shǎo

論 壯 數 多 少

The number of moxibustion cones

《千金》云：凡言壯數者，若丁壯、病根深篤可倍於方數，老少羸弱可減半
（又云：小兒七日以上周年以還不過七壯，炷如雀屎）。扁鵲灸法有至
五百壯、千壯，曹氏灸法有百壯、有五十壯，《小品》諸方亦然。惟《明
堂》本經多云針入六分，灸三壯，更無餘論。故後人不準，惟以病之輕重而
增損之。

Qiān Jīn 《千金》says: When talking about the number of moxibustion cones, [we should] double the number of cones given in medical prescriptions on strong healthy men or when the root of the disease is deep and serious; and halve the number of cones on old, young, and weak men. (It also says: For children seven days old, up to the age of one, burn no more than seven cones of moxibustion. The cone should be the size of a sparrow's dropping). According to the moxibustion methods of Biǎn Què, we usually apply up to five hundred or a thousand cones of moxibustion. According to the moxibustion methods of Master Cáo,[15] we burn a hundred cones or fifty cones of moxibustion; it is the same with the prescriptions in *Xiǎo Pǐn* 《小品》(Short Sketches). Only *Míng Táng* 《明堂》says [things like] needle 6 fēn deep and burn three cones of moxibustion. No other discussions [like this] can be found. So later generations do not have a standard; they increase and decrease [the number of cones] according to the severity of the disease.

凡灸頭頂止於七壯，積至七七壯止（《銅人》）。若治風則灸上星、前頂、
百會，皆至二百壯。

When applying moxibustion on the head, burn up to seven cones of moxibustion; or accumulate up to seven times seven cones and then stop (*Tóng Rén* 《銅人》). Burn up to two hundred cones of moxibustion on Shàng Xīng 上星 (Du 23), Qián Dǐng 前頂 (Du 21), or Bǎi Huì 百會 (Du 20) for wind [diseases].

---

15. Master Cáo refers to Cáo Xī 曹翕 from the state of *Wèi* 魏 during the Three Kingdoms Period. He summarized the methods of moxibustion from the *Qín* 秦 to his time in a book called *Cáo Shì Jiǔ Jīng* 《曹氏灸經》(Moxibustion Classic of Master Cáo). This book has since been lost.

腹背宜灸五百壯，若鳩尾、巨闕亦不宜多。四肢但去風邪不宜多灸，灸多則四肢細而無力（《明上》）。而《千金》於足三里穴乃云多至三二百壯。心俞禁灸，若中風則急灸至百壯。

It is appropriate to burn five hundred cones of moxibustion on the abdomen and back. But it is inappropriate to burn a lot of cones on Jiu Wěi 鳩尾 (Ren 15) and Jù Quē 巨闕 (Ren 14). When applying moxibustion on the four limbs to eliminate wind evils, a lot of cones of moxibustion is not appropriate; otherwise, it will cause thin weak extremities (*Míng Shàng* 《明上》). But *Qiān Jīn* 《千金》 says to burn up to two or three hundred cones of moxibustion on Zú Sān Lǐ 足三里 (ST 36). Moxibustion is contraindicated on Xīn Shù 心俞 (UB 15), but [we should] quickly burn up to a hundred cones of moxibustion for wind stroke.

皆視其病之輕重而用之，不可泥一說，而又不知其有一說也。《下經》只云若是禁穴，《明堂》亦許灸一壯至三壯。恐未盡也。

We should apply the appropriate number of moxa cones based on the severity of the disease. We cannot simply follow one theory and ignore the other theories. Only *Xià Jīng* 《下經》 says whether [a specific point] is contraindicated [for moxibustion]. *Míng Táng* allows the burning of one to three moxa cones on [these contraindicated points]. I am afraid that [this discussion] is not complete.

《千金》云：凡宦游吳蜀，體上常須三兩處灸之，勿令瘡暫差，則瘴癘溫瘧毒瓦斯不能著人，故吳蜀多行灸法。有阿是之法，言人有病，即令捏其上，若里當其處，不問孔穴即得便快。成痛處，即云阿是，灸刺皆驗，故曰阿是穴。

Qiān Jīn says: When government officers visit Wú and Shǔ,[16] they burn moxibustion on two or three places on their body, and do not let the moxa sores heal even temporarily. Thus miasma, pestilence, warm malaria, and toxic qì does not attack them. That is why moxibustion is very popular in Wú and Shǔ. There is also an *ā shì* 阿是 (ouch point) method: If a person is sick, pinch the [affected] area immediately. If it is the correct place, the person will feel better right away, even if it is not a point. The painful site is called *ā shì*. Applying moxibustion or pricking it is very effective. So it is called an *ā shì* point.

---

16. Wú 吳 and Shǔ 蜀 were two of the three countries of the Three Kingdoms Period (220–280 CE). Even though this passage was written later during the *Táng* Dynasty, these names were still used to signify the region. Wú 吳 was in what is now called the Jiāngnán region and Shǔ 蜀 was in the present-day Sìchuān province. In this text, both of these areas were viewed as far from civilization, where good doctors might be scarce and strange diseases await.

2.10
Ài Zhù Dà Xiǎo

艾炷大小

The size of moxa cones

《千金》云：黃帝曰灸不三分，是謂徒冤。炷務大也，小弱乃小作之（又云：小兒七日以上周年以還不過七壯，炷如雀糞）。《明堂下經》云：凡灸欲艾炷根下廣三分，若不三分，即火氣不能遠達，病未能愈。則是艾炷欲其大，惟頭與四肢欲小爾。

Qiān Jīn 《千金》 says: The Yellow Emperor says: If moxa cones are not three fēn wide, then [the patient] suffers in vain. Make sure the cones are big enough; small-size cones are only applied on the young and weak. (It also says: For the children seven days old, up to the age of one, burn no more than seven moxa cones. The cone should be the size of a sparrow's dropping). *Míng Táng Xià Jīng* 《明堂下經》 says: When applying moxibustion, the size of the bottom of the cone must be three fēn wide. If it is less than three fēn, the fire qì cannot reach far and the disease will not be cured. So the size of the cones should be big, except when applied to the head and the four limbs.

至《明堂上經》乃云：艾炷依小竹箸頭作。其病脈粗細狀如細線，但令當脈灸之。雀糞大炷，亦能愈疾。又有一途，如腹內疝瘕痃癖塊伏梁氣等，惟須大艾炷。故《小品》曰：腹背爛燒，四肢則但去風邪而已。如巨闕、鳩尾，雖是胸腹穴，灸之不過四七炷，只依竹箸頭大，但令正當脈灸之。艾炷若大復灸多，其人永無心力。如頭上灸多，令人失精神。臂腳灸多，令人血脈枯竭四肢細而無力。既失精神又加於細，即令人短壽（見承漿穴）。此論甚當，故備著之。

Only *Míng Táng Shàng Jīng* 《明堂上經》 says: Make cones [the size of] the head of a small bamboo chopstick. If the size of a vessel[17] is as narrow as a thin thread when someone is ill, apply moxibustion right on the vessel. Cones the size of a sparrow's dropping can also cure disease. There is another way: If [the patient] has *shān*-mounting, *jiǎ*-conglomerations,[18] *xuán*-strings,

---

17. This could mean blood vessel or it could refer to the channels, as in ancient times the word vessel was frequently used for what we call the channels today.

18. *Shàn jiǎ* 疝瘕 (mounting conglomerations) is a type of *shàn* disorder. Symptoms include burning pain in the lower abdomen and a white discharge from the urethra.

pǐ-aggregations,[19] and deep-lying beam qì[20] in the abdomen, use large cones. So *Xiǎo Pǐn* 小品 (Short Sketches) says: [When applying moxibustion], burn the back and abdomen thoroughly [using more cones]; but on extremities, only a few cones should be applied to eliminate wind evils. Even though Jù Què 巨闕 (Ren 14) and Jiu Wěi 鳩尾 (Ren 15) are the points on abdomen and chest region, no more than four times seven cones the size of the head of bamboo chopstick should be burned. But we need to apply the moxibustion right on the vessel. If large cones are frequently used, the patient will never have heart strength. Burning too many cones on the head makes people lose spirit; burning too many cones on the arms and legs dries up people's blood vessels, thus making their extremities thin and weak. If the patient loses spirit and also has thin [weak extremities], they will not live long (see Chéng Jiāng 承漿 (Ren 24)). This discussion is very important, so I put it here.

2.11
Diǎn Ài Huǒ

點艾火

Lighting the mugwort fire

《下經》云：古來灸病，忌松、柏、枳、橘、榆、棗、桑、竹八木，切宜避之。有火珠曜日以艾承之得火；次有火鏡耀日亦以艾引得火，此火皆良。諸蕃部落用鑌鐵擊挌石得火出，以艾引之。凡人卒難備，即不如無木火清麻油點燈，燈上燒艾莖點灸是也，兼滋潤灸瘡，至愈不疼痛。用蠟燭更佳。

Xià Jīng 《下經》 says: Since ancient times, when treating disease with moxibustion, fire from eight kinds of wood has been contraindicated: pine, cypress, trifoliate orange, orange, elm, jujube, mulberry, and bamboo; avoid using them all. We can use the fire bead[21] to reflect the rays of the sun, holding the mugwort close to receive its fire. Another way is to use a fire mirror [convex lens] to reflex the rays of the sun, holding the mugwort close to conduct fire. These fires are both good.

---

19. *Xuán pǐ* 痃癖 (Strings and aggregations) are two kinds of abdominal masses, usually caused by cold-phlegm accumulation with binding of qì and blood.

20. *Fú liáng qì* 伏梁氣 (deep-lying beam qì) indicates certain kinds of abdominal diseases, usually caused by qì and blood accumulation or stagnation. One is heart accumulation, including the symptoms of masses, distention, and accumulations below the heart with vexation; another is periumbilical swelling and pain; a third is abdominal abscesses.

21. A fire bead is a kind of stone resembling a bead. It is round in shape, the size of egg, white or clear in color, and very shiny. Some sources say it has a colored glaze.

People in various fiefs and tribes make fire by striking a stone [flint] with an iron blade, conducting the fire to the mugwort. But it is difficult for ordinary people to prepare this in a hurry, so they prefer pure sesame oil to wood, lighting a lamp and burning a mugwort stem in its fire. [Then they use the stem to] light the moxa cones. This also moistens the moxa sores so they won't feel any pain while [the moxa sores] heal. Using a candle [to light moxa cones] is better.

《良方》云：凡取火者宜敲石取火（今舟行人以鐵鈍刀擊石穴，以紙灰為火丸，在下承之亦得火），或水精鏡於日得太陽火為妙，天陰則以槐木取火。

Liáng Fāng《良方》says: It is appropriate to strike a stone [flint] to get fire (nowadays the people who live on boats use a blunt iron knife to strike a hollow in a stone, and then use paper ash to make a fire ball below to catch the fire). Or it is wonderful to use a crystal mirror [lens] on a sunny day to obtain the fire of the sun. On cloudy days, use pagoda-tree wood (sophora wood, *huái mù* 槐木) to get fire.

2.12
Zhì Jiǔ Chuāng

治灸瘡

Treating moxa sores

《下經》云：凡著艾得瘡發所患即瘥，不得瘡發其疾不愈。《甲乙經》云：灸瘡不發者，用故履底灸令熱熨之，三日即發。今用赤皮蔥三五莖去青，於糖火中煨熟，拍破熱熨瘡十餘遍，其瘡三日自發。予見人灸不發者，頻用生麻油漬之而發；亦有用皂角煎湯候冷，頻點之而發。亦有恐氣血衰不發，於灸前後煎四物湯服，以此湯滋養氣血故也。蓋不可一概論也。

Xià Jīng《下經》says: Disease will be cured as soon as moxibustion makes sores erupt; otherwise, the patient will not be cured by moxibustion. *Jiǎ Yǐ Jīng*《甲乙經》says: If moxa sores do not erupt, heat up the sole of an old shoe and press it on [the site]; moxa sores will erupt within three days. Nowadays [people] use three or five stalks of red-skinned scallions. After cutting off the green parts, put them in embers and ash, and roast them until they are hot. Pat them to break them open, and apply them on the sores ten or more times while warm. The sores will erupt within three days. I have also seen people smear the area with raw sesame oil frequently when the sores do not erupt, and this works as well. Some cook *zào jiǎo* 皂角 [gleditsia], wait until the decoction cools, then dot [the sores] frequently with the decoction to make the sores erupt. If [one is] concerned that the sores cannot erupt because the qì and blood are debilitated, [then] some take *Sì Wù Tāng* 四物湯 (Four Agents Decoction) to nourish the qì and blood before receiving moxibustion. One cannot treat different matters as the same.

予嘗灸三里各七壯，數日過不發，再各灸兩壯，右足發，左足不發，更灸左足一壯，遂發兩月。亦在人以知取之。若任其自然，則終不發矣。此人事所以當盡也。

I once applied seven cones of moxibustion each on both sides of Sān Lǐ 三里 (ST 36), but moxa sores had not erupted after several days, so I applied two more cones of moxibustion again on each side. The sores on the right leg erupted, but not on the left leg. I applied one more cone of moxibustion on left leg, and then the sores erupted and have been there for two months. We should also do this for patients based on our knowledge. If we leave things to nature, moxa sores might never erupt. So we should try our best.

凡著灸住火，便用赤皮蔥、薄荷，煎湯溫洗瘡周，回約一二尺，令驅逐風氣於瘡口出，兼令經脈往來不滯，自然瘡壞疾愈（今人亦有恐水殺人不用湯淋）。若灸瘡退火痂後，用東南桃枝、青嫩柳皮煎湯溫洗，能護瘡中諸風。若瘡內黑爛，加胡荽煎。若瘡疼不可忍，多時不較，加黃連煎神效。

After the moxibustion is complete, decoct red-skinned scallions and mint; wash all around the moxa sores with the warm decoction. Wash in a one or two chǐ circle to expel the wind qì through the opening of the moxa sores and also to remove obstructions in the channels. The disease will be cured after moxa sores erupt naturally. (Nowadays people are afraid that water can kill them [because of infection], so they do not take showers.) When the [mugwort] fire retreats from the moxa sores and they scab over, decoct peach twig from the southeast [side of the tree] and green tender willow bark. Wash the moxa sores with the warm decoction to shield the sores from any wind strike. If the sores become black and festering inside, *hú suī* 胡荽 [coriander] can be added to the decoction. If there is unbearable pain from the sores and it does not recover for long time, it is divinely effective to add *huáng lián* 黃連 (Coptidis Rhizome Frictum) to the decoction.

凡貼灸瘡，春用柳絮，夏用竹膜，秋用新棉，冬用兔腹上白細毛，貓兒腹毛更佳。今人多以膏藥貼之，日三兩易全不疼。但以膏藥貼則易干爾。若要膿出多而疾除，不貼膏藥尤佳。

Apply the following on moxa sores: use willow catkins in the spring; bamboo membranes in the summer; new cotton in the fall, and fine white fur from a rabbit's abdomen in the winter. The fur from a cat's abdomen is even better. Nowadays, people usually apply a plaster on the sores and change [the plaster] two or three times a day so it is easy to be free of pain, but a plaster dries [the sores] out easily. [In certain situations], it would be better to not use a plaster, if it is important to have more pus exudation, so as to cure the disease [faster].

2.13
Jì Shí Wù

忌食物

Dietary contraindications

既灸，忌豬、魚、熱面、生酒、動風冷物，雞肉最毒，而房勞尤當忌也。

When applying moxibustion, it is contraindicated [to consume] pork, fish, hot noodles, fresh liquor [unheated liquor], cold things that can stir up wind, and especially chicken which has the most toxicity. Sexual taxation is also specifically contraindicated.

《下經》云：灸時不得傷飽、大飢、飲酒、食生硬物，兼忌思慮、憂愁、恚怒、呼罵、呼嗟嘆息等（今下里人灸後亦忌飲水，將水濯手足）。

Xià Jīng《下經》 says: When applying moxibustion, overeating, excessive hunger, drinking alcohol, and eating raw, hard food all should be avoided; excessive thought, anxiety, anger, shouting, and cursing, as well as sighing, etc. also are contraindicated. (Nowadays, among the common people, drinking water, or washing the hands and feet are also contraindicated after applying moxibustion).

2.14
Bì Rén Shén Děng

避人神等

Avoiding the Human Spirit (*Rén Shén* 人神),[22] and so forth

《千金》云：欲行針灸，先知行年宜忌及人神所在，不與禁忌相應即可。故男忌除，女忌破，男忌戊，女忌己。有日神忌，有每月忌，有十二時忌，有四季人神，有十二部人神，有十二部年人神，有九部旁通人神。有雜忌旁通，又有所謂血支血忌之類。凡醫者不能知此避忌，若逢病人厄會，男女氣怯，下手至困。通人達士，豈拘此哉。若遇急卒暴患，不拘此法。許希亦云：若人病卒暴，宜急療。亦不拘此，故後之醫者，亦云卒暴之疾，須速灸療。一日之間，止忌一時是也。

Qiān Jīn 《千金》 says: When applying acupuncture and moxibustion, one should know what to do and what not to do regarding the prediction of a person's luck in a given year, as well as the location of the human spirit. Things will be fine if the contraindications are not offended. So males should avoid *Chú* 除 [eliminate] days and *Wù* 戊 [yáng earth] days, while the females should avoid *Pò* 破 [break] days[23] and *Jǐ* 己 [yīn earth][24] days. There are daily, monthly, and hourly contraindications for the human spirit; there are seasonal, twelve body part, twelve-year cycle, and nine sections of the body contraindications for the human spirit. There are also miscellaneous contraindications, contraindications for what is called the *Xuè Zhī* 血支 [blood branch] and the *Xuè Jì* 血忌 [blood

---

22. *Rén shén* 人神 (human spirit): *Shén* 神 is usually translated as spirit when it applies to what is stored in the heart. Here, this is more like a god or deity that travels thoroughly the human body on a regular time schedule. If you needle the body part where the human spirit currently resides, you can damage this deity, causing a bad outcome. Today, it is a rare practitioner that follows this type of day selection.

23. *Chú* 除 and *Pò* 破: These are two of the twelve on-duty positions in Chinese day selection. The twelve on-duty positions repeat in order, every twelve days and are calculated based on the earthly branch of the current month. Each on-duty position has its own activities that are beneficial or harmful. In Chinese almanacs, an on-duty position is listed for each day. This helps determine the appropriate activities for that day.

24. *Wù* 戊 and *Jǐ* 己: These are the fifth and sixth of the ten heavenly stems [*Tiān Gān* 天干]. In the Chinese calendar, the ten heavenly stems and twelve earthly branches are used to count the hours, days, months, and years. They each have an associated element and yīn-yáng polarity which affect the qì of that time period. For the details, see Volume V of *Zhēn Jiǔ Dà Chéng* 針灸大成 (The Great Compendium of Acupuncture and Moxibustion), translated by Lorraine Wilcox, Appendix A and B.

avoidance],[25] and so forth. If doctors do not know these contraindications, they will have difficulty giving treatment when a patient has bad luck or qì timidity. Those who understand need not be restrained by this. But in urgent and critical conditions, we cannot be restrained by these rules. Xú Xī 許希 also said: If a patient suffers an urgent or critical disease, we should give treatment immediately. We cannot stick to these rules. So doctors in later generations also said to treat urgent and critical diseases immediately. Only prohibitions for the two-hour time periods are followed during the day.

《千金》云：癰疽疔腫，喉痹客忤，尤為急，凡作湯藥不可避凶日，覺病須臾即宜便治。又曰：凡人卒暴得風，或中時氣，凡百所苦，須急救療，漸久後皆難愈。此論甚當。夫急難之際，命在須臾，必待吉日後治，已淪於鬼錄矣。此所以不可拘避忌也。惟平居治病於未形，選天德，月德等日，服藥、針灸可也。

Qiān Jīn《千金》says: Welling-abscesses, flat-abscesses, clove sores and swellings, throat *bì*-impediment, and visiting hostility[26] are especially urgent [diseases]. When they are treated with decoctions these inauspicious days cannot be avoided. If we feel the disease [will change] fast, then it is appropriate to treat right away. It also says: When people suffer sudden wind strike, or are struck by seasonal qì, or the hundred [diseases], they need to be treated immediately. It is more difficult to recover after a long duration. This discussion is very important. During a critical and difficult condition, life is in danger. If we have to wait for an auspicious day to treat, [the patient] will be dead already. So we cannot stick to these contraindications. We can choose a *Tiān Dé* 天德 [heavenly virtue][27] day or a *Yuè Dé* 月德 [lunar virtue] day to give the patient herbs, acupuncture, and moxibustion, only when treating disease in ordinary times.

---

25. *Xuè Zhī* 血支 [blood branch] and *Xuè Jì* 血忌 [blood avoidance]: Days that are contraindicated for acupuncture or other activities where bleeding could occur, based on the Chinese calendar.

26. Visiting hostility is a pediatric disease. Its symptoms include sudden crying, vomiting, diarrhea, abdominal pain, or tugging and slackening after seeing strangers or hearing strange sounds. It is usually due to wind-phlegm attack. Its underlying root is the instability of spirit-qì in children.

27. *Tiān Dé* 天德 [heavenly virtue] and *Yüè Dé* 月德 [lunar virtue]: In ancient China, people calculated these auspicious stars based on comparing the month branch to the day stem.

2.15
Xiàng Tiān Shí

相天時

Observing the weather and time

《千金》云：日正午以後乃可灸，謂陰氣未至，灸無不著。午前平旦穀氣虛，令人癲眩，不可針灸。卒急者不用此例。

Qiān Jīn《千金》says: Apply moxibustion only after midday, because the yīn qì has not come yet. Moxibustion will have remarkable results. Grain qì is vacuous before noon and at dawn, it makes people dizzy and confused. So it is not appropriate to perform acupuncture and moxibustion. But these rules do not apply in urgent conditions.

《下經》云：灸時若遇陰霧、大風雪、猛雨、炎暑、雷電、虹霓暫停，候晴明即再灸。急難亦不拘此。

Xià Jīng《下經》says: Moxibustion should be temporarily stopped when there is fog, strong wind, snowstorms, heavy rain, extreme summer heat, lightning, thunder, rainbows, and rosy clouds. Wait until the day is sunny and bright to apply moxibustion again. These rules also are not applicable in urgent and difficult conditions.

Puncturing the Affected Site (*Ā Shì* Points)
The Effects of Acupuncture and Moxibustion
Abbreviations[28]

---

28. These last three sections are listed in the table of contents, but the text is missing in all existing editions of the book.

Zhēn Jiǔ Zī Shēng Jīng

《針灸資生經·第三》

3.01
Xū Sǔn

虛損

Vacuity Detriment

腦虛冷 、腦衄 、風寒入腦，久遠頭疼等：亦宜灸囟會 。

Vacuity detriment and cold of the brain, spontaneous bleeding of the brain, wind cold invading the brain and chronic headache: It is appropriate to apply moxibustion on Xìn Huì 囟會 (Dū 22).

予年逾壯，萢寒夜觀書，每覺腦冷；飲酒過量，腦亦疼甚。後因灸此穴而愈。有兵士患鼻衄不已，予教令灸此穴即愈。有人久患頭風，亦令灸此穴即愈。但《銅人》、《明堂經》只云主鼻塞、不聞香臭等疾而已。故予書此，以補其治療之闕。然以腦戶不宜針觀之，囟會亦不宜針。《針經》止云八歲以下不宜針，恐未盡也。

[Author's notes:] When I passed my vigorous age [30 or 40 years of age], I suffered cold in the brain while reading books on cold nights. I also had pain in my brain when I drank too much. These symptoms were cured after applying moxibustion on this point. When a soldier suffered incessant nose bleeds, I asked him to apply moxibustion on this point and it cured the symptoms immediately. Someone else suffered head wind[1] for a long time; I also asked him to do moxibustion on this point and the disease was cured. However *Tóng Rén* 《 銅人 》 and *Míng Táng Jīng* 《 明堂經 》 only mention this point to treat nasal congestion, inability to smell, and so forth. So I write this to fill in the missing parts of its use in treatment. If it is inappropriate to needle Nǎo Hù 腦戶 (Dū 17), Xìn Huì (Dū 22) is also inappropriate. *Zhēn Jīng* 《 針經 》 only says that it is inappropriate to needle this point on those who are under the age of eight. I fear that is not all.

凡飲食不思，心腹膨脹，面色萎黃，世謂之脾腎病者：宜灸中脘 。

No desire to eat, inflation in the heart and abdomen, and withered-yellow facial complexion. This is called spleen and kidney disease: it is appropriate to apply moxibustion on Zhōng Wǎn 中脘 (Rèn 12).

---

1. Head wind indicates chronic intermittent headaches. It is usually caused by contraction of wind-cold.

諸葛亮夙興夜寐，罰至二十皆親覽，而所啖食不至數升。司馬仲達知
其將死。既而亮卒，仲達追之。楊儀反旗鳴鼓，若將拒焉。仲達乃
退，不敢逼。百姓為之諺曰：死諸葛走生仲達。仲達聞之，曰：吾便
料生，不便料死故也。其曰料生，蓋料其事多而食不如前，死之兆
也。食不如前，仲達且知諸葛之且死。

[Author's notes:] Zhūgě Liàng[2] got up early and went to sleep very late; he even had to personally attend punishments of twenty strikes [with a thick board]. But he could not eat more than
several *shēng*.[3] Sīmǎ Zhòngdá[4] knew he was about to die. After Zhūgě Liàng was already dead,
Sīmǎ Zhòngdá chased after him [not knowing he was already dead]. Yáng Yí [who was now lead-
ing Zhūgě Liàng's troops] turned around and struck the drum[5] as if he were going to fight. Sīmǎ
Zhòngdá did not dare to force it and retreated. The saying among the people was: A dead Zhūgě
Liàng can drive away a living Sīmǎ Zhòngdá. When [Sīmǎ] Zhòngdá heard this, he said: I can
predict the living, but not the dead. When he said he could "predict the living," it indicated that
he could read the signs that Zhūgě Liàng would die, because Zhūgě [Liàng] was too busy and his
appetite had declined. [Sīmǎ] Zhòngdá knew Zhūgě Liàng would die because he knew Zhūgě
[Liàng] ate less than before.

今人飲食減少，是胃氣將絕，不可久生矣。方且常食堅硬，使愈難克
化；服峻補藥，使脾胃反熱，愈不能食。初不知灸中脘等穴以壯脾
胃，亦惑之甚也。（《難經》論四時，皆以胃氣為本。釋者曰：言五
臟皆以胃氣為本。胃者水穀之府，人須仰胃氣為主也。然則欲全生
者，宜灸胃脘。）

Nowadays, people don't live long because they eat and drink less, so their stomach qì expires. Also,
they often eat hard [things] which are difficult to digest; or they take drastic supplementation herbs
which can lead to heat in the spleen and stomach. Then they cannot eat anymore. In the beginning,
people do not know they can apply the moxibustion on points such as Zhōng Wǎn 中脘 (Rèn
12) to strengthen the spleen and stomach, and their confusion becomes more extreme.

(When *Nàn Jīng* 《難經》 discusses the four seasons, it always considers stomach qì the root.
An explanation says: This says that the stomach is the root of the five viscera. The stomach is the
mansion of water and grains; and people all rely on stomach qì for survival. If someone wants to
maintain his life, it is appropriate to apply moxibustion on Wèi Wǎn 胃脘 (Rèn 12).)

---

2. Zhūgě Liàng 諸葛亮 (181-234) was the prime minister in the state of *Shǔ* 蜀 during the Three
Kingdoms Period (三國時代). He was also a famous author, politician, and military strategist.

3. A *shēng* was about 200 milliliters at the time.

4. Sīmǎ Zhòngdá 司馬仲達 (179-251) was also named Sīmǎ Yí 司馬懿. He was a general and
politician in the state of *Wèi* 魏 during the Three Kingdoms Period (三國時代). He is perhaps best
known for defending *Wèi* from the Northern Expeditions of Zhūgě Liàng 諸葛亮.

5. In ancient China, the phrase "strike the drum" meant ordering an attack.

久冷傷憊臟腑，泄利不止，中風不省人事等疾：宜灸神闕。

Enduring cold damaging and exhausting the viscera, with incessant diarrhea, wind stroke with unconsciousness, and so forth: It is appropriate to apply moxibustion on Shén Quē 神闕 (Rèn 8).

舊傳有人年老而顏如童子者，蓋每歲以鼠糞灸臍中一壯故也。予嘗久患溏利，一夕灸三七壯，則次日不如廁，連數夕灸，則數日不如廁。足見經言主泄利不止之驗也。又予年逾壯，覺左手足無力，偶灸此而愈。後見同官說中風人多灸此，或百壯或三五百壯皆愈，而經不言主中風，何也？

[Author's notes:] It was said in the past that the face of certain old people appear like that of a child. This is because they burn one cone of moxibustion, the size of a mouse dropping on the umbilicus every year. I myself have suffered enduring sloppy stool. If I applied three times seven cones of moxibustion at night, then I wouldn't go to the latrine [suffer diarrhea] the next day. If I applied moxibustion for several nights in a row, then I wouldn't use the latrine for several days. So we can see why the classics said this point is very effective for treating incessant diarrhea. After I passed my vigorous age [30 or 40 years old], I felt weakness in my left hand and foot. When I occasionally applied moxibustion on this point, the disease was cured. Later, I heard my colleagues say they applied moxibustion on this point when someone suffered wind stroke. After they burned a hundred, three hundred, or five hundred cones, the disease was cured. Why didn't the classics mention that it could treat wind stroke?

臟氣虛憊，真氣不足，一切氣疾，久不瘥者：宜灸氣海（《銅》）。

Exhaustion of visceral qì, insufficiency of true qì, and all qì diseases that cannot be cured for long time: It is appropriate to apply moxibustion on Qì Hǎi 氣海 (Rèn 6) (*Tóng*《銅》).

人身有四海，氣海、血海、照海、髓海是也，而氣海為第一。氣海者，元氣之海也。人以元氣為本，元氣不傷，雖疾不害；一傷元氣，無疾而死矣。宜頻灸此穴，以壯元陽。若必待疾作而後灸，恐失之晚也。

[Author's notes:] The human body has four seas: Qì Hǎi 氣海 (Rèn 6 – the sea of qì), Xuè Hǎi 血海 (SP 10 – the sea of blood), Zhào Hǎi 照海 (KI 6 – the shining sea), and Suǐ Hǎi 髓海 (KI 14 – the sea of marrow).[6] The sea of qì is the first [among them]. Qì Hǎi (Rèn 6) is the sea of original qì. Original qì is the root of a person. If original qì is not damaged, even someone suffering from

---

6. Each of these points has the word sea (*hǎi* 海) in its name.

disease won't be harmed [much]. But if original qì is damaged, someone without disease will die. It is appropriate to apply moxibustion on this point frequently to strengthen original yáng. It is too late if moxibustion is only applied after the disease occurs.

腑臟虛乏，下元冷憊等疾：宜灸丹田。

Vacuity and weakness of the organs, cold and vacuity in the lower origin: It is appropriate to apply moxibustion on Dān Tián 丹田 (Cinnabar Field).[7]

人有常言，七七之數，是旁太歲壓本命。六十有一，是太歲壓本命。人值此年，多有不能必者，是固然矣。然傳不云吉人吉其凶者乎。常觀《素問》以六八之數為精髓竭之年，是當節其欲矣。（《千金》云：五十者一月一泄，要之，四十八便當依此。）

[Author's notes:] People often say that the age of 49 [seven times seven][8] is a side-*Tàisuì*[9] that presses against one's own fate (*běn mìng*).[10] At the age of 61, the *Tàisuì* presses against one's own fate (*běn mìng*); when someone is in this year, then something uncertain often occurs. However, it was not passed down that lucky people are lucky during their bad luck. In reading *Sù Wèn* 《素問》, it considered the age of 48 (six times eight) the time when essence and marrow dry out, so people should restrain from sexual indulgence. (*Qiān Jīn* 《千金》 says: A 50 year old person can have sexual activity once a month; to sum it up, they should follow this rule at the age of 48.)

《千金》載《素女論》，六十者閉精勿泄，是欲當絕矣。宜節不知節，宜絕不能絕，坐此而喪生，蓋自取之，豈歲之罪哉？人無罪歲，

---

7. Dān Tián 丹田 (Cinnabar field) is an alternate name for Guān Yuán 關元 (Rèn 4), Zhōng Jí 中極 (Rèn 3) or Shí Mén 石門 (Rèn 5).

8. *Sù Wèn* 《素問》 (Plain Questions) Chapter 1, counts women's life in seven-year periods and men's in eight-year periods.

9. *Tàisuì* 太歲 indicates the star directly opposite to Jupiter. It is a concept of Chinese astrology and is also important in Daosim and Fēng Shuǐ. In Chinese astrology, there are sixty heavenly generals (one for each of the 60 stem-branch combinations) who assist the Jade Emperor in taking charge of the well-being of the Mortal World. Each of these takes charge for one year in the sixty-year cycle. In Daoism, whoever was born in a year that is inauspicious when compared to the current year, perhaps in a year that clashes with the *Tàisuì* 太歲 of the year – these people are advised to have a prayer session with a Daoist Priest to ask for blessings in obtaining peace and good fortune throughout the year. In Fēng Shuǐ, the area of the house corresponding with the position of that year's *Tàisuì* 太歲 is to be left undisturbed, or misfortune will befall the residence.

10. Here, *běn mìng* 本命 indicates the stem-branch combination of a person's year birth. Since the cycle consists of sixty years, the stem-branch combination is the same as the person's birth year at the age sixty-one.

則雖有孽，猶可違矣。所謂吉其凶者如此，雖不灸丹田可也。（丹田可灸七七壯或三五百壯。）

Qiān Jīn《千金》recorded *Sù Nǚ Lùn*《素女論》: People should not discharge essence at the age of 60, which means their desire should expire. If someone does not restrain themselves when they should; or someone does not expire [their desires] when they should; they will die. The patient can only blame themselves, not their age. If someone is not in a year of misfortune, even if they sin, they can still evade [disaster]. This is what is called lucky during bad luck, even if they do not apply moxibustion on Dān Tián 丹田 (Cinnabar Field). (Burn seven times seven cones or three or five hundred cones of moxibustion on Dān Tián (Cinnabar Field).)

陽氣虛憊，失精絕子：宜灸中極。

Exhaustion of yáng qì, seminal loss and infertility: It is appropriate to apply moxibustion on Zhōng Jí 中極 (Rèn 3).

中極一名氣原，蓋氣之原也，人之陽氣虛憊者，可不灸此以實其氣耶？（按《難經》云：丹田名大中極，言丹田取人之身上下四向最為中間也，故名為極。此亦曰中極，其去丹田只一寸，雖未若丹田之最中，然不中不遠矣。）

[Author's notes:] Zhōng Jí (Rèn 3), also named Qì Yuán 氣原, is the origin of qì. When someone suffers exhaustion of yáng qì, we cannot replenish qì without applying moxibustion on this point. (*Nàn Jīng*《難經》says: Dān Tián 丹田 (Cinnabar Field) is also named Dà Zhōng Jí 大中極 (Rèn 4 – great central pole). Dān Tián (Cinnabar Field) is located in the exact center of the four directions of human body, so it is the *jí* 極 (pole). This is also named Zhōng Jí (Rèn 3) and is one cùn away from Dān Tián (Cinnabar Field). Although it is not the exact center like Dān Tián (Cinnabar Field), it is not too far away from the center.)

三里治胃寒，心腹脹滿，胃氣不足，惡聞食臭，腸鳴腹痛，食不化（《銅》）。秦承祖云：諸病皆治。華佗云：療五勞羸瘦，七傷虛乏，胸中瘀血，乳癰。《外臺·明堂》云：人年三十以上，若不灸三里，令氣上衝目（《明下》云眼暗）。《千》云：主陰氣不足，小腹堅，熱病汗不出，口苦壯熱，身反折，口噤，腰痛不可顧，胃氣不足，久泄利，食不化，脅下注滿，不能久立，狂言、狂歌、妄笑、恐怒、大罵、霍亂、遺尿失氣，陽厥淒淒，惡寒云云。凡此等疾，皆刺灸之，多至五百壯，少至二三百壯。

Sān Lǐ 三里 (ST 36) treats stomach cold, distention and fullness of heart and abdomen, insufficiency of stomach qì, aversion to the smell of food, rumbling intestines, abdominal pain and non-transformation of food (*Tóng* 《 銅 》 [11]). Qín Chéngzǔ said: It can treat all diseases. Huá Tuó said: It cures the five taxations, marked emaciation, seven damages, vacuity and lack of strength, static blood in the chest, and mammary welling-abscess. *Wài Tái · Míng Táng* 《 外臺·明堂 》 says: Once over the age of 30, if we do not apply moxibustion on Sān Lǐ (ST 36), it allows the qì to surge up into the eyes (*Míng Xià* 《 明下 》 says: dim vision). *Qiān* 《 千 》 says: It governs insufficiency of yīn qì, hardness of the smaller abdomen, heat disease with absence of sweating, bitter taste in the mouth, vigorous fever, body arched backwards, clenched jaws, lower back pain with inability to turn, insufficiency of stomach qì, enduring diarrhea, non-transformation of food, distention and fullness under the rib-sides, inability to stand for long, manic raving, manic singing, frenetic laughing, fear and anger, violent cursing, sudden turmoil, enuresis and flatus, yáng reversal and aversion to cold. Needle and apply moxibustion on this point to treat all the above diseases. Burn up to five hundred cones of moxibustion at the most, or two or three hundred cones at the least.

《小品》云：四肢但去風邪，不宜多灸，七壯至七七壯止，不得過隨年數。故《銅人》於三里穴止云灸三壯、針五分而已。《明堂上經》乃云日灸七壯，止百壯，亦未為多也。至《千金方》則云多至五百壯，少至二三百壯，何其多耶。要之，日灸七壯，或艾炷甚小，可至二七壯，數日灸至七七壯止。灸瘡既乾，則又報灸之，以合乎若要安，丹田三里不曾乾之說可也。必如《千金》之壯數，恐犯《小品》之所戒也。

[Author's notes:] *Xiǎo Pǐn* 《 小品 》 says: It is inappropriate to apply a lot moxibustion on the four limbs just to eliminate wind evils. Burn seven cones up to seven times seven cones of moxibustion, and no more than the same number of cones as the age of the patient. That is why *Tóng Rén* 《 銅人 》 only mentions burning three cones of moxibustion and needling 5 fēn deep for Sān Lǐ 三里 (ST 36). *Míng Táng Shàng Jīng* 《 明堂上經 》 says: Burn seven cones of moxibustion daily, up to a hundred cones; that is not a lot. But *Qiān Jīn Fāng* 《 千金方 》 says: Burn up to five hundred cones of moxibustion at the most, and two or three hundred cones at the least; that is a lot. To summarize: Burn seven cones of moxibustion daily; or burn two times seven cones if the size of the moxa cone is very small, and up to seven times seven cones in few days. Apply moxibustion again after the moxa sores are dry. This matches the theory of "if you want good health, do not let the Dān Tián 丹田 (cinnabar field) and Sān Lǐ 三里 (ST 36) become dry." If we apply the number of cones stated in *Qiān Jīn* 《 千金 》, I fear it will offend the contraindications in *Xiǎo Pǐn*.

予舊有腳氣疾，遇春則足稍腫，夏中尤甚，至冬腫漸消。偶夏間依《素問》注所說穴之所在，以溫針微刺之，翌日腫消，其神效有如此

---

11. *Tóng* 《 銅 》 should be located in the next parenthesis with the *Míng Xià* 《 明下 》, not here. This was a typographical error.

者。謬刺且爾，況於灸乎。有此疾者，不可不知。此不止治足腫，諸
疾皆治云。

In the past, I suffered the disease of leg qì; my feet were swollen a little bit in the spring, worse in the middle of the summer, and the swelling gradually went away in the winter. In summer, by chance I followed the point location based on the the Annotation of *Sù Wèn* 《 素問 》 and punctured with warm needle [technique]. The swelling dispersed the next day. There are wondrous effects like this. If cross needling can have this effect, how about moxibustion? People should know this if they suffer this disease. It treats not only swelling of the feet, but also all kinds of diseases.

涌泉治心痛不嗜食，婦人無子，男子如蠱，女子如妊娠（《 千 》作如阻 ），
五指端盡痛，足不得履地：宜針灸（《 銅 》）。《 千 》云：主忽忽喜忘，身
體腰脊如解，大便難，小便不利，足中清至膝，咽中痛，不可內食，喑不能
言，衄不止，云云 。

Yǒng Quán 涌泉 (KI 1) treats heart pain, no desire to eat, infertility in women, *gǔ* 蠱 distention in males, [distention] in females that looks like they are pregnant (*Qiān* 《 千 》 says obstruction), pain at the tips of the five toes so that the feet cannot step on the ground: It is appropriate to needle and apply moxibustion [on this point] (*Tóng* 《 銅 》). *Qiān* says: It treats forgetfulness and confusion, [discomfort] in body and low back like they are splitting, difficult defecation, inhibited urination, chills from the center of the feet to the knees, sore pharynx, difficulty swallowing food, loss of voice, incessant bleeding, and so forth.

《 千金 》於諸穴皆分主之，獨於膏肓、三里、涌泉穴特云治雜病。是
三穴者，無所不治也，但《 明堂 》云：若灸，廢人行動爾。既欲愈
疾，雖不行動數日，未為害也。

[Author's notes:] *Qiān Jīn* 《 千金 》 lists the individual indications of the points. But when talking about Gāo Huāng 膏肓 (UB 43), Sān Lǐ 三里 (ST 36), and Yǒng Quán 涌泉 (KI 1), it especially says they treat miscellaneous diseases. That means there is nothing these three points cannot treat. But *Míng Táng* 《 明堂 》 says: People lose mobility when moxibustion is applied on them. If we want to cure disease, even if someone loses his mobility for several days, it is not really harmful.

脾俞治食多身瘦，泄利，體重，四肢不收，腹痛不嗜食（《 銅 》 ）。

Pí Shù 脾俞 (UB 20) treats eating a lot but the body is thin, diarrhea, heavy body, and loss of use of the limbs, abdominal pain and no desire to eat (*Tóng*).

胃俞治胃寒腹脹，不嗜食，羸瘦（《銅》）。

Wèi Shù 胃俞 (UB 21) treats stomach cold, abdominal distention, no desire to eat and marked emaciation (*Tóng* 《銅》).

人之言曰血氣未動者，瘠甚而不害。血氣既竭者，雖肥而死矣。則身之羸瘦，若未足為人之害者。殊不知人之羸瘦，必其飲食不進者也。飲食不進，則無以生榮衛，榮衛無以生，則氣血因之以衰，終於必亡而已。故《難經疏》云：人仰胃氣為主。是人資胃氣以生矣。《五臟論》云：脾不磨食不消。是脾不壯，食無自而消矣。既資胃氣以生，又資脾以消食，其可使脾胃一日不壯哉。必欲脾胃之壯，當灸脾胃俞等穴可也。

[Author's notes:] People say: If blood and qì are not affected, there is no harm even if someone is thin. If blood and qì are exhausted, someone will die, even if they are plump. So marked emaciation alone is not enough to harm people. People hardly realize that the marked emaciation must relate to absence of food intake. Absence of food intake does not allow *yíng* and *wèi* to be engendered; thus it causes debilitation of qì and blood, and finally the person will die. *Nàn Jīng Shū* 《難經疏》 says: People rely on stomach qì as the governing principle; this means people should promote stomach qì in order to live.[12] *Wǔ Zàng Lùn* 《五臟論》 says: If the spleen does not grind, the food will not disperse. So if the spleen is not vigorous, food cannot automatically disperse. People not only depend on stomach qì to survive, but they also rely on the spleen to disperse food. So the spleen and stomach cannot be weak even for one day. One should apply moxibustion on back transport points of spleen and stomach to strengthen the spleen and stomach.

心中風，狂走發癇語悲泣，心胸悶亂，咳唾血：宜針心俞（《銅》）。

Heart wind-strike,[13] frenetic walking, epilepsy, sorrowful speech and weeping, oppression and derangement in the heart and chest, cough and spitting of blood: It is appropriate to needle Xīn Shù 心俞 (UB 15) (*Tóng*).

《難經疏》言：心為臟腑之主，法不受病，病則神去氣竭。故手足為之清（手足節冷），名真心痛，旦發夕死；手足溫者，名厥心痛，可

12. "人仰胃氣為主。是人資胃氣以生矣。 People rely on stomach qì as the governing principle; this means people should *promote* stomach qì in order to *live*." The title of this book comes from this sentence: The Life-Promoting Classic.

13. Heart wind-strike indicates wind invading the heart. Symptoms include fever, inability to get up, lying supine, or lying on the sides.

急治也。故《千金》言：心中風者，急灸心俞百壯，服續命湯。必泥心俞不可灸之說，則無策矣。但心俞雖可針，若刺中心，一日必死，又豈易針耶。必欲無此患，平居當養其心，使之和平，憂愁思慮，不使傷其神，乃策之上。必不免此，亦當服鎮心丹等藥補助，乃其次也。

[Author's notes:] *Nàn Jīng Shū* 《 難經疏 》 says: The heart is the monarch of the organs. Normally, it should not contract disease; if it becomes diseased, the spirit scatters and qì becomes exhausted. If the hands and feet are cold (cold joints in the hands and feet), it is called true heart pain; it comes on in the morning and expires in the evening. If the hands and feet are warm, it is called reversal heart pain; this needs to be treated immediately. *Qiān Jīn* 《 千金 》 says: For heart wind-strike, apply a hundred cones of moxibustion immediately on Xīn Shù 心俞 (UB 15), then take *Xù Mìng Tāng* 續命湯 (Life Prolonging Decoction). If we stick to the theory of "do not apply moxibustion on Xīn Shù (UB 15)," then we do not have any strategy. We can needle Xīn Shù (UB 15), but if the heart is punctured, the patient will die in one day. So this point is not easy to needle. If we do not want to suffer this disease, we should nourish the heart in our daily life, making it calm and harmonized, in order to avoid damage from anxiety, excessive thought, and preoccupation. This is the best strategy. If we cannot avoid [these emotions which damage the heart], we need to take *Zhèn Xīn Dān* 鎮心丹 (Heart Settling Elixir) and so forth to supplement and assist; this is the second choice.

腎俞治虛勞羸瘦，腎虛水臟久冷，小便濁，出精，陰中疼，五勞七傷虛憊，足寒如冰，身腫如水（《銅》）。

Shèn Shù 腎俞 (UB 23) treats vacuity-taxation and marked emaciation, vacuity of the kidneys and enduring coldness of the water viscera, turbid urine, seminal loss, genital pain, the five taxations and the seven damages, vacuity fatigue, icy cold feet, and swollen body that looks like [it is filled with] water (*Tóng* 《 銅 》).

《難經疏》云：夾脊骨有二腎，在左為腎，在右為命門。言命門者，性命之根本也。其穴與臍平，凡灸腎俞者，在平處立，以杖子約量至臍；又以此杖子當背脊骨上量之，知是與臍平處也。然後相去各寸半取其穴，則是腎俞穴也。更以手按其陷中，而後灸之，則不失穴所在矣。凡灸以隨年為壯。灸固有功，亦在人滋養之如何爾。

[Author's notes:] *Nàn Jīng Shū* 《 難經疏 》 says: There are two kidneys, one on each side of the spine; the one on the left is the kidney; the one on the right is Life Gate. Life Gate is the root of life. Its points are level with the umbilicus. When applying moxibustion on Shèn Shù (UB 23), ask the patient to stand on a level place; measure [from the ground up to] the umbilicus with a stick; then measure [from the ground up to] the spine with the same stick to find the site which is level with the umbilicus. Locate the points 1.5 cùn away from the spine. These are Shèn Shù (UB 23). Press the depression, then apply the moxibustion on it; this way the points will not be missed. Burn the same number of cones as the age of the patient. Though moxibustion works, we still need to enrich and nourish the kidneys.

人當愛護丹田。吾既於《既效方》論之詳矣，而妻妾之戕害，蓋未之
及也。君子偕老之序曰：夫人淫亂，失事君子之道，故陳人君之德，
服飾之盛，宜與君子偕老也。宜偕老而不至偕老，夫人之罪多矣。故
詩人以是刺之，意可見也。至於士夫志得意滿，不期驕而驕至，侍妾
數十人，少亦三五輩，淫言藝語，不絕於耳，不能自克，而淫縱其欲
者多矣。為內子者，恬不之怪。人有問之者，則曰自母言之，則為賢
母，自我言之，未免為妒婦人也。人或以此多之，其夫亦以為賢而不
妒，孰知其不妒乃所以為禍之歟。雖然，二南之化，至於無妒忌而
止。今而言此，豈求異於詩人耶？是不然。古人十日一御，荀子彼其
不妒者，蓋使媵妾得備十日一御之數爾。不妒則同，所以不妒則異。
吾故表而出之，以為夫婦之戒，固非求異於詩人也。

People should take good care of the Dān Tián 丹田 (cinnabar field). I have discussed this in detail in *Jì Xiào Fāng* 《既效方》 (Already Effective Formulas), but the damage from wives and concubines has not been thoroughly explained. The preface of [a poem named] *Jūn zǐ xié lǎo* 君子偕老 [Growing Old Together with the King, my Husband][14] says: "The wife was licentious; she failed to serve the King in the proper way. So [the poem] explained that if she was virtuous as the wife of the King, she could wear splendid attire and live with her husband, the king, until death." It is suitable for a husband and wife to live together until death, but this couple could not and the wife was more to blame. Thus, the poet used this poem to mock her [the king's wife]; his intention can be seen. A successful gentleman can unexpectedly become arrogant. He can have dozens or at least three or five concubines. Their obscene words keep coming and lingering in his ears. He cannot control himself; most people like him will indulge in desires without restraint. The wives are calm and do not consider this odd at all. When people ask why, they say: As a mother, we will be virtuous; as a woman, we would rather not be jealous. People praise them because of this, and their husbands think the wives are virtuous and are not jealous. Actually, this attitude can cause trouble; even though the civilization of *Èr Nán* (the Two Souths)[15] had no jealousy, it ended. What I discuss

14. *Jūn zǐ xié lǎo* [Growing Old Together with the King, my Husband] is a poem from *Shī Jīng* 《詩經》 (The Classic of Poetry, also translated variously as the Book of Songs, or the Book of Odes). It is the earliest existing collection of Chinese poems and songs, consisting of 305 poems and songs, many dating from the 10th to the 7th century BCE. In this poem, Jūnzǐ refers to King Wèi Xuān Gōng who reigned 718-700 BCE. The preface is from annotations to *Shī Jīng* made during the Western *Hàn* Dynasty by Máo Hēng 毛亨 and Máo Cháng 毛萇.

15. Èr Nán 二南 (the Two Souths) indicates Shào Nán 召南 and Zhōu Nán 周南. They were two states in ancient China.

today, how could I disagree with the poet? The ancient people had sexual activity every ten days. Xúnzǐ[16] said: The reason for not having jealousy is that the concubines knew the rule of having sexual activity every ten days. Being without jealousy is same, but the reason for it is different.[17] I express my opinion here, not because I disagree with the poet, but to warn couples about this.

曲骨主失精，五臟虛竭：灸五十壯（《千》）。《明下》云：但是虛乏冷極，皆宜灸。

Qū Gǔ 曲骨 (Rèn 2) governs seminal loss, vacuity, and exhaustion of five viscera: Apply fifty cones of moxibustion (*Qiān* 《千》). *Míng Xià* 《明下》 says: It is appropriate to apply moxibustion for vacuity fatigue and extreme cold.

骨髓冷疼，灸上廉七十壯（《千》）。

Cold pain of the marrow: Apply seventy cones of moxibustion on Shàng Lián 上廉 (ST 37) (*Qiān*).

《難經疏·八會》曰：腑會中管，治腑之病。臟會章門，臟病治此。筋會陽陵泉，筋病治此。髓會絕骨，髓病治此。血會膈俞，血病治此。骨會大杼（禁灸），骨病治此。脈會太淵，脈病治此。氣會膻中，氣病治此。然則骨髓有病，當先大杼、絕骨，而後上廉可也。

[Author's notes:] *Nàn Jīng Shū·Bā Huì* 《難經疏·八會》 (Eight Meeting Points) says: The meeting [influential] point of the bowels is Zhōng Guǎn 中管 (Rèn 12), it can treat the diseases of the bowels; the meeting [influential] point of the viscera is Zhāng Mén 章門 (LV 13), it can treat diseases of the viscera; the meeting [influential] point of the sinews is Yáng Líng Quán 陽陵泉 (GB 34), it can treat diseases of the sinews; the meeting [influential] point of the marrow is Jué Gǔ 絕骨 (GB 39), it can treat diseases of the marrow; the meeting [influential] point of the blood is Gé Shù 膈俞 (UB 17), it can treat diseases of the blood; the meeting [influential] point of the bones is Dà Zhù 大杼 (UB 11) (moxibustion is contraindicated), it can treat diseases of the bones; the meeting [influential] point of the vessels is Tài Yuān 太淵 (LU 9), it can treat diseases of the vessels; the meeting [influential] point of the qì is Dàn Zhōng 膻中 (Rèn 17), it can treat diseases of qì. For diseases of the marrow, [treat] Dà Zhù (UB 11) and Jué Gǔ (GB 39) first and then Shàng Lián (ST 37).

16. Xúnzǐ 荀子 (312–230 BC) was a Chinese Confucian philosopher who lived during the Warring States Period and contributed to one of the Hundred Schools of Thought. Xúnzǐ 荀子 believed a person's inborn tendencies needed to be curbed through education and ritual.

17. The two cases mentioned here where there is no jealosy are 1. wives who allow their husbands to have concubines and 2. concubines who know that they can have sex every ten days. In both cases, these women are not jealous, but their reasoning is different.

膀胱、三焦津液少，大小腸寒熱（見腰痛），或三焦寒熱：灸小腸俞五十
壯。三焦、膀胱、腎中熱氣：灸水道隨年（《千》）。膏肓俞主無所不療：
羸瘦虛損，夢中失精，上氣咳逆，發狂健忘等疾。

Insufficient fluid in the urinary bladder and sānjiāo, cold and heat in the large and small intestines (see the section on lower back pain) or sānjiāo: Apply fifty cones of moxibustion on Xiǎo Cháng Shù 小腸俞 (UB 27).

Hot qì in the sānjiāo, urinary bladder and kidneys (*Qiān* 《千》): Burn the same number of cones as the patient's age on Shuǐ Dào 水道 (ST 28).

Gāo Huāng Shù 膏肓俞 (UB 43) treats everything: marked emaciation, seminal loss while dreaming, counterflow qì ascent with cough, mania and forgetfulness, and so forth.

膏肓俞無所不療，而古人不能求其穴。是以晉景公有疾，秦醫曰緩者
視之曰：在肓之上、膏之下，攻之不可，達之不及，藥不至焉，不可
為也。晉侯以為良醫，而孫真人乃笑其拙，為不能尋其穴而灸之也。
若李子豫之赤龍丹，又能治其膏肓上五音下之鬼，無待於灸也。是緩
非特拙於不能灸，亦無殺鬼藥矣。其亦技止於此哉。

[Author's notes:] Gāo Huāng Shù (UB 43) cures everything, but ancient people did not [know how to] find the point. When Jìn Jǐng Gōng 晉景公 (the Duke Jìng 景 of Jìn 晉) was sick, Doctor Huǎn from Qín went to see him and said: The disease is located above *gāo* 膏 (fat below the tip of the heart) and below the *huāng* 肓 (the space below the heart and above the diaphragm). Moxibustion cannot attack it, acupuncture cannot reach it, herbs cannot arrive there; so the disease was not treatable. Duke Jìn thought Huǎn was a good doctor, but Sūn Zhēnrén laughed at his clumsiness, because [Doctor Huǎn] could not find the point and apply moxibustion. It seems that *Chì Lóng Dān* 赤龍丹 (Red Dragon Elixir) from Lǐ Zǐyù[18] can treat ghosts above the Gāo Huāng 膏肓 and below the five tones,[19] so there is no need to wait for moxibustion. Because Huǎn was not good at moxibustion, and there were no herbs to kill ghosts, his skill stopped at this [level].

---

18. Lǐ Zǐyù 李子豫 was a doctor during the *Jìn* (晉) Dynasty.

19. The five notes indicate the five-tone scale in ancient Chinese music. They are *Gōng* 宮, *Shāng* 商, *Jüé* 角, *Zhǐ* 徵, and *Yǔ* 羽. They are equivalent to do, re, mi, sol, and la in the Western music scale. In Chinese medicine each viscera corresponds to one note.

3.02
Jiǔ Èr Shí Zhǒng Gǔ Zhēng

炙二十種骨蒸

Applying moxibustion for twenty kinds of steaming bone [disease][20]

崔知悌序云：骨蒸病者，亦名傳尸，亦謂殗殜，亦稱復連，亦曰無辜。丈夫以精氣為根，女人以血氣為本。無問老少，多染此疾。予嘗三十日灸活十三人，前後瘥者，數逾二百。非止單攻骨蒸，又別療氣療風，或瘴或勞，或邪或癖。病狀既廣，灸活者不可具錄。灸後宜服治勞地黃元，良。

The preface of *Cuī Zhīdī*[21] says: Steaming bone disease[22] is also called *chuán shī* 傳尸 [corpse transmission], or *yè dié* 殗殜 [mild disease with occasional need to lie down], or *fù lián* 復連 [marked emaciation], or *wú gū* 無辜 [marked emaciation in children]. Essence and qì are considered the root in males while the females take blood and qì as their origin. No matter if old or young, people frequently contract this disease. Once, within thirty days I saved thirteen people and totally cured more than two hundred people with moxibustion. I applied moxibustion not only to attack steaming bone disease, but also treat qì and wind [diseases], or miasma, or taxation, or evils, or aggregations. Since the list of symptoms is so broad, all the people who are able to survive after moxibustion cannot be recorded completely. It is very good to take *Zhì Láo Dì Huáng Yuán* 治勞地黃元 (Rehmannia Pill for treating Consumption) after the moxibustion treatment.

凡取四花穴：以稻稈心量口縫如何闊，斷其長多少；以如此長裁紙四方，當中剪小孔。別用長稻稈踏腳下，前取腳大指為止，後取腳曲跧橫紋中為止。斷了卻環在喉結下垂向背後，看稈止處。即以前小孔紙當中安，分為四花，蓋灸紙四角也。又一醫傳一法：先橫量口吻取長短，以所量草就背上三椎骨下直量至草盡處，兩頭用筆點了，再量中

---

20. This chapter is not listed in the main table of contents.

21. Cuī Zhīdī 崔知悌 was a famous doctor of the *Táng* (唐) Dynasty. He was the author of *Gǔ Zhēng Bìng Jiǔ Fāng* 《骨蒸病灸方》 (Moxibustion formulas for steaming bone disease).

22. Steaming bone disease is caused by insufficiency of yīn. It includes the symptoms of tidal fever with morning coolness and nighttime fevers, irritability, disturbed sleep, dark urination, and five center heat. It is usually associated with tuberculosis in Western medicine.

指長短為準。卻將量中指草橫直量兩頭，用筆圈四角，其圈者是穴（不圈不是穴）。可灸七七壯止。

[Author's notes:] To locate the four flowers point: measure the width of the person's mouth with a stalk of straw and break it [at this length]. Cut a square of paper the length of this straw and snip a small hole in the center. Place another long stalk of straw below the foot, and measure from the tip of the big toe in the front to the transverse curved crease [of the knee] at the back of the leg. Break the stalk [at this length] and wrap it around the neck below the Adam's apple, letting the ends of the stalk hang down the back. Place the small hole of the previously made square of paper at the ends of the stalks. Apply moxibustion to the four corners of the paper. This corresponds to the four flowers.

There is another method from a different doctor: measure the width of the mouth with a blade of grass, and place the blade of grass vertically below the third vertebra on the back. Mark the two ends of the blade of grass; then measure the length of the middle finger with another blade of grass as the standard; place this grass transversely [centered on each of the two previous marks]. Mark a circle on the four corners with brush. The points are in the circles (What is outside the circle is not the point). Apply seven times seven cones of moxibustion.

3.03
Láo Zhài (Chuán Shī, Gǔ Zhēng, Léi Shòu)

勞瘵（傳尸　骨蒸　羸瘦）

Consumption
(Corpse-transmission, steaming bones, marked emaciation)

中髎治丈夫五勞七傷六極，腰痛，大便難，小便淋瀝，腹脹下利食泄（《
銅》）。三里治五勞羸瘦，七傷虛乏。《明下》云：五勞虛乏，四肢羸瘦。
肩井治五勞七傷。大椎治五勞七傷，溫瘧痎瘧，氣疰背膊急，頸項強（《
明》上、下同），風勞食氣。肺俞治寒熱喘滿，虛煩口乾，傳尸骨蒸勞，肺
痿咳嗽。《明》云：療肉痛皮癢，傳尸骨蒸肺嗽。魄戶治虛勞肺痿（《明》
云勞損痿黃），五尸走疰，項強。《明下》云：療勞損虛乏。

Zhōng Liáo 中髎 (UB 33) treats[23] the five taxations, the seven damages, and the six extremes,[24] lower back pain, difficult defecation, dribbling urination, abdominal distention, diarrhea, and food damage diarrhea [all] in males (*Tóng* 《銅》).

Sān Lǐ 三里 (ST 36 or LI 10) treats the five taxations, marked emaciation, the seven damages and vacuity-fatigue. *Míng Xià* 《明下》 says: The five taxations, vacuity-fatigue, and marked emaciation of four limbs.

Jiān Jǐng 肩井 (GB 21) treats the five taxations and the seven damages.

Dà Zhuī 大椎 (Dū 14) treats the five taxations and the seven damages, warm malaria, chronic malaria, qì infixation,[25] back and arm tension, stiffness of the neck and nape (*Míng Shàng* 《明上》 and *Xià* 《下》 agree), wind taxation, and consumption of qì.

---

23. From this point on, the word *zhì* 治 "treat" indicates that the text is quoted from *Tóng Rén Tú Jīng* 《銅人圖經》; the word *liáo* 療 "cure" indicates that the text is quoted from *Shèng Huì Fāng* 《聖惠方》; the word *zhǔ* 主 "govern" indicates that the text is quoted from *Qiān Jīn Yào Fāng* 《千金要方》, Volume 30.

24. The six extremes indicate six kinds of extreme vacuity. The six extremes are blood extreme, sinew extreme, flesh extreme, qì extreme, bone extreme, and essence extreme.

25. *Zhù* 疰 (infixation) indicates chronic diseases of long duration and infectious diseases.

Fèi Shù 肺俞 (UB 13) treats [sensations of] cold and heat, panting and fullness, vacuity-vexation, dry mouth, corpse-transmission and steaming bones, lung wilting, and cough. *Míng* 《 明 》 says: It cures flesh pain and itching skin, corpse-transmission, steaming bones, and lung cough.

Pò Hù 魄戶 (UB 42) treats vacuity-fatigue and lung wilting (*Míng* says: taxation and detriment and withered yellowing), five corpse[26] infixation, and neck stiffness. *Míng Xià* 《 明下 》 says: It cures taxation and detriment and vacuity fatigue.

秦承祖云：支正療五勞，四肢力弱虛乏等（《 明下 》）。譩譆療勞損虛乏，不得睡。下焦俞療背痛身熱。曲骨但是虛乏冷極皆灸。氣海療冷病，面黑，肌體羸瘦，四肢力弱，小腹氣積聚，賁豚，腹弱脫陽欲死不知人，五臟氣逆上攻。

Qín Chéngzǔ said: Zhī Zhèng 支正 (SI 7) cures the five taxations and weakness and fatigue of four limbs, etc. (*Míng Xià*).

Yī Xī 譩譆 (UB 45) cures taxation and detriment, vacuity-fatigue, and insomnia.

Xià Jiāo Shù 下焦俞 [Lower Burner Transport][27] cures back pain and body heat.

Applying moxibustion on Qū Gǔ 曲骨 (Rèn 2) treats vacuity fatigue and extreme cold.

Qì Hǎi 氣海 (Rèn 6) treats cold diseases, dark facial complexion, marked emaciation, weakness of four limbs, accumulations and gatherings of qì in smaller abdomen, running-piglet qì, weakness of the abdomen with collapse of yáng and unconsciousness; and counterflow qì of the five viscera attacking upward.

膏肓俞治羸瘦虛損，夢中失精，無所不療（《 銅 》）。腎俞治虛勞羸瘦，耳聾，腎虛水臟久冷（《 明 》有腰痛），心腹膨脹，脅滿引小腹痛，目視眈眈，少氣溺血，小便濁，出精陰疼，五勞七傷虛憊，腳膝拘急（《 明 》有好獨臥），足寒如冰，頭重身熱振栗，腰中四肢淫濼，洞泄食不化，身腫如水。《 明下 》云：療身寒熱，食多身羸瘦，面黃黑，目眈眈，女久積冷氣成勞。

---

26. Five corpse infixation: Flying corpse infixation has wandering pain under the skin and between the muscles, and stabbing pain that occurs randomly; fixed corpse infixation has fullness and distention of the heart and abdomen with stabbing pain that occurs suddenly, also accompanied by panting and qì surging upward into the chest; sinking corpse infixation has colicky pain and distention of the heart and abdomen with panting, and pain and distention attacking the rib-sides; wind corpse infixation has weakened extremities due to wind; in hidden corpse infixation, the disease hides deeply inside the body. There are no symptoms when it is stable; during episodes, prickly pain of the heart and abdomen with panting and distention occur.

27. The location of this point is uncertain.

Gāo Huāng Shù 膏肓俞 (UB 43) treats all [kinds of conditions such as] marked emaciation, vacuity-detriment, and seminal loss while dreaming, there is nothing it does not cure. (*Tóng* 《銅》).

Shèn Shù 腎俞 (UB 23) treats vacuity fatigue with marked emaciation, deafness, kidney vacuity and enduring coldness of the water viscera (*Míng* 《明》 has lower back pain), inflation in heart and abdomen, rib-side fullness with pain radiating to the smaller abdomen, blurred vision, qì shortage and bloody urine, cloudy urine, seminal loss and genital pain, the five taxations and the seven damages, vacuity fatigue, tension of knees and feet (*Míng* also has somnolence), icy cold feet, heaviness of the head and body heat with shivering, soreness and weakness of the low back and four limbs, throughflux diarrhea and non-transformation of food, and swollen body as if it is filled with water. *Míng Xià* 《明下》 says: It treats [sensations of] cold and heat of the body, eating a lot with marked emaciation, yellow and dark facial complexion, blurred vision and taxation in women caused by enduring accumulation of cold qì.

腦空治勞疾，贏瘦，體熱，頸項強。章門治傷飽，身黃贏瘦。漏谷治食不為肌膚。下管治日漸贏瘦（見痞癖）。下管（見腹脹）、胃俞（見虛損）、脾俞、下廉（見飧泄）治贏瘦。

Nǎo Kōng 腦空 (GB 19) treats taxation diseases, marked emaciation, hot body, and stiffness of the neck and nape.

Zhāng Mén 章門 (LV 13) treats damage from overeating, yellow body, and marked emaciation.

Lòu Gǔ 漏谷 (SP 7) treats [the condition of food that is] eaten does not become flesh and skin.

Xià Guǎn 下管 (Rèn 10) treats gradual marked emaciation (see the section on strings and aggregations).

Xià Guǎn (Rèn 10) (see the section on abdominal fullness), Wèi Shù 胃俞 (UB 21) (see the section on vacuity detriment), Pí Shù 脾俞 (UB 20), and Xià Lián 下廉 (ST 39 or LI 8) (see the section on swill diarrhea) treats marked emaciation.

小兒贏瘦，食飲少、不生肌膚：灸胃俞一壯（《明下》）。

Marked emaciation, loss of appetite, and [food] does not generate flesh and skin in children: Apply one cone of moxibustion on Wèi Shù 胃俞 (UB 21) (*Míng Xià* 《明下》).

灸勞法：其狀手足心熱，多盜汗，精神困頓，骨節疼寒；初發咳嗽，漸吐膿血；肌瘦面黃，減食少力。令身正直，用草子，男左女右，自腳中指尖量過腳心下，向上至曲䐐大紋處截斷。卻將此草自鼻尖量，從頭正中（須分開頭

心發貼肉量）至脊，以草盡處用墨點記 。別用草一條，令病患自然合口量闊
狹截斷，卻將此草於墨點上平折兩頭盡處量穴 。灸時隨年多灸一壯（ 如年三
十，灸三十一 ），累效（《 集效 》）。

Moxibustion method for taxation: The symptoms include heat in the palms and soles, night sweat-ing, spirit exhaustion, and cold painful joints. There is cough in the beginning; then it gradually develops into spitting of blood and pus, thin muscles, yellow facial complexion, loss of appetite and weakness. Let the patient stand up straight. Using the left side on males and the right side on fe-males, measure with a straw from the tip of middle toe, through the sole, up to the big curved crease [of the knee]. Cut the straw and use it to measure from the tip of the nose to the spine, through the midline of the head (parting the hair on the vertex and measuring on the flesh [scalp]). Mark the site at the end of the straw with ink. Ask the patient to close his mouth naturally, use another straw to measure the width of his mouth, and cut it. Place this straw horizontally on the ink-marked spot, laying the two ends flat. The point is located at the ends of the straw. Apply the same number of the cones as the patient's age and add one more (for age 30, apply thirty-one cones of moxibustion). It has cumulative effects (*Jí Xiào* 《 集效 》).

羸瘦固瘵疾， 自有寒熱等證， 宜隨證醫治。若素來清癯者， 非有疾
也。惟病後瘦甚， 久不復常， 謂之形脫。與夫平昔充肥， 忽爾羸瘦，
飲食減少者， 或有他疾乘之， 則難救療。須辨之於早， 而著艾可也。
然仲景論六極， 必曰：精極令人氣少無力， 漸漸內虛， 身無潤澤， 翁
翁羸瘦， 眼無精光， 且云八味腎氣差六極。而差五勞則是八味丸所當
服（仲景常服， 或常服去附子加五味子）。而腎俞等穴， 尤所當灸
也。

[Author's notes:] Marked emaciation is certainly a consumptive disease, but it also has cold and heat patterns. It is appropriate to treat according to the differentiation. If the patient has always been thin, that is not this disease; this is only if the patient becomes thin after illness and cannot return to normal for a long time. It is called shedding of the physical body [marked emaciation]. For example, if the patient was always fat, but suddenly became markedly emaciated with decreased food intake; or if other diseases are attacking, it is then difficult to treat. We should make an early diagnosis and apply moxibustion. When [Zhāng] Zhòngjǐng discussed the six extremes he said: Essence extreme causes qì shortage and weakness in people, and then there is gradual development of internal vacuity, absence of body moisture, severe marked emaciation and lack of spirit in eyes. *Bā Wèi Shèn Qì* [*Wán*] 八味腎氣 [丸] (Eight Ingredients for Kidney Qì Pill) cures the Six Extremes, while *Bā Wèi Wán* 八味丸 (Eight Ingredients Pill) cures the five taxations ([Zhāng] Zhòngjǐng usually gave this; or removed the *fù zǐ* 附子 (Aconiti Radix) and added *wǔ wèi zǐ* 五味子 (Schisandrae Fructus). It is appropriate to apply moxibustion on Shèn Shù 腎俞 (UB 23).

脾俞、大腸俞主腹中氣脹，引脊痛。食多身羸瘦，名曰食晦：先取脾俞，後取季肋。五臟六腑心腹滿，腰背痛，飲食吐逆，寒熱往來，小便不利，羸瘦少氣：灸三焦俞隨年（《千》）。

Pí Shù 脾俞 (UB 20) and Dà Cháng Shù 大腸俞 (UB 25) govern qì distention of the abdomen with pain radiating to the spine.

[When] someone eats a lot, but has marked emaciation, this is called *shí huì* 食晦: Treat Pí Shù (UB 20) first, then Jì Xié 季脅 (LV 13).

Fullness of the heart and abdomen, lower and upper back pain, overeating, counterflow vomiting, alternating [sensations of] cold and heat, inhibited urination, marked emaciation and qì shortage: Apply the same number of cones of moxibustion as the age of the patient on Sān Jiāo Shù 三焦俞 (UB 22) (*Qiān* 《千》).

3.04
Shèn Xū (Shèn Qì, Xiǎo Cháng Qì)

腎虛（腎氣　小腸氣）

Kidney vacuity
(Kidney qì, small intestine qì[28])

腎俞治腎虛水臟久冷（《銅》見勞，《明》同 ）。中膂俞治腎虛消渴（ 見渴 ）。陽蹻療腎氣（《明》 ）。下廉療小腸氣不足，面無顏色 。

Shèn Shù 腎俞 (UB 23) treats kidney vacuity and enduring coldness in the water viscus (see the section on taxation in *Tóng* 《銅》; *Míng* 《明》 agrees).

Zhōng Lǚ Shù 中膂俞 (UB 29) treats kidney vacuity and wasting-thirst [diabetes mellitus] (see the section on thirst [Wasting-thirst disorder]).

Yáng Qiāo 陽蹻 (UB 62) cures kidney qì (*Míng*).

Xià Lián 下廉 (ST 39 or LI 8) cures insufficient qì of the small intestine and pale facial complexion.

灸小腸氣疝癖氣，發時腹痛若刀刺不可忍者：並婦女本藏氣血癖，走疰刺痛，或坐臥不得，或大小便不通，可思飲食：於左右腳下下第二指第一節曲紋中心，各灸十壯，每壯如赤豆大 。甚驗（《集效》 ）。（一云：治寒病腎腸氣發，牽連外腎大痛，腫硬如石。）

Applying moxibustion for small intestine qì with strings and aggregations of qì, initially with unbearable abdominal pain like the stabbing of a knife; plus females with qì and blood aggregations in the viscera, wandering infixation with pricking pain, or inability to sit or lie down, or difficult defecation and urination, but with a desire to eat: Apply ten cones of moxibustion on the center of the first curved crease under the second toe of the left and right feet.[29] Burn cones the size of a red bean. This is very effective (*Jí Xiào* 《集效》). (One source says: This treats cold disease with kidney

---

28. The text in parenthesis is added based on the main table of contents.
29. This would be located on the plantar side of the toe. It is not certain whether this is the first crease moving distally or proximally, but it seems to be the proximal crease.

and intestine qì disorders, as well as severe pain radiating to the external kidneys [male genitals] which are swollen and hard like a stone.)

治小腸氣方甚多，未必皆效。《耆域方》奪命散、《良方》蒼猝散皆已試之效者。有一兵患小腸氣，依此方灸足第二指下文五壯，略效而再發，恐壯數未多也。予以鎮靈丹十粒與之，令早晚服五粒而愈。灸固捷於藥，若灸不得穴，又不如藥相當者見效之速。且灸且藥，方為當爾。近傳一立聖散，用全干蠍七枚、縮砂仁三七枚、炒茴香一錢為末，分三服，熱酒調下和滓空心服。此疾是小腸受熱，蘊積不散，久而成疾，服此立效。雖未試用，以其說有理，故附於此。

There are a lot of formulas to treat small intestine qì, but not all of them are effective. *Duó Mìng Sǎn* 奪命散 (Life Clutching Powder) from *Qí Yù Fāng*《耆域方》(Formulas from *Qí Yù*) and *Cāng Cù Sǎn* 蒼猝散 (Urgency Powder) from *Liáng Fāng*《良方》are tested and are effective. There was a soldier who suffered small intestine qì; I followed the above method and applied five cones of moxibustion on the crease under his second toes. It had some effect but the disorder relapsed. I am afraid that I did not burn enough cones. So I gave him 10 pieces of *Zhèn Líng Dān* 鎮靈丹 (Settle the Spirit Elixir) and asked him to take five pieces each time in the morning and evening. The disease was cured. Though moxibustion is better than herbs, if it is not applied on the right points, it won't have the same rapid effect as herbs. The most appropriate method is to combine moxibustion and herbs together. Recently, people have been talking about a *Lì Shèng Sǎn* 立聖散 which is made from the powder of seven pieces of dried *quán xiē* 全蝎 (scorpions), 3-7 pieces *suō shā rén* 縮砂仁 (Amomi Villosi Semen seu Fructus) and 1 *qián* [3 grams] of fried *huí xiāng* 茴香 (Foeniculi Fructus). Divide the powder into three portions, mix [one portion] with warm liquor, then drink it along with the dregs on an empty stomach. This disease is caused by heat attacking small intestine and accumulating for a long time. It is effective immediately upon taking this powder. I have not tried it yet, but the theory is reasonable, so I attach it here.

有士人年少，覓灸夢遺。為點腎俞酸痛，其令灸而愈。則不拘老少，腎皆虛也。古人云：百病皆生於心。又云：百病皆生於腎。心勞生百病，人皆知之，腎虛亦生百病，人未知也。蓋天一生水，地二生火，腎水不上升，則心火不下降，茲病所由生也。人不可不養心，不愛護腎乎。

A young man asked for moxibustion for seminal emissions with dreams. I palpated *Shèn Shù* 腎俞 (UB 23) on him, and it was sore. After applying moxibustion, the disease was cured. The kidneys [can be] vacuous no matter how old or young. People in ancient times said: The hundred diseases arise out of the heart. The hundred diseases also arise out of the kidneys. People all knew that heart taxation could cause the hundred diseases, but they did not know that kidney vacuity also can cause the hundred diseases. Heaven-one generates water while earth-two generates fire; if kidney-water cannot rise upward, then heart-fire will fail to bear down, thus this is the source of the diseases that are generated. So people should nourish the heart and protect the kidneys.

3.05
Xiāo Kě (Xiāo Shèn Xiāo Zhōng)

消渴（消腎　消中）

Wasting-thirst
(Kidney wasting, center wasting)

商丘主煩中渴（《千》）。意舍主消渴，身熱面目黃（《明》同）。承漿（《明下》云飲水不休）、意舍、關衝、然谷主消渴嗜飲。隱白主飲渴。勞宮主苦渴食不下。曲池主寒熱渴。行間、太衝主嗌乾善渴（並《千》）。

Shāng Qiū 商丘 (SP 5) governs vexation and thirst (*Qiān* 《千》).

Yì Shě 意舍 (UB 49) governs wasting-thirst, generalized fever, and yellow face and eyes (*Míng* 《明》 agrees).

Chéng Jiāng 承漿 (Rèn 24) (*Míng Xià* 《明下》 says incessant drinking of water), Yì Shě (UB 49), Guān Chōng 關衝 (SJ 1) and Rán Gǔ 然谷 (KI 2) govern wasting-thirst, and fondness for drinking [fluids].

Yǐn Bái 隱白 (SP 1) governs thirsty drinking.

Láo Gōng 勞宮 (PC 8) governs severe thirst and difficulty getting food down.

Qū Chí 曲池 (LI 11) governs thirst with desire for cold or hot drinks.

Xíng Jiān 行間 (LV 2) and Tài Chōng 太衝 (LV 3) govern dry throat with tendency to drink [fluids] (all in *Qiān*).

意舍（見腹脹）、中膂俞治腎虛消渴，汗不出（《明》作汗出），腰脊不得俯仰，腹脹脅痛（《銅》）。兌端治小便黃，舌乾消渴。然谷治舌縱煩滿消渴。水溝治消渴飲水無度（《明》同）。陽綱療消渴（《明下》見腸鳴）。

Yì Shě 意舍 (UB 49) (see the section on abdominal fullness) and Zhǒng Lǚ Shù 中膂俞 (UB 29) treats kidney vacuity, wasting-thirst, absence of sweating (*Míng*《明》says sweating), inability to bend the lumbar spine forward and backward, abdominal distention, and rib-side pain (*Tóng*《銅》).

Duì Duān 兌端 (Dū 27) treats yellow urine, dry tongue, and wasting-thirst.

Rán Gǔ 然谷 (KI 2) treats protracted tongue, vexation, fullness, and wasting-thirst.

Shuǐ Gōu 水溝 (Dū 26) treats wasting-thirst and drinking water without limit (*Míng* agrees).

Yáng Gāng 陽綱 (UB 48) cures wasting-thirst (see the section on rumbling intestines in *Míng Xià*《明下》)

古方載渴病有三，曰消渴，曰消中，曰消腎。消腎，最忌房事。李祠部必云腎虛則消渴，消中亦當忌也。張仲景云：宜服八味丸，或服之不效者，不去附子也。有同舍患此，人教服去附子加五味子八味元，即效。有同官患此，予教服《千金》枸杞湯，效。

[Author's notes:] Ancient medical books have three thirsting disorders: wasting-thirst, center wasting, and kidney wasting. Bedroom activities are most contraindicated for kidney wasting. Officer Lǐ of the Ministry of Sacrifices said kidney vacuity results in wasting-thirst. People who have center wasting also need to shun [bedroom activities]. Zhāng Zhòngjǐng said: It is appropriate to take *Bā Wèi Wán* 八味丸 (Eight Ingredients Pill). Do not remove *fù zǐ* 附子 (Aconiti Radix) if it is not effective. A friend suffered this, and someone asked him to take [this pill], but to remove the fù zǐ and add *wǔ wèi zǐ* 五味子 (Schisandrae Fructus). It worked right away. A co-officer suffered this too, and I asked him to take *Gǒu Qí Tāng* 枸杞湯 (Lycium Decoction) from *Qiān Jīn*《千金》. It was effective.

坡文載眉山張醫治楊穎臣渴病（見坡）：麝香當門子，酒漬作十元。取枳枸（俗謂雞距子，亦曰癩漢指頭），作湯，飲之愈。張云：消渴消中，皆脾衰而腎敗，土不能勝水，腎液不上溯，乃成此疾。今診楊脾極巨，脈熱而腎衰，當由果實過度，虛熱在脾，故飲食兼人而多飲水。水多故溺多，非消渴也。麝香能敗酒，瓜果近輒不植；屋外有枳枸木，屋中釀酒不熟；故以二物去酒果毒。其論渴有理。故載於此。

[Sū Dōng] Pō [蘇東]坡 recorded what Master Zhāng from Méi Shān used to treat Yáng Yǐngchén 楊穎臣, who had thirsting disease (see Pō 坡): Soak 10 pieces of granular musk in liquor and decoct *zhǐ gǒu* 枳枸[30] in it (this is usually called *jī jù zǐ* 雞距子 [chicken claw], also

---

30. *Zhǐ gǒu* 枳枸 is also called *zhǐ jǔ zǐ* 枳椇子 (Turnjujube) [Hovenia Acerba Lindl]. This fruit

named *lài hàn zhǐ tóu* 癩漢指頭 [fingers of leprosy patient]). Drink the decoction and the disease will be cured. Master Zhāng said: Wasting-thirst and center wasting are both due to spleen debilitation and vanquished kidneys. Earth cannot overcome the water; kidney fluid cannot flow upward, and this leads to the disease. Now when checked, Yáng [Yǐngchén]'s spleen was extremely large, the vessel was hot, and his kidneys were debilitated. He ate too much - there was vacuity heat in his spleen, so he ate and drank more than [normal] people. If someone drinks a lot and urinates a lot it is not wasting-thirst. Musk can ruin liquor and fruit trees cannot be planted nearby. If there is a *zhǐ gǒu* 枳枸 tree outside the house, liquor won't mature inside the house. So these two things can remove the toxicity of liquor and fruit. This discussion of thirsting is reasonable, so I attached it here.

凡消渴經百日以上，不得灸刺。灸刺則於瘡上漏膿水不歇，遂致癰疽羸瘦而死。亦忌有所誤傷。初得患者，可如方刺灸。若灸諸陰而不愈，宜灸諸陽（詳見《千金》，有數十穴）。

Do not apply acupuncture and moxibustion on people who suffer wasting-thirst for more than a hundred days. There will be sores with incessant discharge of pus after acupuncture and moxibustion; this will lead to abscesses, as well as marked emaciation. People die from these diseases. Accidental injury should also be avoided. During the beginning stage of [the disease], we can follow above methods and apply acupuncture and moxibustion. If it is not cured after applying moxibustion on the various yīn [aspects of the body], then try it on the various yáng [aspects] (See the details in *Qiān Jīn* 《千金》. There are several tens of points).

---

enters the spleen and heart channels. It can be used to treat vexation, feeling hot, thirst, vomiting, and drunkenness.

3.06

Yīn Wěi Suō (Liǎng Wán Qiān)

陰痿縮（兩丸騫）

Wilted and retracted genitals
(Defects of both testicles [sinking and retracting])

陰谷主陰痿，小腹急引陰內廉痛（《千》）。大赫、然谷主精溢上縮。太衝主兩丸騫縮，腹堅不得臥（《甲》云：臍環痛，陰騫兩丸縮）。石門主小腹堅痛，下引陰中，不得小便，兩丸騫。陰交主腹膜堅，痛引陰中，不得小便，兩丸騫。陰縮：灸中封。大赫（見失精）、中封主痿厥（見疝）。曲泉主不尿，陰痿。

Yīn Gǔ 陰谷 (KI 10) governs genital wilting and tension of the smaller abdomen with pain radiating to the medial aspect of the genitals (*Qiān* 《千》).

Dà Hè 大赫 (KI 12) and Rán Gǔ 然谷 (KI 2) govern seminal spillage and upward retraction [of the genitals].

Tài Chōng 太衝 (LV 3) governs retraction of the two testicles and abdominal hardness with inability to lie down (*Jiǎ* 《甲》 says: pain around the umbilicus and retraction of the genitals and both testicles).

Shí Mén 石門 (Rèn 5) governs hardness and pain in the smaller abdomen radiating to the genitals, inability to urinate, and retraction of both testicles.

Yīn Jiāo 陰交 (Rèn 7) governs abdominal fullness and hardness with pain radiating to the genitals, inability to urinate, and retraction of both testicles.

Retracted genitals: Apply moxibustion on Zhōng Fēng 中封 (LV 4).

Dà Hè (KI 12) (see the section on [treating dream] emissions) and Zhōng Fēng (LV 4) (see the section on prominent *shàn*-mounting) govern wilting and reversal diseases.

Qū Quán 曲泉 (LV 8) governs anuria and retracted genitals.

氣衝治陰痿莖痛（《千》同），兩丸騫，痛不可忍（《銅》）。五樞（見疝）、歸來治卵縮（見陰痛）。

Qì Chōng 氣衝 (ST 30) treats retracted genitals, pain of the penis (*Qiān* 《千》 agrees), and both testicles retracted with unbearable pain (*Tóng* 《銅》).

Wǔ Shū 五樞 (GB 27) (see the section on prominent *shàn*-mounting) and Guī Lái 歸來 (ST 29) treat retracted testicles (see the section on pain of the penis).

筋攣陰縮入腹，相引痛：灸中封五十壯，或不滿五十壯。老少加減。又云：此二穴，喉腫，厥逆，五臟所苦，鼓脹，並主之。

Hypertonicity of the sinews causes retraction of the genitals into the abdomen, as well as pulling pain: Apply fifty cones of moxibustion on Zhōng Fēng 中封 (LV 4) or Bù Mǎn 不滿.[31] Modify [the number of cones] according to the age. It is also said: These two points also govern swollen throat, reverse counterflow, what the five viscera suffer,[32] and drum distention.

31. The location of point Bù Mǎn 不滿 is unknown.

32. *What the five viscera suffer* indicates the disorders each organ can suffer. The liver suffers from tension, the heart suffers from slackening, the spleen suffers from dampness, the kidneys suffer from dryness, and the lungs suffer from qì rising.

3.07
Yīn Tǐng Chū

陰挺出

Vaginal protrusion
(Prolapsed uterus)

大敦主陰挺出 。少府主陰挺長（《千》並見疝 ）。上髎（《千》見絕子 ）治婦人陰挺出不禁（《銅》）。陰蹻 、照海（ 見淋 ）、水泉（ 見月事 ）、曲泉（ 見瘕癖，《千》同 ）治婦人陰挺出 。

Dà Dūn 大敦 (LV 1) governs vaginal protrusion (prolapsed uterus).

Shào Fǔ 少府 (HT 8) governs the vagina protruding a long way out (also see the section on *shàn*-mounting in *Qiān*《千》).

Shàng Liáo 上髎 (UB 31) (see the section on infertility in *Qiān*) treats vaginal protrusion (*Tóng*《銅》).

Yīn Qiāo 陰蹻 (KI 6 or KI 8), Zhào Hǎi 照海 (KI 6) (see the section on dribbling and dribbling urinary block), Shuǐ Quán 水泉 (KI 5) (see the section on menstruation), and Qū Quán 曲泉 (LV 8) (see the discussion of strings and aggregations; *Qiān* agrees) treat vaginal protrusion.

陰蹻（ 見淋瀝 ）療陰挺出（《明》）。

Yīn Qiāo (KI 6 or KI 8) (see the section on dribbling) cures vaginal protrusion (*Míng*《明》).

3.08
Zhuǎn Bāo

轉胞

Shifted bladder[33]

涌泉主胞轉（《千》見淋）。關元主婦人胞轉不得尿（見無子，又主胞閉
塞。《銅》云：治胞轉不得尿。）。腰痛小便不利，苦胞轉：灸中極七壯（
小兒同），又灸十五椎，或臍下一寸或四寸，隨年。凡飽食訖忍小便，或走
馬，或忍小便入房，或大走，皆致胞轉，臍下急滿不通（方見《千金》）。
凡尿不在胞囊中，為胞屈僻，津液不通。蔥葉除尖頭，內陰莖孔中深三寸，
微用口吹，胞脹津通，愈。

Yǒng Quán 涌泉 (KI 1) governs shifted bladder (see the section on dribbling in *Qiān* 《千》).

Guān Yuán 關元 (Rèn 4) governs shifted bladder with anuria (see the section on infertility; it also governs blockage of the bladder. *Tóng* 《銅》 says: It treats shifted bladder with anuria).

Lower back pain and inhibited urination, suffering shifted bladder: Apply seven cones (same for children) of moxibustion on Zhōng Jí 中極 (Rèn 3), or burn the same number of cones as the age of the patient on the fifteenth vertebra, or 1 cùn or 4 cùn below the umbilicus.

Shifted bladder can be caused by any of the following: Holding in urine after eating or when riding a horse, or holding in urination during sexual activity, or when running; with acute fullness and obstruction below the umbilicus (see the formulas in *Qiān Jīn* 《千金》). Whenever urine is not inside the bladder sac, the bladder is crooked and deviated, and the fluids [meaning urine] will be blocked.[34] Use a scallion leaf, remove the tip, and insert it 3 cùn into the penis. Blow [through the scallion] softly to inflate the bladder and then the fluids [urine] will flow freely; thus the disorder will be cured.

---

33. Shifted bladder refers to urinary disorders during pregnancy. The symptoms are: difficult, frequent urination and dribbling urination or retention of urine.
34. This sentence is difficult to understand.

3.09

Yīn Jīng Téng

陰莖疼

Pain of the penis

曲泉（見疝）、行間主癃閉，莖中痛（《千》）。氣衝主陰痿莖痛。列缺（見失精）、陰陵泉、少府主陰痛。歸來主賁豚卵上入引莖痛。

Qū Quán 曲泉 (LV 8) (see the section on prominent *shàn*-mounting) and Xíng Jiān 行間 (LV 2) govern dribbling urinary block and pain of the penis (*Qiān*《千》).

Qì Chōng 氣衝 (ST 30) governs genital wilting and pain of the penis.

Liè Quē 列缺 (LU 7) (see the section on [treating dream] emissions), Yīn Líng Quán 陰陵泉 (SP 9), and Shào Fǔ 少府 (HT 8) govern genital pain.

Guī Lái 歸來 (ST 29) governs running piglet disorder and testicles retracted upward with pain radiating to the penis.

歸來治小腹賁豚，卵縮莖痛（《銅》）。橫骨治陰器縱伸痛（見淋）。水道治小腹滿，引陰痛（見小腹滿）。氣衝治莖痛（見陰痿）。會陰治陰中諸病，前後相引痛，不得大小便，陰端寒衝心。大敦治陰頭痛（見疝）。腎俞（見勞）、志室（見陰腫）、陰谷（見溺難）、太衝（見小便不利）治陰痛。

Guī Lái (ST 29) treats running piglet in the smaller abdomen, retracted testicles, and pain of the penis (*Tóng*《銅》).

Héng Gǔ 橫骨 (KI 11) treats painful erections (see the section on dribbling and dribbling urinary block).

Shuǐ Dào 水道 (ST 28) treats fullness of the smaller abdomen with pain radiating to the penis (see the section on fullness of the smaller abdomen).

Qì Chōng (ST 30) treats pain of the penis (see the section on wilted and retracted genitals).

Huì Yīn 會陰 (Rèn 1) treats all diseases of the genitals and pulling pain in anterior and posterior [yīn – the genitals and the anus], difficult defecation and urination, and cold in the tip of the penis that surges up into the heart.

Dà Dūn 大敦 (LV 1) treats pain of the tip of the penis (see the section on prominent *shàn*-mounting).

Shèn Shù 腎俞 (UB 23) (see the section on taxation), Zhì Shì 志室 (UB 52) (see the section on genital swelling), Yīn Gǔ 陰谷 (KI 10) (see the section on difficult urination), and Tài Chōng 太衝 (LV 3) (see the section on inhibited urination) treat genital pain.

《千金翼》云：七傷為病，小便赤熱，乍數時難，或時傷多，或如針刺，陰下常濕，陰痿消小，精清而少，連連獨泄，陰端寒冷，莖中疼痛云云（當早服藥, 著艾 ）。莖中痛：灸行間三十壯 。

Qiān Jīn Yì 《千金翼》 says: Because of the seven damages, hot red urine, [along with] urinary frequency, or difficult urination, or copious urine, or a pricking feeling, wet genital region, wilted shrunken genitals, clear scant semen, constant spermatorrhea, cold in the tip of the penis, pain of the penis, and so forth (it is better to take herbs and apply moxibustion early). For pain of the penis: Apply thirty cones of moxibustion on Xíng Jiān 行間 (LV 2).

3.10
Páng Guāng Qì

膀胱氣

Bladder qì[35]

章門療膀胱氣癖疝，瘕氣，膀胱氣痛狀如雷聲，積聚氣（《明》）。岐伯灸膀胱氣攻衝兩脅，時臍下鳴，陰卵入腹：灸臍下六寸兩旁各寸六分三七壯。五樞療膀胱氣攻兩脅，（《下》）。

Zhāng Mén 章門 (LV 13) cures bladder qì, aggregations, *shàn*-mounting, conglomeration qì, pain from bladder qì with the condition of thunderous sounds, and qì accumulations and gatherings (*Míng*《明》).

Qí Bó [prescribed] moxibustion for bladder qì surging upward and attacking both rib-sides, rumbling below the umbilicus, and testicles retracted into the abdomen: Apply three times seven cones of moxibustion on the site 6 cùn below the umbilicus and 1.6 cùn to the sides.[36]

Wǔ Shū 五樞 (GB 27) cures bladder qì attacking both rib-sides (*Xià*《下》).

膀胱冷，灸之如腎虛法（《千》）。膀胱、三焦津液少，大小腸寒熱（見腰痛），或三焦寒熱：灸小腸俞五十壯。三焦、膀胱、腎中熱氣：灸水道隨年壯。水道治小腹滿，引陰中痛，腰背急，膀胱有寒，三焦結熱，小便不利。

Cold in the bladder: Follow the methods for applying moxibustion to treat kidney vacuity (*Qiān*《千》).

Fluid insufficiency in the bladder and sānjiāo, with cold and heat in the large intestine, small intestine (see the section on lower back pain) and sānjiāo: Apply fifty cones of moxibustion on Xiǎo Cháng Shù 小腸俞 (UB 27).

---

35. Bladder qì indicates two disorders. One is pain and swelling of smaller abdomen with urinary difficulty. It is also an alternate name for *shàn*-mounting. According to the author's notes below, this section discusses *shàn*-mounting.

36. This is an unnamed non-channel point.

Hot qì in the sānjiāo, bladder, and kidneys: Burn the same number of cones as the patient's age on Shuǐ Dào 水道 (ST 28).

Shuǐ Dào (ST 28) treats fullness of the smaller abdomen with pain radiating to the genitals, lower and upper back tension, cold in the bladder, accumulation of heat in the sānjiāo and inhibited urination.

《千金》云：氣衝主癲。《明堂》云：氣衝療癀疝，是癀疝，即癲也。《必用》云：治水癲偏大，上下不定，疼不可忍，俗呼為膀胱氣。是膀胱氣即癲疝也。然太倉公診命婦云：疝氣客於膀胱，難於前後溲而溺赤，又不可便認膀胱氣為疝氣云。

[Author's notes:] *Qiān Jīn* 《千金》 says: Qì Chōng 氣衝 (ST 30) governs prominent [*tuí shàn* 癀疝 mounting]. *Míng Táng* 《明堂》 says: Qì Chōng (ST 30) cures prominent *shàn*-mounting [*tuí shàn* 癀疝 mounting].[37] Prominent *shàn*-mounting [*tuí shàn* 癀疝 mounting] means *tuí shàn* 癲疝 mounting. *Bì Yòng* 《必用》 says: [Qì Chōng (ST 30)] treats what is called bladder qì, with unilateral enlargement of watery prominent [*shàn*-mounting] moving up and down with unbearable pain. So bladder qì is prominent *shàn*-mounting. Tài Cānggōng[38] diagnosed a noble woman[39] saying: *Shàn*-mounting qì stays in the bladder, causing difficult urination and defecation with reddish urine. In that case, we cannot say bladder qì is *shàn*-mounting qì.

37. In this note, the author tells us that *tuí shàn* 癀疝 (mounting) is a synonym for *tuí shàn* 癲疝 (mounting). Note that the characters and the tones are different, even if the rest of the Pinyin is the same. Prominent *shàn*-mounting is a type of *shàn*-mounting qì with symptoms such as swollen scrotum and a slippery pulse at the left *guān* (liver) position.

38. Tài Cānggōng 太倉公 is another name for Chúnyú Yì 淳於意.

39. *Mìng fù* 命婦 (noble woman) was a title or rank given to certain women in ancient China by the emperor.

3.11
Yīn Hàn (Shī Yǎng)

陰汗（濕癢）

Genital sweating
(Damp itching)

會陽治陽氣虛乏，陰汗濕（《銅》）。魚際（見寒熱）療陰汗（《明》）。《千》云：主陰濕，腹中餘疾。中極、陰蹻、腰尻交、陰交、曲泉主陰癢（《千》）。會陰主陰頭寒。少府主陰癢（見疝）。

Huì Yáng 會陽 (UB 35) treats yáng qì vacuity and dampness from genital sweating (*Tóng*《銅》).

Yú Jì 魚際 (LU 10) (see the section on [sensations of] cold and heat) cures genital sweating (*Míng*《明》). *Qiān*《千》 says: It governs dampness of the genitals and other diseases in the abdomen.

Zhōng Jí 中極 (Rèn 3), Yīn Qiāo 陰蹻 (KI 6 or KI 8), Yāo Kāo Jiāo 腰尻交 (UB 34), Yīn Jiāo 陰交 (Rèn 7), and Qū Quán 曲泉 (LV 8) govern genital itching (*Qiān*).

Huì Yīn 會陰 (Rèn 1) governs cold in the tip of the penis.

Shào Fǔ 少府 (HT 8) governs genital itching (see the section on prominent *shàn*-mounting).

仲景論七傷曰：一、陰汗，二、精寒，三、精清，四、精少，五、囊下濕癢，六、小便數，七、夜夢陰人。然則陰汗、陰濕癢者，蓋七傷之數也，可不早治之乎？（有人作文字則氣濕，亦心氣使然，心腎相為表里故也）。《千金翼》敍虛損云：疾之所起，生自五勞，即生六極（詳見寒熱），復生七傷。一陰寒，二陰痿，三里急，四精連連不絕，五精少囊濕，六精清，七小便數。（其病小便赤熱，或如針刺，陰痿小，陰下常濕，精清而少云云。論與仲景少異，故載之於此。）

[Author's notes:] When [Zhāng] Zhòngjǐng discussed the seven damages, he said: first, genital sweating; second, cold semen; third, clear semen; fourth, scant semen; fifth, damp itching in the scrotum; sixth, frequent urination; seventh, dreaming of yīn people [ghosts]. So genital sweating and genital damp itching are [two of] the seven damages; why don't people get treatment earlier? (*When people write, qì becomes dampness. This is caused by heart qì; the heart and the kidneys are exteriorly and interiorly related.)[40]

When *Qiān Jīn Yì* 《千金翼》 discussed vacuity detriment, it said: Diseases that arise come from the five taxations which generate the six extremes (see the details in the section on [sensations of] cold and heat), and then the seven damages. First is genital cold; second is genital wilting; third is internal tension; fourth is incessant semen [spermatorrhea]; fifth is scant semen with dampness in the scrotum; sixth is clear semen; seventh is frequent urination. (*[The symptoms of] these diseases include: hot red urine, or needles pricking [a sensation during urination], wilted small genitals, wet genital region, clear scant semen, and so forth. There is a little difference between this discussion and Zhāng Zhòngjǐng's, so I attached it here.)

3.12
Yīn Zhǒng (Yīn Chuāng)

陰腫 （陰瘡）

Genital swelling
(Genital sores)

曲泉（見無子）、陰蹻（見漏下）、大敦、氣衝（見疝）主陰腫（《千》）。志室、胞肓療陰痛下腫。崑崙在外踝後跟骨上治陰腫。《明下》云：內崑崙在內踝後五分筋骨間，療小兒陰腫。灸三壯。曲泉治陰腫㾴痛（見風勞）。氣衝治婦人陰腫（見月事），又療陰腫（《明下》見疝）。膀胱俞治陰生瘡（見便赤）。

Qū Quán 曲泉 (LV 8) (see the section on infertility), Yīn Qiāo 陰蹻 (KI 6 or KI 8) (see the section on spotting of blood), Dà Dūn 大敦 (LV 1), and Qì Chōng 氣衝 (ST 30) (see the section on prominent *shàn*-mounting) govern genital swelling (*Qiān* 《千》).

Zhì Shì 志室 (UB 52) and Bāo Huāng 胞肓 (UB 53) cure genital pain and swelling (*Míng* 《明》).

Kūn Lún 崑崙 (UB 60) is located on the heel, posterior to the lateral malleolus. It treats genital swelling (*Tóng* 《銅》). *Míng Xià* 《明下》 says: Inner Kūn Lún 內崑崙 is located in the

---

40. This passage in parenthesis seems misplaced.

sinews and bones, 5 fēn posterior to the medial malleolus. It treats genital swelling in children. Burn three cones of moxibustion.

Qū Quán 曲泉 (LV 8) treats genital swelling and leg pain (see the section on wind taxation).

Qì Chōng 氣衝 (ST 30) treats genital swelling in women (see the section on menstruation); it also governs genital swelling (see the section on prominent *shàn*-mounting in *Míng Xià* 《明下》).

Páng Guāng Shù 膀胱俞 (UB 28) treats genital sores (see the section on bloody stool).

有人陰腫，醫以赤土塗之，令服八味丸而愈。一小兒陰腫，醫亦以赤土塗之愈（今人用寫字油柱木用）。若久病而陰腫，病已不可救，宜速灸水分穴。蓋水分能分水穀，水穀不分故陰腫。不特陰腫，它處亦腫也。尤宜急服禹餘糧丸云（見《既效方》）。

[Author's notes:] Someone suffered genital swelling, so the doctor applied red soil on it and asked them to take *Bā Wèi Wán* 八味丸 (Eight Ingredient Pill). The disease was cured. When a child suffered genital swelling, the doctor also applied red soil on it. The disease was cured (nowadays, people use *Xiě Zì Yóu Zhù Mù* 寫字油柱木[41]). If someone suffers chronic disease with genital swelling, the disease is not curable. We should apply moxibustion on Shuǐ Fēn 水分 (Rèn 9) immediately. Shuǐ Fēn (Rèn 9) can separate water and grains; when water and grains cannot separate, genital swelling is formed. The swelling is not only in the genitals, but also in other places. People should take *Yú Yú Liáng Wán* 禹餘糧丸 (Limonite Pill) immediately (see *Jì Xiào Fāng* 《既效方》).

---

41. This substance is unknown today.

3.13
Xiǎo Fù Tòng

小腹痛

Pain of the smaller abdomen

陰蹻療小腹偏痛，嘔逆嗜臥（《明》）。中極療小腹痛，積聚堅如石，小便
不利，失精絕子，面黯（《下》）。

Yīn Qiāo 陰蹻 (KI 6 or KI 8) cures unilateral pain in smaller abdomen, retching counterflow, and somnolence (*Míng* 《明》).

Zhōng Jí 中極 (Rèn 3) cures pain of the smaller abdomen, accumulations and gatherings that are hard as a stone, inhibited urination, seminal loss and infertility, and dark facial complexion (*Xià* 《下》).

腎俞、復溜、中封、承筋、陰包、承山、大敦主小腹痛（《千》）。石門、
商丘主小腹堅痛，下引陰中。石門、水分主小腹拘急痛。涌泉主風入腹中，
小腹痛。臍中等主小腹疝氣痛（見疝）。太溪主小腹熱而偏痛。

Shèn Shù 腎俞 (UB 23), Fù Liū 復溜 (KI 7), Zhōng Fēng 中封 (LV 4), Chéng Jīn 承筋 (UB 56), Yīn Bāo 陰包 (LV 9), Chéng Shān 承山 (UB 57), and Dà Dūn 大敦 (LV 1) govern pain of the smaller abdomen (*Qiān* 《千》).

Shí Mén 石門 (Rèn 5) and Shāng Qiū 商丘 (SP 5) govern hardness and pain in the smaller abdomen radiating to the genitals.

Shí Mén (Rèn 5) and Shuǐ Fēn 水分 (Rèn 9) govern hypertonicity and pain of the smaller abdomen.

Yǒng Quán 涌泉 (KI 1) governs wind entering the abdomen and pain of the smaller abdomen.

Qí Zhōng 臍中 (Rèn 8) and so forth govern pain of the smaller abdomen due to *shàn*-mounting qì (see the section on prominent *shàn*-mounting).

Tài Xī 太溪 (KI 3) governs heat and unilateral pain of the smaller abdomen.

肝俞（見咳逆）、小腸俞（見便赤）、蠡溝、照海（見疝）、下廉（見飧泄）、丘墟、（見腋腫）、中都（見腸鳴）治小腹痛（《銅》）。

Gān Shù 肝俞 (UB 18) (see the section on coughing counterflow), Xiǎo Cháng Shù 小腸俞 (UB 27) (see the section on bloody stool), Lí Gōu 蠡溝 (LV 5), Zhào Hǎi 照海 (KI 6) (see the section on prominent *shàn*-mounting), Xià Lián 下廉 (ST 39) (see the section on swill diarrhea), Qiū Xū 丘墟 (GB 40) (see the section on swelling of the axilla), and Zhōng Dū 中都 (LV 6) (see the section on rumbling intestines) treat pain of the smaller abdomen (*Tóng* 《銅》).

太衝治腰引小腹痛。帶脈治婦人小腹堅痛，月脈不調，帶下赤白，里急瘛瘲。五樞主小腹痛（見疝）。曲泉主女子小腹腫（無子），婦人陰痛，引心下。（小腹絞痛：灸膝外邊上去一寸宛宛中。《千翼》）

Tài Chōng 太衝 (LV 3) treats low back pain radiating to the smaller abdomen.

Dài Mài 帶脈 (GB 26) treats hardness and pain of the smaller abdomen in women, monthly vessel irregularities, red and white vaginal discharge, abdominal tension, and tugging and slackening.

Wǔ Shū 五樞 (GB 27) governs pain of the smaller abdomen (see the section on prominent *shàn*-mounting).

Qū Quán 曲泉 (LV 8) governs swelling of the smaller abdomen (see the section on infertility) in women and genital pain radiating to the region below the heart in women. (*Gripping pain of the smaller abdomen: Apply moxibustion in the depression on the lateral aspect 1 cùn above the knee. *Qiān Yì* 《千翼》.)

3.14
Xiǎo Fù Zhàng Mǎn

小腹脹滿

Distention and fullness of the smaller abdomen

大巨治小腹脹滿，煩渴，瘄疝，偏枯、四肢不舉（《銅》）。曲骨治小腹脹滿，小便淋澀不通，瘄疝、小腹痛。然谷治小腹脹（見疝）。幽門治小腹脹滿，嘔沫吐涎喜唾。京門（見腸鳴）、蠡溝（見疝）、中封治小腹腫（見瘧）。胞肓治小腹堅急（見腹痛）。水道治小腹滿，引陰中痛，腰背強急，膀胱有寒，三焦結熱，小便不利。大敦治小腹痛，中熱、喜寐。小便不利，小腹脹滿，虛乏：灸小腸俞隨年（《千》）。五臟虛勞，小腹弦急脹熱：灸腎俞五十壯，老小損之。若虛冷，可百壯。委中主小腹堅腫。

Dà Jù 大巨 (ST 27) treats distention and fullness of the smaller abdomen, vexation and thirst, prominent *shàn*-mounting, hemilateral withering, and inability to lift the four limbs (*Tóng* 《銅》).

Qū Gǔ 曲骨 (Rèn 2) treats distention and fullness of the smaller abdomen, dribbling and difficult urination with stoppage, prominent *shàn*-mounting, and pain of the smaller abdomen.

Rán Gǔ 然谷 (KI 2) treats distention of the smaller abdomen (see *shàn*-mounting).

Yōu Mén 幽門 (KI 21) treats distention and fullness of the smaller abdomen, retching of foam, vomiting of drool, and frequent spitting.

Jīng Mén 京門 (GB 25) (see the section on rumbling intestines), Lí Gōu 蠡溝 (LV 5) (see the section on prominent *shàn*-mounting), and Zhōng Fēng 中封 (LV 4) treat swelling of the smaller abdomen (see the section on malaria).

Bāo Huāng 胞肓 (UB 53) treats hardness and tension of the smaller abdomen (see the section on abdominal pain).

Shuǐ Dào 水道 (ST 28) treats abdominal fullness with pain radiating to the genitals, stiffness of the lower and upper back, cold in the bladder, heat bind in the sānjiāo, and inhibited urination.

Dà Dūn 大敦 (LV 1) treats pain of the smaller abdomen with heat attacking and somnolence.

Inhibited urination, distention, and fullness of the smaller abdomen, vacuity and lack [of strength]: Apply moxibustion on Xiǎo Cháng Shù 小腸俞 (UB 27). Burn the same number of cones as the age of the patient *Qiān* 《 千 》.

Vacuity of the five viscera, taxation; bowstring tension, fullness, and heat of the smaller abdomen: Apply fifty cones of moxibustion on Shèn Shù 腎俞 (UB 23). Reduce [the number of cones] in old and young people. Burn a hundred cones of moxibustion for vacuity cold.

Wěi Zhōng 委中 (UB 40) governs hardness and swelling of the smaller abdomen.

銅人云：小腸俞治小便赤澀淋瀝，小腹痛。《千金》亦云：治小腹脹滿。此治小腹脹痛要穴也。若灸不效，方灸其它穴云。

[Author's notes:] *Tóng Rén* 《 銅人 》 says: Xiǎo Cháng Shù 小腸俞 (UB 27) treats rough voiding, dribbling of reddish urine, and pain of the smaller abdomen. *Qiān Jīn* 《 千金 》 also says: It treats distention and fullness of the smaller abdomen. This is an important point to treat distention and pain of the smaller abdomen. If there is no effect after applying moxibustion on this point, then burn moxibustion on other points.

3.15

Tuí Shàn (Zhū Shàn Qì, Tāi Shàn, Hán Shàn, Cù Shàn)

癩疝（諸疝氣　胎疝　寒疝　卒疝）

Prominent *shàn*-mounting
(All *shàn* qì, fetal *shàn*, cold *shàn*, sudden *shàn*)

《必用方》云：治水癩偏大，上下不定，疼不可忍，俗呼為膀胱氣。
用煅過牡蠣二兩、炮乾薑一兩，為末塗病處，即愈。則是水癩，即膀
胱氣也。《千金》云：氣衝主癩。《明堂下經》云：治癪疝。則是
癩，即癪疝也。恐人惑其名而誤治之，故為之辨。

[Author's notes:] *Bì Yòng Fāng* 《必用方》 says: To treat what is called bladder qì, with unilateral enlargement of watery prominent [*shàn*-mounting], moving up and down with unbearable pain: Powder 2 *liǎng*[42] of calcined *mǔ lì* 牡蠣 (ostreae concha calcinatum) and 1 *liǎng* of blast-fried *gān jiāng* 乾薑 (zingiberis rhizome praeparatum); then apply it on the affected area. The disease will be cured. This watery prominent [*shàn*-mounting] is bladder qì. The *Qiān Jīn* 《千金》 says: Qì Chōng 氣衝 (ST 30) governs prominent [*tuí shàn* 癩疝 mounting]. *Míng Táng Xià Jīng* 《明堂下經》 says: It treats prominent *shàn*-mounting [*tuí shàn* 癪疝 mounting]. So [*tuí shàn* 癪疝 mounting] is the same as *tuí shàn* 癩疝 mounting. I am afraid that people are confused about the name and give the wrong treatment, so I differentiate it here.[43]

曲泉主癪疝，陰跳，痛引臍中（《千》）。中都、合陽、中郄、關元、大
巨、交信、中封、太衝、地機主癩疝。中封主癩疝，癃暴痛，痿厥。少府主
陰痛，實時挺長，寒熱，陰暴痛遺尿，偏虛則暴癢氣逆，卒疝、小便不利。
衝門主婦人陰疝。

Qū Quán 曲泉 (LV 8) governs prominent *shàn*-mounting and twitching genitals with [pain] radiating to the center of the umbilicus (*Qiān* 《千》).

---

42. A *liǎng* 兩 is a unit of weight. During the *Sòng* Dynasty (when this was written), 1 *liǎng* equaled 37.3 grams; today 1 *liǎng* equals 31.25 grams and is often rounded off to 30 grams.

43. In this note, the author repeats that *tuí shàn* 癪疝 (mounting) is a synonym for *tuí shàn* 癩疝 (mounting). Note that the characters and the tones are different, even if the rest of the Pinyin is the same. See above.

Zhōng Dū 中都 (LV 6), Hé Yáng 合陽 (UB 55), Zhōng Xì 中郄 (UB 40), Guān Yuán 關元 (Rèn 4), Dà Jù 大巨 (ST 27), Jiāo Xìn 交信 (KI 8), Zhōng Fēng 中封 (LV 4), Tài Chōng 太衝 (LV 3), and Dì Jī 地機 (SP 8) govern prominent *shàn*-mounting.

Zhōng Fēng (LV 4) governs prominent *shàn*-mounting, dribbling blockage with violent pain, and wilting reversal.

Shào Fǔ 少府 (HT 8) governs genital pain, persistent erection, [sensations of] cold and heat, violent pain of the genitals and enuresis during repletion; violent itching, qì counterflow, sudden *shàn*-mounting, and inhibited urination during vacuity.

Chōng Mén 衝門 (SP 12) governs genital *shàn*-mounting in women.

商丘主陰股內痛，氣癃狐疝走上下，引小腹痛，不可俯仰。巨闕主狐疝。太衝主狐疝，嘔厥。肩井旁肩解與臂相接處主偏癲。氣衝主癲，陰腫痛。中管主衝疝，冒死不知人。交信主氣癃癲疝陰急，股樞胻內廉痛。臍中、石門、天樞、氣海主小腹疝氣游行，五臟疝繞臍，衝胸不得息（並《千》）。

Shāng Qiū 商丘 (SP 5) governs pain of the medial aspect of the groin, qì welling-abscess,[44] foxy *shàn*-mounting moving up and down, with pain radiating into the smaller abdomen, and inability to bend forward and backward.

Jù Quē 巨闕 (Rèn 14) governs foxy *shàn*-mounting.

Tài Chōng 太衝 (LV 3) governs foxy *shàn*-mounting, vomiting, and reversal.

[The point which is located] lateral to Jiān Jǐng 肩井 (GB 21) and on the junction of the shoulder joint and arm governs unilateral prominent *shàn*-mounting.

Qì Chōng 氣衝 (ST 30) governs prominent *shàn*-mounting, genital swelling, and pain.

Zhōng Guǎn 中管 (Rèn 12) governs surging *shàn*-mounting and unconsciousness.

Jiāo Xìn 交信 (KI 8) governs qì dribbling blockage, prominent *shàn*-mounting and genital tension, and pain of the medial aspect of the knee joint and [thigh] muscle.

Qí Zhōng 臍中 (Rèn 8), Shí Mén 石門 (Rèn 5), Tiān Shū 天樞 (ST 25), and Qì Hǎi 氣海 (Rèn 6) govern wandering *shàn*-mounting of the smaller abdomen, with *shàn*-mounting of the five viscera winding around the umbilicus, surging into the chest, and causing inability to breathe (along with *Qiān* 《千》).

---

44. Qì welling-abscess indicates a welling-abscess with swelling in the throat. It is usually caused by toxic heat. Here, this may indicate a similar disease but in the genital region.

臍疝繞臍痛，衝胸不得息：灸臍中 。臍疝繞臍痛：石門主之 。臍疝繞臍痛，時止：天樞主之 。又主氣疝煩嘔（《千》云：主氣疝嘔），面腫賁豚（並《甲》）。氣衝主癲（《明下》作癀疝），陰腫痛，陰痿莖中痛，兩丸蹇痛，不可仰臥 。五樞主陰疝，兩丸上入小腹痛 。《明下》云：主陰疝小腹痛 。陰交 、石門 、太衝主兩丸蹇（ 見陰縮 ）。

Umbilical *shàn*-mounting with pain winding around the umbilicus, surging into the chest and causing inability to breathe: Apply moxibustion on Qí Zhōng 臍中 (Rèn 8).

Shí Mén 石門 (Rèn 5) governs umbilical *shàn*-mounting with pain winding around the umbilicus.

Tiān Shū 天樞 (ST 25) governs umbilical *shàn*-mounting with pain winding around the umbilicus; the pain may stop temporarily. It also governs qì *shàn*-mounting, vexation and vomiting (*Qiān* 《千》 says: It governs qì *shàn*-mounting and vomiting), facial swelling, and running piglet qì (*Jiǎ* 《甲》 agrees).

Qì Chōng 氣衝 (ST 30) governs *Tuí* 癲 (*Míng Xià* 《明下》 says: prominent *shàn*-mounting), genital swelling and pain, genital wilting and pain of the penis, retraction and pain of both testicles, and inability to lie face up.

Wǔ Shū 五樞 (GB 27) governs genital *shàn*-mounting and both testicles retracted upward into the smaller abdominal with pain. *Míng Xià* says: It governs genital *shàn*-mounting and pain of the smaller abdomen.

Yīn Jiāo 陰交 (Rèn 7), Shí Mén (Rèn 5), and Tài Chōng 太衝 (LV 3) govern retraction of both testicles (see the section on wilted and retracted genitals).

交信（ 見淋 ）、中都（ 見腸鳴 ）、大巨 、曲骨（ 見小腹 ）治癀疝（《銅》）。曲泉治丈夫癀疝，陰股痛，小便難，腹脅支滿，癃閉，少氣泄利，四肢不舉，實即身熱目眩痛，汗不出，目䀮䀮，膝痛筋攣，不可屈伸 。

Jiāo Xìn 交信 (KI 8) (see the section on dribbling), Zhōng Dū 中都 (LV 6) (see the section on rumbling intestines), Dà Jù 大巨 (ST 27), and Qū Gǔ 曲骨 (Rèn 2) (see the section on [distention and fullness of] the smaller abdomen) treat prominent *shàn*-mounting (*Tóng* 《銅》).

Qū Quán 曲泉 (LV 8) treats prominent *shàn*-mounting in men, pain of the groin, urinary difficulty, propping fullness of the abdomen and rib-sides, dribbling urinary block, qì shortage, diarrhea, inability to lift the four limbs. In repletion, there is body heat with dizzy vision and eye pain, absence of sweating, diminished vision, knee pain and hypertonicity of the sinews, and inability to bend and stretch.

《千金》曰：癲有四種。腸癲卵脹，難灸。氣癲、水癲，針灸易治。卵偏大、上入腹：灸三陰交隨年。卵偏大癲病：灸關元百壯，或大敦隨年壯，或橫骨邊二七壯，夾莖是（詳見《千金》）。

Qiān Jīn《千金》says: There are four types of prominent *shàn*-mounting. With intestinal *shàn*-mounting, the testicles are distended and it is difficult to apply moxibustion. *Qì shàn*-mounting and water *shàn*-mounting are easy to treat with acupuncture and moxibustion. Unilateral enlargement of a testicle that is retracted upward into the abdomen: Apply the same number of cones of moxibustion as the age of the patient on Sān Yīn Jiāo 三陰交 (SP 6). Unilateral enlargement of a testicle and prominent *shàn*-mounting: Apply a hundred cones of moxibustion on Guān Yuán 關元 (Rèn 4), or apply the same number of cones of moxibustion as the patient's age on Dà Dūn 大敦 (LV 1), or apply two times seven cones of moxibustion on the lateral side of Héng Gǔ 橫骨 (KI 11) and alongside the penis (for the details, see *Qiān Jīn*).

築賓治小兒胎疝（《明下》同），痛不得乳。小兒胎疝，卵偏重：灸囊後縫十字紋當上三壯，春較夏灸，秋較冬灸。

Zhù Bīn 筑賓 (KI 9) treats fetal *shàn*-mounting in children (*Míng Xià*《明下》agrees), pain, and inability to drink [breast] milk.

Fetal *shàn*-mounting in children with unilateral heaviness of a testicle: Apply three cones of moxibustion on the cross-like crease at the seam on the back of the scrotum. Apply moxibustion in summer if the disease improves in the spring, or burn moxibustion in winter if the disease improves in the fall.

太衝主女子疝及小腹腫，溏泄，癃，遺尿，陰痛，面黑，目眥痛，漏血（《千》）。蠡溝主女子疝，赤白淫下，時多時少，暴腹痛。陰交、石門主疝（見無子）。小兒氣癲：灸足厥陰大敦，左灸右，右灸左，各一壯。太倉公診司空命婦曰：疝氣客於膀胱，難於前後，溲而溺赤：灸其足厥陰脈左右各一所，即不遺溺而溲清（更為火齊湯，飲之而疝氣散）。陰市、肝俞療寒疝，下至腰腳如冷水，水傷諸疝，按之在膝上伏兔下寒痛，腹脹滿，厥少氣。《明下》云：卒疝，小腹痛，力痿氣少，伏兔中寒，腰如冷水。《銅》云：寒疝小腹脹，腰以下伏兔上，寒如冷水。

Tài Chōng 太衝 (LV 3) governs *shàn*-mounting in women and swelling of the smaller abdomen, sloppy diarrhea, dribbling block, enuresis, genital pain, dark facial complexion, pain of the canthus, and spotting of blood (*Qiān*《千》).

Lí Gōu 蠡溝 (LV 5) governs *shàn*-mounting in women, varying amount of mixed white and red ooze [leucorrhea], and violent abdominal pain.

Yīn Jiāo 陰交 (Rèn 7) and Shí Mén 石門 (Rèn 5) govern *shàn*-mounting (see the section on infertility).

Qì tuí [*shàn*-mounting] in children: Apply one cone of moxibustion on Dà Dūn 大敦 (LV 1) of the foot juéyīn. Burn moxibustion on the right side when the disease is on the left; or burn moxibustion on the left side when it is on the right.

Tài Cānggōng diagnosed a noble woman of the ministry of public works, and said: *Shàn*-mounting qì has invaded the bladder, so it is difficult for her to defecate and urinate and the urine is red. Apply moxibustion on a site on the left and right foot juéyīn vessel. Then the enuresis will go away and the urine will become clear (furthermore, the *shàn*-mounting will disperse when *Huǒ Jì Tāng* 火齊湯 (Fire Decoction) is taken.)

Yīn Shì 陰市 (ST 33) and Gān Shù 肝俞 (UB 18) cure cold *shàn*-mounting with coldness down the lower back and legs that feels like [the back was soaked in] cold water, water damage and various *shàn*-mounting, cold pain above the knees and below the crouching rabbit [anterior thigh] when pressed, distension and fullness of the abdomen, reversal, and qì shortage. *Míng Xià* 《 明 下 》 says: Sudden *shàn*-mounting with pain of the smaller abdomen, lack of strength, shortness of qì, cold in the crouching rabbit [anterior thigh], and coldness in the low back as if [it were soaked in] cold water. *Tóng* 《 銅 》 says: Cold *shàn*-mounting with distention in the smaller abdomen and coldness below the low back and above crouching rabbit [anterior thigh] as if [it were soaked in] cold water.

合陽治寒疝陰偏痛（ 《 銅 》 ）。然谷治寒疝小腹脹，上搶胸脅 。次髎治疝氣下墜，腰脊痛不得轉搖，急引陰器痛不可忍，腰下至足不仁，背膝寒，小便赤淋，心下堅脹 。太溪 、行間（ 見白濁 ）、肓俞（ 見腹脹 ）、肝俞治寒疝（見咳，《 明 》同 ）。陰交治寒疝，引小腹痛，腰膝拘攣 。五樞治男子寒疝，卵上入小腹痛 。中封治寒疝引腰中痛，或身微熱 。大敦主寒疝陰挺出（ 見《 下 》 ）。

Hé Yáng 合陽 (UB 55) treats cold *shàn*-mounting and unilateral pain of the genitals (*Tóng*).

Rán Gǔ 然谷 (KI 2) treats cold *shàn*-mounting with distension of the smaller abdominal that rushes upward to the chest and rib-sides.

Cì Liáo 次髎 (UB 32) treats *shàn*-mounting with downward sagging [of the testicles], acute unbearable pain of the low back and spine that radiates to the genitals with inability to turn to the side, numbness from the low back down to the feet, cold in the interstices of the back, dribbling red urine, and hardness and distention below the heart.

Tài Xī 太溪 (KI 3), Xíng Jiān 行間 (LV 2) (see the section on white turbidity), Huāng Shù 肓俞 (KI 16) (see the section on abdominal distension), and Gān Shù 肝俞 (UB 18) treat cold *shàn*-mounting (see the section on cough; *Míng* 《 明 》 agrees).

217

Yīn Jiāo 陰交 (Rèn 7) treats cold *shàn*-mounting with pulling pain in smaller abdomen, and hypertonicity of the low back and knees.

Wǔ Shū 五樞 (GB 27) treats cold *shàn*-mounting in men and testicles retracted upward into the smaller abdomen with pain.

Zhōng Fēng 中封 (LV 4) treats cold *shàn*-mounting with pain that radiates to the low back or slight generalized heat.

Dà Dūn 大敦 (LV 1) cures cold *shàn*-mounting and vaginal protrusion (see *Xià*《下》).

舍弟少，戲舉重，得偏墜之疾。有客人為當關元兩旁相去各三寸青脈上灸七壯，即愈。王彥賓患小腸氣，亦如此灸之愈（餘見膀胱）。

[Author's notes:] My younger brother was a weight lifter when he was young, but then he suffered unilateral sagging disease. A guest applied seven cones of moxibustion on the green vessels 3 cùn lateral to the Guān Yuán 關元 (Rèn 4) and the disease was cured. Wáng Yànbīng suffered small intestine qì; it also was cured after applying the same method of moxibustion (for the rest, see the section on the urinary bladder).

金門（見尸厥）、丘墟（見腋腫）治暴疝痛。大敦治卒疝，小便數遺溺，陰頭中，心痛汗出，陰上入腹，陰偏大，腹臍中痛，悒悒不樂，病左取右，病右取左。蠡溝治卒疝，小腹腫，時小腹暴痛，小便不利如癃閉，數噫恐悸，少氣不足，腹痛，悒悒不樂，咽中悶如有息肉，背拘急不可俯仰。太衝治小兒卒疝，嘔逆發寒，咽乾胕腫，內踝前痛淫濼，胕酸腋下腫。《明下》云：療卒疝，小腹痛，小便不利如淋。照海治卒疝，小腹痛，嘔吐，嗜臥。

Jīn Mén 金門 (UB 63) (see the section on deathlike reversal) and Qiū Xū 丘墟 (GB 40) (see the section on swelling of the axilla) treat violent *shàn*-mounting pain.

Dà Dūn (LV 1) treats sudden *shàn*-mounting, frequent urination and enuresis, pain of the tip of the penis, heart pain with sweating, retraction of the genitals upward into the abdomen, unilateral enlargement of the genitals, pain of the abdomen and umbilicus, and unhappiness. Treat on the right side when the disease is on the left; or treat on the left side when the disease is on the right.

Lí Gōu 蠡溝 (LV 5) treats sudden *shàn*-mounting, swelling of the smaller abdomen, frequent violent pain of the smaller abdomen, inhibited urination like dribbling urinary block, frequent belching, fear with palpitations, qì shortage, abdominal pain and unhappiness, oppressed feeling in the throat like there are polyps, and hypertonicity of the back with inability to bend forward and backward.

Tài Chōng 太衝 (LV 3) treats sudden *shàn*-mounting in children, vomiting counterflow and chills; dry throat, skin swelling, pain and weakness in the anterior aspect of the medial malleolus, leg soreness and swelling of the axilla. *Míng Xià*《明下》says: [Tài Chōng 太衝 (LV 3)] cures sudden *shàn*-mounting, pain of the smaller abdomen, and inhibited urination similar to *lín*-strangury.

Zhào Hǎi 照海 (KI 6) treats sudden *shàn*-mounting, pain of the smaller abdomen, vomiting and retching, and somnolence.

陰蹻療卒疝，小腹痛（《上》同）。左取右，右取左，立已（《明》）。蠡溝療卒疝，小股腫，小便不利（交儀同），臍下積氣如卵石，足寒脛酸屈伸難（《下》）。石門療卒疝繞臍痛。關元療卒（《銅》作暴，《千》同）疝小腹痛，轉胞不得小便。陷谷療卒疝小腹痛。交信（見淋）療卒疝。華佗療卒陰卵偏大：取足大指去甲五分內側白肉際，灸三壯，炷如半棗核。左取右，右取左。

Yīn Qiāo 陰蹻 (KI 6 or KI 8) cures sudden *shàn*-mounting and pain of the smaller abdomen (*Shàng*《上》agrees). Treat the right for diseases of the left side; treat the left for disease of the right; the disease will be cured immediately (*Míng*《明》).

Lí Gōu 蠡溝 (LV 5) cures sudden *shàn*-mounting, mild swelling of the thighs, inhibited urination (*Jiāo Yí* 交儀 agrees), pebble-like qì accumulations below the umbilicus, cold feet, and sore lower legs with difficulty bending and stretching (*Xià*《下》).

Shí Mén 石門 (Rèn 5) cures sudden *shàn*-mounting, and pain around the umbilicus.

Guān Yuán 關元 (Rèn 4) cures sudden (*Tóng*《銅》says violent; *Qiān*《千》agrees) *shàn*-mounting, pain of the smaller abdomen, shifted bladder, and inability to urinate.

Xiàn Gǔ 陷谷 (ST 43) cures sudden *shàn*-mounting and pain of the smaller abdomen.

Jiāo Xìn 交信 (KI 8) (see the section on dribbling) cures sudden *shàn*-mounting.

Huá Tuó's treatment of sudden unilateral enlargement of a testicle: Apply three cones of moxibustion 5 fēn away from the nail of the big toe at the medial border of the white flesh. Use cones the size of half a date pit. Treat the right for disease of the left; treat the left for disease of the right.

照海主四肢淫濼，身悶，陰暴起疝（《千》）。大敦主卒疝暴痛，陰跳上入腹，寒疝，陰挺出偏大腫，臍腹中悒悒不樂，小便難而痛。灸刺立已，左取右，右取左（《甲》云：照海主之）。

Zhào Hǎi (KI 6) governs pain and weakness of the four limbs, generalized oppression, and sudden *shàn*-mounting of the genitals (*Qiān*).

Dà Dūn 大敦 (LV 1) governs sudden *shàn*-mounting with violent pain, genitals retracting upward into the abdomen, cold *shàn*-mounting, erection with unilateral enlargement and swelling, discom-

219

fort in the umbilicus and abdomen, and difficult painful urination. The disease will be cured right after treatment with acupuncture and moxibustion. Treat the right for diseases of the left; treat the left for the disease of the right (*Jiǎ* 《甲》 says: Zhào Hǎi 照海 (KI 6) governs [this disease]).

3.16
Shàn Jiǎ (Yú Jiàn Xuán Pǐ)

疝瘕（餘見痃癖）

Shàn-mounting and conglomerations
(for the rest, see the section on strings and aggregations)

陰陵泉治疝瘕，小便不利，氣淋（《銅》）。《千》云：主婦人疝瘕，按之如以湯沃股內至腰，飧泄，陰痛，小腹痛堅急，下濕，不嗜食。

Yīn Líng Quán 陰陵泉 (SP 9) treats *shàn*-mounting and conglomerations, inhibited urination and qì *lín*-strangury (*Tóng* 《銅》). *Qiān* 《千》 says: It governs *shàn*-mounting and conglomerations in women; when pressed, it feels like hot water washing from the medial aspect of the genitals to the low back, with swill diarrhea, genital pain, pain, hardness and tension of the smaller abdomen, dampness below [in the genitals], and no desire to eat.

太溪主胞中有大疝瘕積聚，與陰相引（《千》）。太陰郄、衝門主疝瘕陰疝。四滿主臍下疝積（《甲》云：胞中有血）。石門主腹滿疝積。四滿（見積聚）、中極治疝瘕。府舍治疝癖（見脾疼）。

Tài Xī 太溪 (KI 3) governs great *shàn*-mounting, conglomerations, accumulations, and gatherings in the bladder that radiate [pain] to the genitals (*Qiān*).

Tài Yīn Xī 太陰郄 [Dì Jī 地機 (SP 8)] and Chōng Mén 衝門 (SP 12) govern *shàn*-mounting, conglomerations, and genital *shàn*-mounting.[45]

Sì Mǎn 四滿 (KI 14) governs *shàn*-mounting and accumulations under the umbilicus (*Jiǎ* 《甲》 says: blood inside the bladder).

---

45. Genital *shàn* 陰疝 [*shàn*-mounting] is one type of *shàn* usually caused by cold attacking the liver and kidneys. In males, the symptoms include sudden retraction of the testicles into the abdomen with acute abdominal pain, and swelling of the scrotum and testicles.

Shí Mén 石門 (Rèn 5) governs abdominal fullness and *shàn*-mounting accumulations.

Sì Mǎn 四滿 (KI 14) (see the section on accumulations and gatherings) and Zhōng Jí 中極 (Rèn 3) treat *shàn*-mounting and conglomerations.

Fǔ Shě 府舍 (SP 13) treats *shàn*-mounting and aggregations (see the section on spleen pain).

瘕聚：灸氣海 、天樞百壯（ 並見腹脹 ）。丘墟主大疝腹堅 。關元治瘕聚（ 見赤白帶 ）。帶下：灸間使三十 。又淋，小便赤，尿道痛，臍下結塊如覆盆，或因食得，或因產得，惡露不下，遂成疝瘕，或因月事不調，血結成塊，皆針之（ 《 千翼 》 ）。

Conglomerations and gatherings: Apply a hundred cones of moxibustion on Qì Hǎi 氣海 (Rèn 6) and Tiān Shū 天樞 (ST 25) (also see the section on abdominal fullness).

Qiū Xū 丘墟 (GB 40) governs great *shàn*-mounting and abdominal hardness.

Guān Yuán 關元 (Rèn 4) treats conglomerations and gatherings (see the section on red and white vaginal discharge).

Vaginal discharge: Apply thirty cones of moxibustion on Jiān Shǐ 間使 (PC 5). It also treats *lín*-strangury, reddish urine, pain of the urethra, a lump that appears like an overturned basin below the umbilicus which may be caused by eating or by retention of lochia after childbirth, followed by formation of *shàn*-mounting and conglomerations; or the blood accumulates into a lump because of irregular menstruation. For all of these, needle [Jiān Shǐ (PC 5)] (*Qiān Yì* 《 千翼 》).

3.17
Lín Lóng (Lín Lì, Yú Jiàn Xiǎo Biàn Bù Tōng)

淋癃（淋瀝　餘見小便不通）

Lín-strangury and dribbling urinary block
(Dribbling; for the rest, see the section on urinary stoppage)

關元主胞閉塞，小便不通，勞熱石淋。又主石淋，臍下三十六疾，不得小便，並灸足太陽。懸鐘主五淋。大敦、氣門主五淋不得尿。氣衝主腹中滿熱，淋閉不得尿。交信主氣淋。復溜主血淋。《明下》云：療五淋，小便如散灰色。關元、涌泉主胞轉氣淋。長強、小腸俞主淋癃。關元、陰陵泉主腎病不可俯仰，氣癃。

Guān Yuán 關元 (Rèn 4) governs blockage of the bladder, urinary stoppage, taxation heat and stone lín-strangury. It also governs stone lín-strangury, the thirty-six diseases below the umbilicus, and inability to urinate. Also apply moxibustion on [Guān Yuán (Rèn 4)] and Foot Tàiyáng 足太陽 (UB 60).

Xuán Zhōng 懸鐘 (GB 39) governs the five lín-stranguries.

Dà Dūn 大敦 (LV 1) and Qì Mén 氣門 (non-channel)[46] govern the five lín-stranguries and inability to urinate.

Qì Chōng 氣衝 (ST 30) governs fullness and heat in abdomen, dribbling, and urinary block.

Jiāo Xìn 交信 (KI 8) governs qì lín-strangury.

Fù Liū 復溜 (KI 7) governs bloody lín-strangury. Míng Xià《明下》says: It cures the five lín-stranguries and urine that is like scattered ash.

Guān Yuán (Rèn 4) and Yǒng Quán 涌泉 (KI 1) govern shifted bladder and qì lín-strangury.

Cháng Qiáng 長強 (Dū 1) and Xiǎo Cháng Shù 小腸俞 (UB 27) govern lín-strangury and dribbling urinary block.

Guān Yuán (Rèn 4) and Yīn Líng Quán 陰陵泉 (SP 9) govern kidney disease, inability to bend forward and backward, and dribbling qì block.

---

46. Qì Mén 氣門 is located 3 cùn lateral to Guān Yuán 關元 (Rèn 4).

曲泉主癃閉 。行間主癃閉，莖中痛 。然谷主癩疝 。

Qū Quán 曲泉 (LV 8) governs dribbling urinary block.

Xíng Jiān 行間 (LV 2) governs dribbling urinary block and pain of the penis.

Rán Gǔ 然谷 (KI 2) governs prominent *shàn*-mounting.

曲骨主小腹脹，血癃，小便難 。胞肓 、秩邊主癃閉下重，不得小便 。陰蹻主女子淋（ 《 明 》云：療諸淋，見淋瀝 ）。

Qū Gǔ 曲骨 (Rèn 2) governs distention in smaller abdomen, bloody dribbling block, and difficult urination.

Bāo Huāng 胞肓 (UB 53) and Zhì Biān 秩邊 (UB 54) govern dribbling urinary block, lower body heaviness and inability to urine.

Yīn Qiāo 陰蹻 (KI 6 or KI 8) governs *lín*-strangury in women (*Míng* 《 明 》 says: It cures all *lín*-stranguries. See the section on dribbling)

石門療氣淋，小便黃（ 《 下 》 ）。長強療五淋 。曲骨療五淋，小便黃 。至陰療小便淋，失精（ 《 下 》 ）。

Shí Mén 石門 (Rèn 5) cures qì *lín*-strangury and yellow urine (*Xià* 《 下 》).

Cháng Qiáng 長強 (Dū 1) cures the five *lín*-stranguries.

Qū Gǔ (Rèn 2) cures the five *lín*-stranguries and yellow urine.

Zhì Yīn 至陰 (UB 67) cures dribbling urination and seminal loss (*Xià*).

中極治五淋，小便赤澀（ 《 明下 》又云：尿道痛 ），失精，臍下結如覆杯，陽氣虛憊，（ 《 銅 》 ）。復溜治五淋，小便如散火 。次髎治赤淋（ 見便不利 ）。然谷 、曲骨治淋瀝（ 見小腹痛 ）。太衝治淋 。陰陵泉治氣淋，寒熱不節 。

Zhōng Jí 中極 (Rèn 3) treats the five *lín*-stranguries, inhibited urination with red urine (*Míng Xià* 《 明下 》 also says pain of the urethra), seminal loss, gatherings below the umbilicus that appear like an overturned cup, and exhaustion of yáng qì (*Tóng* 《 銅 》).

Fù Liū 復溜 (KI 7) treats the five *lín*-stranguries and urine that seems like scattered fire.

Cì Liáo 次髎 (UB 32) treats red *lín*-strangury (see the section on inhibited urination).

Rán Gǔ 然谷 (KI 2) and Qū Gǔ 曲骨 (Rèn 2) treat dribbling (see the section on pain of the smaller abdomen).

Tài Chōng 太衝 (LV 3) treats *lín*-strangury.

Yīn Líng Quán 陰陵泉 (SP 9) treats qì *lín*-strangury and irregular [sensations of] cold and heat.

交信治氣淋，瘄疝，陰急，股引腨內廉骨痛。《明》云：療氣淋，卒疝，大小便難。箕門治淋，遺溺，鼠蹊腫痛，小便不通。大鐘治實則小便淋閉，洒洒腰脊強痛，大便秘澀，嗜臥口中熱；虛則嘔逆多寒，欲閉戶而處，少氣不足，胸脹喘息，舌乾，咽中食噎不得下，善驚恐不樂，喉鳴咳唾血。

Jiāo Xìn 交信 (KI 8) treats qì *lín*-strangury, prominent *shàn*-mounting, genital tension, pain of the thighs radiating to the medial aspect of the calf. *Míng*《明》says: It treats qì *lín*-strangury, sudden *shàn*-mounting, and difficult defecation and urination.

Jī Mén 箕門 (SP 11) treats *lín*-strangury, enuresis, swelling and pain of the groin, and urinary stoppage.

Dà Zhōng 大鐘 (KI 4) treats dribbling urinary block, cold pain and stiffness of the back, constipation, somnolence, and heat in the mouth in repletion; it also treats retching, coldness, liking to stay at home, qì shortage, distention of the chest, panting, dry tongue, food choking the throat with inability to swallow, susceptibility to fright, fear and sadness, throat rales, cough, and spitting of blood in vacuity.

氣淋：灸關元五十壯，或鹽著臍中灸三壯（《千》）。石淋：灸關元、或氣門、或大敦各三十壯。勞淋：灸足太陰百壯。血淋：灸丹田、或復溜各隨年。五淋不小便：中封二七壯，或大敦七壯（餘見《千金》）。

Qì *lín*-strangury: Apply fifty cones of moxibustion on Guān Yuán 關元 (Rèn 4), or apply three cones of salt-moxibustion on Qí Zhōng 臍中 (Rèn 8) (*Qiān*《千》).

Stone *lín*-strangury: Apply thirty cones of moxibustion on Guān Yuán (Rèn 4), or Qì Mén 氣門 (non-channel), or Dà Dūn 大敦 (LV 1).

Taxation *lín*-strangury: Apply a hundred cones of moxibustion on foot tàiyīn 足太陰.[47]

Blood *lín*-strangury: Apply the same number of cones of moxibustion as the age of the patient on Dān Tián 丹田 (cinnabar field) (Rèn 4 or Rèn 5) or Fù Liū 復溜 (KI 7).

---

47. Before the Six Dynasties 六朝 (222-589), foot tàiyīn 足太陰 indicated a point that is located in the depression on the border of white flesh posterior to the medial malleolus; after the *Táng* (唐) Dynasty, it was conflated with Sān Yīn Jiāo 三陰交 (SP 6).

The five *lín*-stranguries with inability to urinate: Apply two times seven cones on Zhōng Fēng 中封 (LV 4); or seven cones on Dà Dūn 大敦 (LV 1) (for the rest, see the section in *Qiān Jīn* 《千金》).

水泉治女小便淋瀝。委陽、志室（見陰痛）、中髎治小便淋瀝。陰蹻療婦人淋瀝，陰挺出（《銅》同），四肢淫濼，心悶，及諸淋（《明》）。關元（《明》同）治不覺遺瀝（《銅》見臍痛）。小腸俞治淋瀝（見小便赤）。

Shuǐ Quán 水泉 (KI 5) treats dribbling urination in women.

Wěi Yáng 委陽 (UB 39), Zhì Shì 志室 (UB 52) (see the section on pain of the penis), and Zhōng Liáo 中髎 (UB 33) treat dribbling urination.

Yīn Qiāo 陰蹻 (KI 6 or KI 8) cures dribbling [urination] in women, vaginal protrusion [prolapsed uterus] (*Tóng* 《銅》 agrees), pain and weakness of the four limbs, a feeling of oppression of the heart, and all *lín*-stranguries (*Míng* 《明》).

Guān Yuán 關元 (Rèn 4) (*Míng* agrees) treats uncontrollable dribbling [incontinence] (see the section on umbilical pain in *Tóng*).

Xiǎo Cháng Shù 小腸俞 (UB 27) treats dribbling (see the discussion of red urine).

予壯年寓學，忽有遺瀝之患，因閱方書，見有用五倍子末酒調服者，服之而愈。藥若相投，豈在多品？而亦無事於灸也，故附著於此。若欲治淋疾，則有王不留行子，神效。彭侍郎以治張道士，服三粒愈（見《既效方》）。有婦人患淋，臥病久之，服諸藥愈甚。其夫入夜來告急，予令取此花葉十余葉，令研細煎服，翌朝再來，云病已減八分，再與數葉煎服，即愈（一名剪金花，一名金盞銀臺）。

[Author's notes:] When I was middle aged, I studied at home and suddenly suffered dribbling after urination. So I read a medical book that said to mix powdered *wǔ bèi zǐ* 五倍子 (Galla Chinensis Galla) with liquor. I was cured after I took it. When the herb matches [the condition], using a lot of herbs is unnecessary. This is also unrelated to moxibustion, so I attached it here. When treating *lín*-strangury disease, *wáng bù liú xíng zǐ* seeds 王不留行子 (Vaccariae Semen) have magical effects. Vice Director Péng used three pieces to treat Daoist Priest Zhāng and cure his disease (see *Jì Xiào Fāng* 《既效方》). There was a lady who suffered *lín*-strangury and had been in bed for a long time; the disease became worse after she took herbs. Her husband came to me in the night for emergency help. I asked him to get 10 leaves of this flower [*wáng bù liú xíng* (Vaccariae)], grind them into a fine powder, boil it, and [let the wife] drink it. He came the next morning and said the disease had improved by 80 percent already. I gave his wife more leaves to cook and drink, and the disease was cured (this plant (Vaccariae) is also named *jiǎn jīn huā* 剪金花 or *jīn zǎn yín tái* 金盞銀臺).

3.18

Xiǎo Biàn Nán (Bù Tōng, Bù Lì)

小便難（不通　不利）

Difficult urination
(Stoppage and inhibition)

涌泉療小便不通（《明》）。曲骨療婦人小便不通（《下》見帶下）。曲泉主陰跳，痛引莖中，不得尿（《千》）。陰交、石門、委陽主小腹堅痛引陰中，不得小便。關元主三十六疾不得小便。氣衝主淋閉不得尿。大敦主小便難而痛（《甲》云：照海主之）。橫骨、大巨、期門主小腹滿，小便難，陰下縱。

Yǒng Quán 涌泉 (KI 1) cures urinary stoppage (*Míng* 《明》).

Qū Gǔ 曲骨 (Rèn 2) cures urinary stoppage in women (see section on vaginal discharge in *Xià* 《下》).

Qū Quán 曲泉 (LV 8) governs twitching genitals with pain radiating to the penis and inability to urinate (*Qiān* 《千》).

Yīn Jiāo 陰交 (Rèn 7), Shí Mén 石門 (Rèn 5), and Wěi Yáng 委陽 (UB 39) govern hardness and pain in the smaller abdomen with pain radiating to the genitals and inability to urinate.

Guān Yuán 關元 (Rèn 4) governs the thirty-six diseases with inability to urinate.

Qì Chōng 氣衝 (ST 30) governs *lín*-strangury, dribbling urinary block, and inability to urinate.

Dà Dūn 大敦 (LV 1) governs painful and difficult urination (*Jiǎ* 《甲》 says: Zhào Hǎi 照海 (KI 6) governs all these symptoms).

Héng Gǔ 橫骨 (KI 11), Dà Jù 大巨 (ST 27), and Qī Mén 期門 (LV 14) govern fullness of the smaller abdomen, difficult urination, and yīn protraction (persistent erection or prolapsed uterus).

陰谷、大敦、箕門、委中、委陽主陰跳遺，小便難。中封、行間主振寒溲白，尿難痛。曲骨主小腹脹，血癃小便難。列缺主小便熱痛。

Yīn Gǔ 陰谷 (KI 10), Dà Dūn 大敦 (LV 1), Jī Mén 箕門 (SP 11), Wěi Zhōng 委中 (UB 40), and Wěi Yáng 委陽 (UB 39) govern twitching genitals, enuresis and difficult urination.

Zhōng Fēng 中封 (LV 4) and Xíng Jiān 行間 (LV 2) govern quivering with cold, white cloudy urine, and painful difficult urination.

Qū Gǔ 曲骨 (Rèn 2) governs distension of the smaller abdomen, bloody dribbling block, and difficult urination.

Liè Quē 列缺 (LU 7) governs hot painful urination.

中極等（ 見失精 ）、承扶 、屈骨端主小便不利（ 見大便不禁 ）。少府 、三里主小便不利癃 。陰陵泉主心下滿 ，寒中 ，小便不利 。胞肓等（ 見淋 ）、石門 、關元 、陰交 、中極（ 並見無子 ）、曲骨（ 見帶下 ）主不得小便 。京門主溢飲 ，水道不通 ，溺黃 。

Zhōng Jí 中極 (Rèn 3) and so forth (see the section on treating dream emissions), Chéng Fú 承扶 (UB 36), and Qū Gǔ Duān 屈骨端 (Rèn 2 or KI 11) govern inhibited urination (see the section on fecal incontinence).

Shào Fǔ 少府 (HT 8) and Sān Lǐ 三里 (ST 36 or LI 10) govern inhibited urination and dribbling block.

Yīn Líng Quán 陰陵泉 (SP 9) governs fullness below the heart, cold strike, and inhibited urination.

Bāo Huāng 胞肓 (UB 53), and so forth (see the section on dribbling), Shí Mén 石門 (Rèn 5), Guān Yuán 關元 (Rèn 4), Yīn Jiāo 陰交 (Rèn 7), Zhōng Jí (Rèn 3) (for all, see the section on infertility), and Qū Gǔ (Rèn 2) (see the discussion of vaginal discharge) govern inability to urinate.

Jīng Mén 京門 (GB 25) governs spillage rheum, blockage of the water passages, and yellow urine.

太衝治腰引小腹痛 ，小便不利 ，狀如淋（ 《明 》同 ）、瘕疝 ，小腹腫 ，溏泄 ，遺溺 ，陰痛 ，面目蒼色 ，胸脅支滿 ，足寒 ，大便難（ 《銅 》）。水道治膀胱寒 ，三焦熱 ，小便不利（ 見小腹痛 ）。會陰治小便難 ，竅中熱（ 《千 》同 ），皮痛 ，陰端寒衝心 。橫骨治腹脹小便難 ，陰器縱伸痛 。

Tài Chōng 太衝 (LV 3) treats low back pain radiating to the smaller abdomen, inhibited urination similar to *lín*-strangury (*Míng* 《 明 》 agrees), prominent *shàn*-mounting, swelling of the smaller abdomen, sloppy diarrhea, enuresis, genital pain, pale facial complexion, propping fullness of the chest and rib-sides, cold feet, and difficult defecation (*Tóng* 《 銅 》).

Shuǐ Dào 水道 (ST 28) treats cold in the bladder, heat in the sānjiāo, and inhibited urination (see the section on pain of the smaller abdomen).

Huì Yīn 會陰 (Rèn 1) treats difficult urination, heat in the orifice [urethra] (Qiān 《千》 agrees), skin pain, and cold in the tip of the penis that surges into the heart.

Héng Gǔ 橫骨 (KI 11) treats distension of the abdomen, difficult urination, and painful protraction of the genitals.

陰包（見腰）、至陰、陰陵泉（見疝）、地機（見水腫）、三陰交（見疢癖）治小便不利。箕門（見淋）治小便不通。陰谷治煩逆溺難，小腹急，引陰痛，股內廉痛。五里治腸中滿，熱閉不得溺。行間治溺難（見白濁）。

Yīn Bāo 陰包 (LV 9) (see the section on the low back), Zhì Yīn 至陰 (UB 67), Yīn Líng Quán 陰陵泉 (SP 9) (see the section on prominent *shàn*-mounting), Dì Jī 地機 (SP 8) (see the section on edema), and Sān Yīn Jiāo 三陰交 (SP 6) (see the section on strings and aggregations) treat inhibited urination.

Jī Mén 箕門 (SP 11) (see the section on dribbling) treats urinary stoppage.

Yīn Gǔ 陰谷 (KI 10) treats vexation, counterflow, difficult urination, tension of the smaller abdomen with pain radiating to the genitals, and pain on medial aspect of the thigh.

Wǔ Lǐ 五里 (LV 10) treats fullness of the intestines, heat blockage, and inability to urinate.

Xíng Jiān 行間 (LV 2) treats difficult urination (see the section on white turbidity).

有人小便淋澀不通，甚以為苦。予令摘王不留行葉（詳見淋瀝），研細煎服，即愈。（黃芪椎破，水煎數沸服，治大小便不通立效。亦有多煎蔥湯，浸臍以下，得通。）

[Author's notes:] Someone suffered a lot from dribbling and inhibited urination with urinary stoppage. I asked him to pick leaves from *wáng bù liú xíng* 王不留行 (Vaccariae) (see the details under dribbling), finely grind them, decoct, and drink it. The disease was cured. (Break up *huáng qí* 黃芪 (Astragalus) [with a mortar and pestle], boil in water for several rollings, and then drink it; stoppage of defecation and urination will be cured immediately. Also, decoct scallions and soak [the body] below the umbilicus to unblock the blockage.)

3.19
Xiǎo Biàn Wǔ Sè

小便五色

The five colors of urine

腎俞主小便難，赤濁，骨寒熱（《千》）。前谷、委中主尿赤難。上廉、下廉主小便難、黃。凡尿青，取井；黃取俞，赤取滎，白取經，黑取合。承漿主小便赤黃，或時不禁。

Shèn Shù 腎俞 (UB 23) governs difficult urination and red turbid urine with [sensations of] cold and heat in the bones (*Qiān* 《千》).

Qián Gǔ 前谷 (SI 2) and Wěi Zhōng 委中 (UB 40) govern painful urination with red urine.

Shàng Lián 上廉 (ST 37) and Xià Lián 下廉 (ST 39) govern difficult urination with yellow urine. Use the *jīng*-well points to treat green urine; use the *shù*-stream points to treat yellow urine; use the *yíng*-spring points to treat red urine; use the *jīng*-river points to treat white [or pale] urine; use the *hé*-sea points to treat black [or dark] urine.

Chéng Jiāng 承漿 (Rèn 24) governs dark yellow urine, or enuresis.

完骨、小腸俞、白環俞、陽綱、膀胱俞主小便赤黃。中管主小腸有熱，尿黃。關元主腎病，氣癃尿黃。京門（又見下不通）、照海主尿黃，水道不通。大陵主目赤，小便如血。關元主傷中尿血。

Wán Gǔ 完骨 (GB 12), Xiǎo Cháng Shù 小腸俞 (UB 27), Bái Huán Shù 白環俞 (UB 30), Yáng Gāng 陽綱 (UB 48), and Páng Guāng Shù 膀胱俞 (UB 28) govern dark yellow urine.

Zhōng Guǎn 中管 (Rèn 12) governs small intestine heat and yellow urine.

Guān Yuán 關元 (Rèn 4) governs kidney disease, qì urinary block, and yellow urine.

Jīng Mén 京門 (GB 25) (also see the section on lower body stoppage in *Xià* 《下》) and Zhào Hǎi 照海 (KI 6) govern yellow urine and blockage of the water passages.

Dà Líng 大陵 (PC 7) governs red eyes and urine that looks like blood.

Guān Yuán 關元 (Rèn 4) governs visceral damage with bloody urine.

大陵治小便如血。關元（《明下》同）治溺血（見臍痛）。下管療小便赤（《明》見腹堅）。陰交治臍下熱，小便赤，氣痛如刀攪，作塊如覆杯。

Dà Líng 大陵 (PC 7) treats urine that looks like blood.

Guān Yuán (Rèn 4) (*Míng Xià* 《明下》 agrees) treats bloody urine (see the section on umbilical pain).

Xià Guǎn 下管 (Rèn 10) cures reddish urine (see the section on hardness of the abdomen in *Míng* 《明》).

Yīn Jiāo 陰交 (Rèn 7) treats heat below the umbilicus, red urine, qì pain that feels like a knife is stirring, and lumps that appear like an overturned cup.

陰蹻療尿黃水，小腹熱，咽乾。《下》云：療小便難。小腸俞療治小便赤澀，小腸緊急。太溪、關元（見賁豚）、白環俞療小便黃（《下》）。

Yīn Qiāo 陰蹻 (KI 6 or KI 8) cures yellow urine, heat in the abdomen, and dry throat. *Xià* 《下》 says: It cures difficult urination.

Xiǎo Cháng Shù 小腸俞 (UB 27) cures inhibited urination with red urine, and tension of the small intestine.

Tài Xī 太溪 (KI 3), Guān Yuán 關元 (Rèn 4) (see the section on running piglet), and Bái Huán Shù 白環俞 (UB 30) cure yellow urine (*Xià*).

小腸俞治小便赤澀淋瀝，小腹痛（《銅》）。膀胱俞治小便赤澀，遺溺，陰生瘡，少氣，脛寒拘急，不得屈伸。上廉治小便難，赤黃。太溪（見傷寒無汗）、兌端（見渴）陰谷（見腹脹）、下廉治溺黃。魂門治小便赤黃。關元（見臍痛）、秩邊（見腰痛）、氣海、陽綱治小便赤澀（見腹脹）。下脘治小便赤（見腹痛）。大敦主尿血，灸三壯。（千）

Xiǎo Cháng Shù 小腸俞 (UB 27) treats inhibited dribbling urination with red urine and pain of the smaller abdomen (*Tóng* 《銅》).

Páng Guāng Shù 膀胱俞 (UB 28) treats inhibited urination with red urine, enuresis, genital sores, qì shortage, cold and hypertonicity of the lower legs, and inability to flex and stretch.

Shàng Lián 上廉 (ST 37) treats difficult urination and red-yellow urine.

Tài Xī 太溪 (KI 3) (see the section on cold damage with absence of sweating), Duì Duān 兌端 (Dū 27) (see the section on wasting-thirst), Yīn Gǔ 陰谷 (KI 10) (see the section on abdominal fullness), and Xià Lián 下廉 (ST 39) treat yellow urine.

Hún Mén 魂門 (UB 47) treats dark yellow urine.

Guān Yuán 關元 (Rèn 4) (see the section on umbilical pain), Zhì Biān 秩邊 (UB 54) (see the section on lower back pain), Qì Hǎi 氣海 (Rèn 6), and Yáng Gāng 陽綱 (UB 48) treat inhibited urination with red urine (see the section on abdominal fullness).

Xià Wǎn 下脘 (Rèn 10) treats red urine (see the section on abdominal pain).

Dà Dūn 大敦 (LV 1) cures bloody urine. Apply three cones of moxibustion (*Qiān* 《千》).

小便有五色，惟赤白色者多，赤色多因酒得之，宜服《本事方》清心丸（予教人服，效）。白色乃下元冷，宜服補藥著灸。腎俞、關元、小腸俞、膀胱俞等，皆要穴也。近有患小便出血者，人教酒與水煎苦荬菜根服，即愈。

[Author's notes:] There are five colors of urine, but red and white [pale] urine are the most common. Red urine is usually caused by liquor. It is appropriate to take *Qīng Xīn Wán* 清心丸 (Heart Clearing Pill) from [*Pǔ Jì*] *Běn Shì Fāng* 《本事方》 (I have asked people to take it and it is effective). White urine is caused by cold in lower origin [affecting kidney yáng]. It is appropriate to take supplementing herbs or apply moxibustion on important points like Shèn Shù 腎俞 (UB 23), Xiǎo Cháng Shù 小腸俞 (UB 27), Páng Guāng Shù 膀胱俞 (UB 28), and so forth. Recently, there was patient who suffered bloody urine; someone taught him to cook the root of *kǔ mǎi cài* 苦荬菜 (Ixeris Denticulatae Herba) in liquor and water. The disease was cured immediately after the patient drank this decoction.

3.20
Zhì Mèng Yí Shī Jīng (Bái Zhuó)

治夢遺失精（白濁）

Treatment of dream emissions
(White turbidity)

虛勞尿精：灸第七椎兩旁各三十壯（《千》）；或曲泉百壯。虛勞白濁：灸
脾俞百壯，或三焦俞、腎俞、章門各百壯。夢失精，小便濁難：灸腎俞百
壯。夢泄精：灸中封五十。男子夢與人交，精泄：灸三陰交五十。

Vacuity-taxation and spermaturia: Apply thirty cones of moxibustion on the site that is lateral to the seventh vertebra (*Qiān* 《 千 》) or a hundred cones on Qū Quán 曲泉 (LV 8).

Vacuity-taxation and white turbidity: Apply a hundred cones of moxibustion on Pí Shù 脾俞 (UB 20) or Sān Jiāo Shù 三焦俞 (UB 22), Shèn Shù 腎俞 (UB 23), and Zhāng Mén 章門 (LV 13).

Seminal emission with dreaming and difficult urination with turbid urine: Apply a hundred cones of moxibustion on Shèn Shù (UB 23).

Dream ejaculation: Apply fifty cones of moxibustion on Zhōng Fēng 中封 (LV 4).

Men dreaming of intercourse with ejaculation: Apply fifty cones of moxibustion on Sān Yīn Jiāo 三陰交 (SP 6).

失精陰縮：灸中封五十。陰痛溺血精出：灸列缺俞五十。失精五臟虛竭：灸
曲骨端五十。失精，陰縮莖痛：灸大赫三十。失精，膝脛痛冷：灸曲泉百
壯。腰脊冷疼，溺濁：灸脾募百壯（ 並《千》）。

Seminal loss and retracted genitals: Apply fifty cones of moxibustion on Zhōng Fēng (LV 4).

Genital pain, bloody urine, and seminal loss: Apply fifty cones of moxibustion on Liè Quē 列缺 (LU 7).

Seminal loss with exhaustion of the five viscera: Apply fifty cones of moxibustion on Qū Gǔ Duān 屈骨端 (Rèn 2 or KI 11).

Seminal loss, retracted genitals, and pain of the penis: Apply thirty cones of moxibustion on Dà Hè 大赫 (KI 12).

Seminal loss with pain and coldness of the knees and lower legs: Apply fifty cones of moxibustion on Qū Quán 曲泉 (LV 8).

Cold pain of the spine and turbid urine: Apply a hundred cones of moxibustion on Pí Shù 脾俞 (UB 20) (along with *Qiān* 《千》).

白濁漏精：灸大椎骨 、尾龜骨並中間共三穴以繩量大椎至尾龜骨折中取中間穴（ 別附 ）。太衝 、中封 、地機主精不足，（ 《千》 ）。中極 、蠡溝 、漏谷 、承扶 、至陰主小便不利，失精（ 《明下》同 ）。

White turbidity and leakage of semen: Apply moxibustion on the three points of *Dà Zhuī Gǔ* 大椎骨 (C7), *Wěi Guī Gǔ* 尾龜骨 (Coccyx) and the point in between. Use a rope to measure from *Dà Zhuī [Gǔ]* (C7) to *Wěi Guī Gǔ* (Coccyx), then fold it in half to locate the point in the middle (also see the attachment).[48]

Tài Chōng 太衝 (LV 3), Zhōng Fēng 中封 (LV 4), and Dì Jī 地機 (SP 8) govern insufficient semen (*Qiān*).

Zhōng Jí 中極 (Rèn 3), Lí Gōu 蠡溝 (LV 5), Lòu Gǔ 漏谷 (SP 7), Chéng Fú 承扶 (UB 36), and Zhì Yīn 至陰 (UB 67) govern inhibited urination and seminal loss (*Míng Xià* 《明下》 agrees).

志室治失精，小便淋瀝 。然谷主精溢（ 大赫同 ），胻酸不能久立，足一寒一熱 。行間治溺難，白濁，寒疝，小腹腫 。腎俞治溺血，便濁，出精（ 《銅》見勞療 ）。膏肓俞治夢失精（ 見勞 ）。至陰 、曲泉（ 見風勞 ）、中極（ 明下同 ）治失精（ 見淋 ）。志室治下腫失精 。

Zhì Shì 志室 (UB 52) treats seminal loss and dribbling urination.

Rán Gǔ 然谷 (KI 2) treats seminal spillage (the same as Dà Hè (KI 12)), leg soreness, and inability to stand for long, with one foot cold and the other hot.

Xíng Jiān 行間 (LV 2) treats difficult urination, white turbidity, cold *shàn*-mounting and swelling of the smaller abdomen.

Shèn Shù 腎俞 (UB 23) treats bloody urine, turbid urine, and seminal loss (see the section on consumption in *Tóng* 《銅》).

---

48. There is no appendix or attachment to this section, so the meaning is unclear.

Gāo Huāng Shù 膏肓俞 (UB 43) treats seminal emission with dreaming (see the section on taxation).

Zhì Yīn 至陰 (UB 67), Qū Quán 曲泉 (LV 8) (see the section on wind taxation), and Zhōng Jí 中極 (Rèn 3) (*Míng Xià*《明下》agrees) treat seminal loss (see the section on dribbling).

Zhì Shì 志室 (UB 52) treats genital swelling and seminal loss.

夢泄精：灸三陰交二七壯，夢斷神良（《千》）。虛勞尿精：陽陵泉或陰陵泉隨年壯，或十椎、十九椎旁三十壯。耳聾，腰痛，失精，食少，膝以下清（云云）：當灸京門五十壯，十四椎百壯。

Dream ejaculation: When two times seven cones of moxibustion are applied on Sān Yīn Jiāo 三陰交 (SP 6), the dreaming stops and the spirit becomes good (*Qiān*《千》).

Vacuity-taxation and spermaturia: Apply moxibustion on Yáng Líng Quán 陽陵泉 (GB 34) or Yīn Líng Quán 陰陵泉 (SP 9). Burn the same number of the cones as the age of the patient; or apply thirty cones of moxibustion on the site that is lateral to the tenth and nineteenth vertebrae.

Deafness, lower back pain, seminal loss, eating less, cold below the knees (and so forth): Apply fifty cones of moxibustion on Jīng Mén 京門 (GB 25) and a hundred cones of moxibustion on the fourteenth vertebra.

《五臟論》曰：心有三孔，藏精汁三合（《千》同），則人之遺漏，其因於心乎？心動則遺漏從之。欲免此患，要養其心，使不動可也。其次，則邪念或起，必早抑之。至游居士云："不愁念起，只恐覺遲"是也。服藥針灸，斯為下矣，然猶愈於不為也。

Wǔ Zàng Lùn《五臟論》 says: The heart has three holes and stores three *gě*[49] of essence (*Qiān* agrees). Is the leakage [of essence] in a person due to the heart? When the heart stirs, leakage follows. If we want to avoid this disease, we must nourish the heart and make it stable. Secondly, we should restrain evil thoughts earlier. Just like Hermit Yóu said: Do not worry about thoughts arising; only fear realizing it too late. Taking herbs and receiving acupuncture-moxibustion are the second choice, but it is better than doing nothing.

---

49. *Gě* 合: A unit of measurement equal to 1/10 of a *shēng* 升 (a unit of dry measurement for grain, equal to about 664 milliliters in the *Sòng* Dynasty).

3.21
Dà Biàn Bù Tōng

大便不通

Fecal stoppage
(Constipation)

大鐘 、中窌 、石門 、承山 、太衝 、中管 、太溪 、承筋主大便難（《千》）。崑崙主不得大便 。肓俞主大便乾，腹中切痛 。石關主大便閉，寒氣結，心堅滿 。

Dà Zhōng 大鐘 (KI 4), Zhōng Liáo 中窌 (UB 33), Shí Mén 石門 (Rèn 5), Chéng Shān 承山 (UB 57), Tài Chōng 太衝 (LV 3), Zhōng Guǎn 中管 (Rèn 12), Tài Xī 太溪 (KI 3), and Chéng Jīn 承筋 (UB 56) govern difficult defecation (*Qiān*《千》).

Kūn Lún 崑崙 (UB 60) governs inability to defecate.

Huāng Shù 肓俞 (KI 16) governs dry stool and cutting pain of the abdomen.

Shí Guān 石關 (KI 18) governs fecal blockage and cold qì bind with hardness and fullness of the heart.

承山（ 見轉筋 ）、太溪（ 見傷寒無汗 ）治大便難（ 《銅》 ）。大鐘（ 《銅》見淋 ）、石關治大便秘澀 。肓俞治大便燥（ 見腰痛 ）。中注治小腹有熱，大便堅燥不利 。太白治腰痛大便難 。太衝治足寒大便難 。

Chéng Shān 承山 (UB 57) (see the section on [cholera with] cramping) and Tài Xī 太溪 (KI 3) (see the section on cold damage with absence of sweating) treat difficult defecation (*Tóng*《銅》).

Dà Zhōng (KI 4) (see the section on dribbling in *Tóng*) and Shí Guān (KI 18) treat constipation.

Huāng Shù (KI 16) treats dry stool (see the section on lower back pain).

Zhōng Zhù 中注 (KI 15) treats heat in the abdomen and inhibited defecation with hard dry stool.

Tài Bái 太白 (SP 3) treats lower back pain and difficult defecation.

Tài Chōng 太衝 (LV 3) treats cold feet and difficult defecation.

石關、膀胱俞療腹痛大便難（《明下》）。大便難：灸七椎旁各一寸七壯（《千》）；又承筋三壯。大便不通：大敦四壯。大便閉塞，氣結，心堅滿：石門百壯（餘見《千金》）。腹中有積，大便秘：巴豆肉為餅，置臍中，灸三壯，即通，神效。耆域蜜兌治大便秘（詳見《既效》）。

Shí Guān 石關 (KI 18) and Páng Guāng Shù 膀胱俞 (UB 28) cure abdominal pain and difficult defecation (*Míng Xià*《明下》).

Difficult defecation: Apply seven cones of moxibustion on [the site] 1 cùn lateral to the seventh vertebra (*Qiān*《千》), or three cones of moxibustion on Chéng Jīn 承筋 (UB 56).

Fecal stoppage [constipation]: Apply four cones of moxibustion on Dà Dūn 大敦 (LV 1).

Fecal block and qì bind with hardness and fullness of the heart: Apply a hundred cones of moxibustion on Shí Mén 石門 (Rèn 5) (for the rest see *Qiān Jīn*《千金》).

Accumulations in the abdomen and constipation: Make a cake of *bā dòu* 巴豆 (Crotonis Fructus), put it on the center of the umbilicus, and apply three cones of moxibustion on top. This is divinely effective.

Add honey from *Qí Yù* [*Fāng*] 耆域 [方] to treat constipation (for the details, see *Jì Xiào Fāng*《既效方》).

3.22
Dà Xiǎo Biàn Bù Tōng

大小便不通

Stoppage of urination and defecation

豐隆主大小便澀難（《明》同）。長強（《明下》同）、小腸俞主大小便難，淋癃。胞肓主癃閉下重，大小便難。

Fēng Lóng 豐隆 (ST 40) governs rough difficult urination and defecation.

Cháng Qiáng 長強 (Dū 1) (*Míng Xià*《明下》agrees) and Xiǎo Cháng Shù 小腸俞 (UB 27) govern difficult urination and defecation, *lín*-strangury, and dribbling block.

Bāo Huāng 胞肓 (UB 53) governs dribbling urinary block, lower body heaviness, and difficult urination and defecation.

水道主三焦約，大小便不通（又云主婦人）。營衝四穴主大小便不利。太溪主大便難，尿黃。中注、浮郄主小腹熱，大便堅。

Shuǐ Dào 水道 (ST 28) governs constrained sānjiāo *yuē*[50] with stoppage of urination and defecation (It also says: It governs women's [diseases]).

Yíng Chōng 營衝 (non-channel),[51] four points, govern inhibited urination and defecation.

Tài Xī 太溪 (KI 3) governs difficult defecation and yellow urine.

Zhōng Zhù 中注 (KI 15) and Fú Xī 浮郄 (UB 38) govern heat in the abdomen and hard stool.

白環俞（見腰脊）、承扶（見痔）、大腸俞治大小便不利（《銅》見腹脹）。會陰治不得大小便（見陰痛，《千》同）。浮郄治小腸熱，大腸結（見筋急）。膀胱俞療大小便難，尿赤（《明》）。交信療大小便難。

50. Sānjiāo yuē 三焦約 (constrained sānjiāo) is a disease. The symptoms include swelling and pain of smaller abdomen with inability to urinate and defecate. It caused by evils, especially wind attacking the sānjiāo.

51. Yíng Chōng 營衝 is located on the vessel in the depression anterior and posterior to the medial malleolus. There are two points on each side.

Bái Huán Shù 白環俞 (UB 30) (see the section on [pain of the] low back and spine), Chéng Fú 承扶 (UB 36) (see the section on hemorrhoids), and Dà Cháng Shù 大腸俞 (UB 25) treat inhibited urination and defecation (see the section on abdominal fullness in *Tóng* 《銅》).

Huì Yīn 會陰 (Rèn 1) treats inability to urinate and defecate (see the section on pain of the genitals, *Qiān* 《千》 agrees).

Fú Xī 浮郄 (UB 38) treats heat of the small intestine and binding of the large intestine (see the section on tension of the sinews).

Páng Guāng Shù 膀胱俞 (UB 28) cures difficult urination and defecation with reddish urine (*Míng* 《明》).

Jiāo Xìn 交信 (KI 8) cures difficult urination and defecation.

一卒傷寒，大小便不通。予與五苓散而皆通。五苓固利小便矣，而大便亦通者，津液生故也。或小便通而大便尚不通，宜用蜜兌道之。（《必用方》：婦人老人大便秘，用麻子、蘇子煮粥食，最佳。）

[Author' notes:] A soldier suffered cold damage with stoppage of urination and defecation. I gave him *Wǔ Líng Sǎn* 五苓散 (Poria Five Powder) and unblocked the stoppage. Though *Wǔ Líng [Sǎn]* (Poria Five Powder) benefits urination, it also frees the bowel movement because it generates fluids. If the urine is freed, but stool is still blocked, add honey to conduct it. (*Bì Yòng Fāng* 《必用方》 says: Constipation in older people and women: Make gruel with *má zǐ* 麻子 [cannabis fructus] and *sū zǐ* 蘇子 [perillae fructus]. This is the best.)

3.23
Xiǎo Biàn Bù Jìn (Yí Niào Fù)

小便不禁（遺尿附）

Incontinence of urine
(attached: enuresis)

便黃
229
疝
220
淋
222
傷寒
661
便赤
253
小便
226
腰脊
551
心煩
335
腰痛
545

承漿主小便不禁（見便黃）。關元（又主婦人小便數，泄不止）、涌泉主小便數。少府主陰暴痛遺尿（《千》）。關門、中府（《甲》作委中）、神門主遺尿。陰陵泉、陽陵泉主失禁遺尿不自知。太衝主女遺尿（見疝）。

Chéng Jiāng 承漿 (Rèn 24) governs incontinence of urine (see the discussion of yellow urine).

Guān Yuán 關元 (Rèn 4) (also governs frequent urination and incessant diarrhea in women) and Yǒng Quán 涌泉 (KI 1) govern frequent urination.

Shào Fǔ 少府 (HT 8) governs violent pain of the genitals and enuresis (*Qiān* 《千》).

Guān Mén 關門 (ST 22), Zhōng Fǔ 中府 (LU 1) (*Jiǎ* 《甲》 says Wěi Zhōng 委中 (UB 40)), and Shén Mén 神門 (HT 7) govern enuresis.

Yīn Líng Quán 陰陵泉 (SP 9) and Yáng Líng Quán 陽陵泉 (GB 34) govern incontinence of urine and enuresis.

Tài Chōng 太衝 (LV 3) governs enuresis in women (see the section on prominent *shàn*-mounting).

關門治遺溺善滿（《銅》）。箕門（見淋）、通里（見傷寒，《千》同）、大敦（見疝）、膀胱俞（見便赤）、太衝（見小便不利）、委中（見腰脊）、神門治遺溺（見心煩）。陰包治遺溺不禁（見腰痛）。

Guān Mén 關門 (ST 22) treats enuresis and fullness (*Tóng* 《銅》).

Jī Mén 箕門 (SP 11) (see the section on dribbling), Tōng Lǐ 通里 (HT 5) (see the section on cold damage; *Qiān* agrees), Dà Dūn 大敦 (LV 1) (see the section on prominent *shàn*-mounting), Páng Guāng Shù 膀胱俞 (UB 28) (see the discussion of reddish urine), Tài Chōng 太衝 (LV 3) (see the section on inhibited urination), Wěi Zhōng 委中 (UB 40) (see the section on [pain of] the low back and spine), and Shén Mén 神門 (HT 7) treat enuresis (see the section on vexation of the heart [and fullness]).

Yīn Bāo 陰包 (LV 9) treats enuresis and incontinence of urine (see the section on lower back pain).

遺溺：灸陽陵泉或足陽明，各隨年（《千》）。遺溺失禁，出不自知：灸陰陵泉隨年 。小便失禁：灸大敦，或行間七壯 。尿床：灸臍下橫文七壯 。婦人遺尿：灸橫骨七壯 。小兒遺尿：灸臍下寸半隨年，又灸大敦三壯（ 餘見《千金》）。曲泉 、陰谷 、陰陵泉 、復溜，（ 此諸穴斷小便利大佳 。不損陽氣，亦云止遺尿 ）。

Enuresis: Apply moxibustion on Yáng Líng Quán 陽陵泉 (GB 34) or Foot Yángmíng 足陽明 (ST 42). Burn the same number of cones as the age of the patient (*Qiān* 《千》).

Enuresis and incontinence of urine, uncontrollable urination: Apply the same number of cones of moxibustion as the age of the patient on Yīn Líng Quán 陰陵泉 (SP 9).

Incontinence of urine: Apply seven cones of moxibustion on Dà Dūn 大敦 (LV 1) or Xíng Jiān 行間 (LV 2).

Bedwetting: Apply seven cones of moxibustion on the crease below the umbilicus.

Enuresis in women: Apply seven cones of moxibustion on Héng Gǔ 橫骨 (KI 11).

Enuresis in children: Apply the same number of cones of moxibustion as the age of the patient on [the site] 1.5 cùn below the umbilicus; also apply three cones of moxibustion on Dà Dūn 大敦 (LV 1) (for the rest, see *Qiān Jīn* 《千金》).

Qū Quán 曲泉 (LV 8), Yīn Gǔ 陰谷 (KI 10), Yīn Líng Quán 陰陵泉 (SP 9), and Fù Liū 復溜 (KI 7) (it is very good to use all these points to stop frequent urination. They do not damage yáng qì, and are also said to stop enuresis).

3.24
Dà Biàn Bù Jìn (Yú Jiàn Xiè Xiè)

大便不禁（餘見泄瀉）

Fecal incontinence
(for the rest, see the section on diarrhea)

大腸俞 、次髎主大小便利 。陽綱主大便不節（《 明 》同 ），腸鳴泄注，小便
赤黃 。承扶主尻中腫，大便直出，陰胞有寒，小便不利。屈骨端主大便泄
數，小便不利，並灸天樞。丹田主泄利不禁，小腹絞痛 。

Dà Cháng Shù 大腸俞 (UB 25) and Cì Liáo 次髎 (UB 32) govern uninhibited bowel movement and urination.

Yáng Gāng 陽綱 (UB 48) governs irregular defecation (*Míng*《 明 》agrees), rumbling intestines, outpour diarrhea, and dark yellow urine.

Chéng Fú 承扶 (UB 36) governs swelling of the sacrum, the stool comes out directly [incontinence], cold in the uterus, and inhibited urination.

Qū Gǔ Duān 屈骨端 (Rèn 2) governs frequent diarrhea and inhibited urination; also apply moxibustion on Tiān Shū 天樞 (ST 25).

Dān Tián 丹田 [cinnabar field] governs diarrhea and [fecal] incontinence with gripping pain of the smaller abdomen.

關元療泄痢虛脹，小便難（《 明 》）。魂門治大便不節（《 銅 》）。老小大
便失禁：灸兩足大指去甲一寸三壯，又灸大指岐間各三壯（《 千 》。 ）三里
主霍亂遺矢 。大便不禁，病亦惄矣：神闕 、石門 、丹田 、屈骨端等，皆是穴
處，宜速灸之 。

Guān Yuán 關元 (Rèn 4) cures diarrhea, dysentery, vacuity distention, and difficult urination (*Míng*).

Hún Mén 魂門 (UB 47) treats irregular defecation (*Tóng*《 銅 》).

Fecal incontinence in the elderly and children: Apply three cones of moxibustion on [the site], 1 cùn away from the nail of both big toes; also burn three cones of moxibustion on [the site] between the juncture of the big toe (*Qiān*《千》).

Sān Lǐ 三里 (ST 36) governs sudden turmoil disorder and fecal incontinence.

Fecal incontinence, the patient is sick and weak: Shén Quē 神闕 (Rèn 8), Shí Mén 石門 (Rèn 5), and Dān Tián 丹田 (Cinnabar Field)), Qū Gǔ Duān 屈骨端 (Rèn 2), and so forth are all points [to treat this]. It is appropriate to apply moxibustion immediately.

予頃患脾泄，醫謂有積，以冷藥利之，大便不禁。服鎮靈丹十余丸，午夜各數丸而愈。今人服此丹三五丸不效，則不服，是以一勺水救輿薪火也，可乎哉？

[Author's notes:] I had spleen diarrhea a little while ago, the doctor said it was because of accumulations and drained it with cold herbs to induce fecal incontinence. I took more than ten pills of *Zhèn Líng Dān* 鎮靈丹 (Settle the Spirit Elixir) and several more pills at midnight. The disease was cured. Nowadays people stop taking this after three or five pills but it is ineffective. This is just like using a spoon of water to put out the fire in a whole cart of firewood. Is that possible?

3.25
Xiè Xiè (Yú Jiàn Tù Xiè)

泄瀉（餘見吐瀉）

Diarrhea
(for the rest, see the section on vomiting and diarrhea)

曲泉治泄利，四肢不舉（《銅》見疝 ）。腹結治腹寒泄利（ 見臍痛 ）。神闕
治泄利不止，小兒奶利不絕，腹大，繞臍痛。氣穴治婦人泄利不止（ 見月
事 ）。陽綱治大便泄利。意舍治大便滑泄（ 並見腹脹 ）。梁門治大腸滑泄，
穀不化（ 見積氣 ）。

Qū Quán 曲泉 (LV 8) treats diarrhea and inability to lift the four limbs (see the section on prominent *shàn*-mounting in *Tóng* 《銅》).

Fù Jié 腹結 (SP 14) treats cold in the abdomen and diarrhea (see the section on umbilical pain).

Shén Quē 神闕 (Rèn 8) treats incessant diarrhea, incessant diarrhea due to drinking milk in children, abdomen enlargement, and pain around the umbilicus.

Qì Xué 氣穴 (KI 13) treats incessant diarrhea in women (see the section on menstruation).

Yáng Gāng 陽綱 (UB 48) treats diarrhea.

Yì Shě 意舍 (UB 49) treats efflux diarrhea (see the section on abdominal fullness).

Liáng Mén 梁門 (ST 21) treats efflux diarrhea and non-transformation of grains [food] (see the section on accumulation of qì).

關門治泄利不欲食（ 見積氣 ）。天樞治泄利食不化。三焦俞治水穀不化，欲
泄注（ 見腹脹 ）。懸樞治水穀不化，下利（ 見積聚 ）。脊中治溫病，積聚下
利。中髎治腹脹下利，食泄。脾俞治泄利（ 見腹脹 ）。膀胱俞治泄利腹痛。
大腸俞 、腎俞治洞泄，食不化（ 見勞瘵 ）。

Guān Mén 關門 (ST 22) treats diarrhea with no desire to eat (see the section on accumulation of qì).

Tiān Shū 天樞 (ST 25) treats diarrhea with non-transformation of food.

Sān Jiāo Shù 三焦俞 (UB 22) treats non-transformation of grains and water [food] and outpour diarrhea (see the section on abdominal fullness).

Xuán Shù 懸俞 (Dū 5) treats non-transformation of grains and water [food] and diarrhea (see the section on accumulations and gatherings).

Jǐ Zhōng 脊中 (Dū 6) treats warm disease, accumulations and gatherings, and diarrhea.

Zhōng Liáo 中髎 (UB 33) treats abdominal distention, diarrhea, and food damage diarrhea.

Pí Shù 脾俞 (UB 20) treats diarrhea (see the section on abdominal fullness).

Páng Guāng Shù 膀胱俞 (UB 28) treats diarrhea and abdominal pain.

Dà Cháng Shù 大腸俞 (UB 25) and Shèn Shù 腎俞 (UB 23) treat throughflux diarrhea and non-transformation of food (see the section on consumption).

會陽治腹中冷氣，泄利不止。京門治小腹急腫，腸鳴洞泄，髎樞引痛。三間治腹滿腸鳴，洞泄。然谷治兒洞泄（見口噤）。關元療腹泄不止（《明下》見賁豚）。京門、然谷、陰陵泉主洞泄不化（《千》）。腎俞、章門主寒中，洞泄不化。京門、崑崙主洞泄，體痛。長強主頭重，洞泄。《明下》云：洞泄不禁。

Huì Yáng 會陽 (UB 35) treats cold qì in the abdomen with incessant diarrhea.

Jīng Mén 京門 (GB 25) treats acute swelling of the smaller abdomen, rumbling intestines, throughflux diarrhea, and pain radiating to the pelvic bone pivot [sacrum].[52]

Sān Jiān 三間 (LI 3) treats abdominal fullness, rumbling intestines, and throughflux diarrhea.

Rán Gǔ 然谷 (KI 2) treats throughflux diarrhea in children (see the section on clenched jaws).

Guān Yuán 關元 (Rèn 4) cures incessant diarrhea (see the section on running piglet in *Míng Xià* 《明下》).

Jīng Mén (GB 25), Rán Gǔ (KI 2), and Yīn Líng Quán 陰陵泉 (SP 9) govern throughflux diarrhea and non-transformation [of grains] (*Qiān* 《千》).

Shèn Shù (UB 23) and Zhāng Mén 章門 (LV 13) govern cold strike, throughflux diarrhea, and non-transformation [of grains].

Jīng Mén 京門 (GB 25) and Kūn Lún 崑崙 (UB 60) govern throughflux diarrhea and body pain.

---

52. It is unclear whether this refers to the hip joint or the sacrum.

Cháng Qiáng 長強 (Dū 1) governs heaviness of the head and throughflux diarrhea. *Míng Xià* 《明下》 says: incessant throughflux diarrhea.

陰陵泉、隱白主胸中熱，暴泄。大腸俞主腸鳴腹䐜腫，暴泄。三焦俞、小腸俞、下窌、意舍、章門主腸鳴腹脹欲泄注。會陽主腹中有寒泄注，腸澼便血。束骨主腸澼泄。天樞主冬月重感於寒則泄，當臍痛，腸胃間游氣切痛。若心腹痛而後泄，此寒氣客於腸間（ 云云 ）：灸關元百壯，服當歸縮砂湯（《指》）。

Yīn Líng Quán 陰陵泉 (SP 9) and Yǐn Bái 隱白 (SP 1) govern heat in the chest and violent diarrhea.

Dà Cháng Shù 大腸俞 (UB 25) governs rumbling intestines, abdominal distention, and violent diarrhea.

Sān Jiāo Shù 三焦俞 (UB 22), Xiǎo Cháng Shù 小腸俞 (UB 27), Xià Liáo 下窌 (UB 34), Yì Shě 意舍 (UB 49), and Zhāng Mén 章門 (LV 13) govern rumbling intestines, abdominal distention and outpour diarrhea.

Huì Yáng 會陽 (UB 35) governs cold in the abdomen, outpour diarrhea, intestinal afflux, and bloody stool.

Shù Gǔ 束骨 (UB 65) governs intestinal afflux and diarrhea.

Tiān Shū 天樞 (ST 25) governs diarrhea caused by cold attack in the winter, pain right in the umbilicus, and moving qì with cutting pain of the intestines and stomach.

Pain of the heart [region] and abdomen first, followed by diarrhea: This is cold qì settling in the intestines (and so forth): Apply a hundred cones of moxibustion on Guān Yuán 關元 (Rèn 4) and take *Dāng Guī Suō Shā Tāng* 當歸縮砂湯 (Tangkuei and Vietnamese Amomum Decoction) (*Zhǐ* 《指》).

泄瀉宜先灸臍中，次灸關元等穴。

[Author's notes:] For diarrhea, first apply moxibustion in the center of the umbilicus, then on Guān Yuán 關元 (Rèn 4) and so forth.

3.26
Sūn Xiè

飧泄

Swill diarrhea

中窌主腹脹飧泄。下廉治小腹痛飧泄，次指間痛，唇乾，涎出不覺，不得汗出，毛髮焦，脫肉少氣，胃中熱，不嗜食。上廉（見脅痛）治飧泄。陰陵泉主婦人飧泄（見疝瘕）。

Zhōng Liáo 中窌 (UB 33) governs abdominal distention and swill diarrhea.

Xià Lián 下廉 (ST 39) treats pain of the smaller abdomen, swill diarrhea, pain of the index finger, dry lips, uncontrollable drooling, absence of sweating, parched hair, emaciated flesh, qì shortage, heat in the stomach, and no desire to eat.

Shàng Lián 上廉 (ST 37) (see the section on pain of the [chest and] rib-sides) treats swill diarrhea.

Yīn Líng Quán 陰陵泉 (SP 9) treats swill diarrhea in women (see the section on *shàn*-mounting and conglomerations).

《素問》言春傷於風，夏必飧泄。苟知傷於風而得之，則藥自可治，雖不著艾，未為害也。

[Author's notes:] *Sù Wèn*《 素問 》says: When damaged by wind in the spring, swill diarrhea will occur in summer. When damaged by wind, herbs can treat it. Even if moxibustion is not applied, it will not cause harm.

《本事方》云：飧泄者，食穀不化也。春時木旺，肝生風邪，淫於脾經，至夏引冷當風，故多飧泄。宜芎藭丸：芎藭、神麴、白朮、附子等分，細末，糊丸梧子大，每服三五十丸，米飲下。治脾濕而泄者，萬無不中，其用芎除濕有理，故載於此。

Běn Shì Fāng《本事方》 says: Swill diarrhea is diarrhea with untransformed food [in the stool]. Wood is effulgent in the spring, so liver generates wind evils and invades the spleen channel. When exposed to wind and attacked by cold in the summer, people develop swill diarrhea. It is appropriate to take *Xiōng Qióng*[53] *Wán* 芎窮丸 (Chuān Xiōng Pill): Grind equal portions of *xiōng qióng* 芎窮 (Chuān Xiōng root), *shén qū* 神曲 (Medicated Leaven), *bái zhǔ* 白术 (Atractylodes), and *fù zǐ* 附子 (Aconite) and so forth into a fine powder, then use paste to make it into pills the size of the fruit of the phoenix tree. Take thirty or fifty pills with rice. This treats diarrhea due to spleen dampness and never misses. It is reasonable to use *xiōng* [*qióng*] (Chuān Xiōng root) to expel dampness, so I attach this here.

3.27
Táng Xiè

溏泄

Sloppy diarrhea

三陰交治溏泄食不化（《銅》見腹脹）。地機（見水腫）治溏泄。地機主溏瘕，腹痛，藏痺。太衝等主溏泄（見痢）。

Sān Yīn Jiāo 三陰交 (SP 6) treats sloppy diarrhea with non-transformation of food (see the section on abdominal fullness in *Tóng*《銅》).

Dì Jī 地機 (SP 8) (see the section on edema) treats sloppy diarrhea.

Dì Jī (SP 8) governs sloppy [diarrhea] with conglomerations, abdominal pain, and viscera bì-impediment (*Qiān*《千》).

Tài Chōng 太衝 (LV 3), and so forth govern sloppy diarrhea (see the section on dysentery).

予嘗患痺疼，既愈而溏利者久之。因灸臍中，遂不登圊。連三日灸之，三夕不登圊。若灸溏泄，臍中第一，三陰交等穴，乃其次也。

[Author's notes:] I had pain from *bì*-impediment; after it was cured I suffered sloppy diarrhea for a long time. When I applied moxibustion on the center of my umbilicus, I did not have to use the la-

---

53. *Xiōng qióng* is another name for *chuān xiōng* 川芎.

trine. I kept applying moxibustion for three days, and then I did not go to the latrine for three days. If we want to treat sloppy diarrhea with moxibustion, the first choice is the center of the umbilicus; Sān Yīn Jiāo 三陰交 (SP 6) and other points are the second choice.

《本事方》云：一親每五更初必溏痢一次者數月。有人云：此名腎泄，腎感陰氣而然。服五味子散愈（五味子二兩，吳茱萸半兩，細粒綠色者，並炒香熟為末，每服兩錢，陳米飲下）。其論溏利有理，故附載之。

Běn Shì Fāng 《本事方》 says: A relative once suffered sloppy diarrhea during the fifth-watch [4-6 am] for several months. People called this kidney diarrhea, which is caused by yīn qì attacking the kidneys. He took *Wǔ Wèi Zǐ Sǎn* 五味子散 (Schisandrae Powder) (2 *liǎng* of *wǔ wèi zǐ* 五味子 (Schisandrae Fructus) and 0.5 *liǎng* of *wú zhū yú* 吳茱萸 (Evodiae Fructus) using small green pieces, stir-fried until fragrant, then ground into a powder. Each time swallow 2 *qián* with aged rice drink). This discussion of sloppy diarrhea made sense, so I attached it here.

予舊患溏利，每天曉必如廁。人教贖豆附丸。服即愈。其方不可得也，它年再患此，只用薑煎附子加豆蔻服，愈。

[Authors' notes:] I suffered sloppy diarrhea in the past. I had to go to the latrine every morning. People told me to buy *Dòu Fù Wán* 豆附丸 (Tsaoko and Aconite Pill). It was cured after I took the pills. [Later] I could not get the formula, so when I had same disease another year, I cooked ginger-fried *fù zǐ* 附子 (Acontite) and added *dòu kòu* 豆蔻. It also cured the disease.

3.28
Lì (Yú Jiàn Xiè)

痢（餘見瀉）

Dysentery
(for the rest, see section on diarrhea)

《素問》言泄痢有五種：一曰胃泄，飲食不化而色黃，胃與脾合故黃
也；二曰脾泄，腹脹而注泄無休，又上逆嘔，此為寒熱之患也；三曰
大腸泄，食畢腸鳴切痛，而痢白色，大腸與肺合故白也；四曰小腸
泄，身瘦而便膿血，小腸與心合，心主血也；五曰大瘕泄，里急後
重，數至圊不能便，莖中痛，此腎泄也。諸家方有二十餘種，此唯言
五種，蓋舉其綱也。

[Author's notes:] *Sù Wèn* 《素問》talks about five types of diarrhea: The first one is called stomach diarrhea with non-transformation of food [as seen from the stool] and yellow color. Stomach and spleen are interconnected, so the color is yellow; the second one is called spleen diarrhea with abdominal distention and incessant outpour diarrhea, qì counterflowing upward, and vomiting. It is caused by cold and heat; the third one is called large intestine diarrhea with rumbling intestines, cutting pain [in the intestines] after eating, and dysentery with white stool. Large intestine and the lungs are interconnected, so the color is white; the fourth one is called small intestine diarrhea with emaciated body, and stools containing pus and blood. Small intestine and the heart are interconnected, and the heart governs the blood; the fifth is called great conglomeration diarrhea with abdominal tension and rectal heaviness [tenesmus], frequent trips to the latrine but inability to defecate, and pain of the penis. This is kidney diarrhea. There are over twenty [types of diarrhea] from all the medical books, but only five are mentioned here to go over the key points.

《必用方》亦有赤白瘕蠱之別。其大概則臟腑寒也。廩丘公所謂諸下
悉寒是也。數予治人痢，惟與以鎮靈丹，無有不效。或未效，更加丸
數，則效矣。若蠱利，則用柏葉、黃連煎服（見《既效》）。諸痢惟
耆域方用厚朴、罌粟殼末最佳。後人又加木香、黃連、陳皮等分，甘
草拌之，黃穀葉數片、薑、棗、烏梅水煎。予嘗用之驗，故載於此。
然痢本無惡證，而有患此而死者，或者世醫以痢為熱病，多服冷藥故
也。若其急難，亦當灼艾，不可專用藥云。

Bì Yòng Fāng 《 必用方 》 also mentioned the difference between red and white *gān* 疳 or *gǔ* 蠱 diseases. The general idea is that they are caused by cold in the viscera. The saying of Master Lǐn Qīu[54] is that "all diarrhea belongs to cold." When I treat dysentery, I only use *Zhèn Líng Dān* 鎮靈丹 (Settle Spirit Elixir) which is always effective. If it does not take effect, adding more pills will work. If it is diarrhea from *gǔ*, decoct and drink *bǎi yè* 柏葉 (Platycladi Cacumen) and *huáng lián* 黃連 (Coptidis Rhizoma) (see *Jì Xiào [Fāng]* 《 既效[方]》). For all dysentery disorders, the [combination of] *hòu pò* 厚樸 (Radix Magnoliae Officnalis) and *yīng sù ké* 罌粟殼 (Papaveris Pericarpium) in *Qí Yù Fāng* 耆域方 (Formula from Qí Yù) works the best. Later generations have added equal portions of *mù xiāng* 木香 (Aucklandiae Radix), *huáng lián* (Coptidis Rhizoma) and *chén pí* 陳皮(Citri Reticulatae Pericapium), mixed with *gān cǎo* 甘草 (Glycyrrhizae); then decoct it with several leaves of yellow grain, ginger, dates and *wū méi* 烏梅 (Mume Fructus). I tried this and it is effective, so I attach it here. Originally, there were no malign signs of dysentery. If people die from dysentery, it is probably because doctors nowadays think dysentery is a heat disease and treat it with cold herbs. If there is urgency and difficulty, we should also burn moxibustion in addition to the herbs.

復溜主腸澼，便膿血，泄痢後重，腹痛如痙狀（《千》）。交信主泄痢赤白（《銅》同）漏血。太衝、曲泉主溏泄，痢注下血。小腸俞主泄痢膿血五色，重下腫痛。丹田主泄痢不禁，小腹絞痛。關元、太溪主泄痢不止。

Fù Liū 復溜 (KI 7) governs intestinal afflux, stools containing pus and blood, diarrhea with rectal heaviness, and abdominal pain like tetany (*Qiān* 《 千 》).

Jiāo Xìn 交信 (KI 8) governs diarrhea with mixed red and white stool (*Tóng* 《 銅 》 agrees), and spotting of blood.

Tài Chōng 太衝 (LV 3) and Qū Quán 曲泉 (LV 8) govern sloppy diarrhea, and outpour diarrhea with precipitation of blood.

Xiǎo Cháng Shù 小腸俞 (UB 27) governs five-colored diarrhea with blood and pus, frequent diarrhea, and [rectal] swelling and pain.

Dān Tián 丹田 [cinnabar field] governs incessant diarrhea with gripping pain of the smaller abdomen.

Guān Yuán 關元 (Rèn 4) , Tài Xī 太溪 (KI 3) govern incessant diarrhea.

脾俞主泄痢不食，食不生肌。五樞主婦人赤白，里急瘕瘀。曲泉治泄水，下利膿血（《銅》見風勞）。中膂俞治腸冷赤白痢（《明》同）。膀胱俞療泄

---

54. Lǐn Qīugōng 廩丘公 [Master Lǐn Qīu] refers to Cáo Xī 曹翕, a doctor during the *Jìn* (晋) Dynasty.

痢，腹痛（《明》）。脊俞療溫病，積聚下痢（《銅》作下利）。關元療泄
痢（見大便不禁）。

Pí Shù 脾俞 (UB 20) governs diarrhea, inability to eat, or eating but without engendering flesh.

Wǔ Shū 五樞 (GB 27) governs mixed white and red [stool] in women, abdominal tension, and tugging and slackening.

Qū Quán 曲泉 (LV 8) treats diarrhea with watery [stool]; or blood and pus (see the section on wind taxation in *Tóng* 《銅》).

Zhōng Lǚ Shù 中膂俞 (UB 29) treats intestinal coldness and red and white dysentery (*Míng* 《明》 agrees).

Páng Guāng Shù 膀胱俞 (UB 28) cures diarrhea and abdominal pain (*Míng*).

Jǐ Shù 脊俞 (Dū 6) cures warm disease, accumulations and gatherings, and dysentery (*Tóng* says diarrhea).

Guān Yuán 關元 (Rèn 4) cures diarrhea (see the discussion of fecal incontinence).

小兒痢下赤白，秋末脫肛，每廁腹痛不可忍：灸十二椎下節間，
名接脊穴一
壯。黃帝療小兒疳痢脫肛，體瘦渴飲，形容瘦悴，諸藥不瘥：灸尾翠骨上三
寸骨陷間三壯。岐伯云：三伏內用桃水浴孩子，午正時當日灸之，用青帛
拭，似見疳蟲隨汗出，神效。小兒秋深冷痢不止：灸臍下二寸、三寸間動脈
中三壯。

Children with white and red dysentery, prolapsed rectum in the late fall, and unbearable abdominal pain when using the latrine: Apply one cone of moxibustion on the *Jiā Jǐ* point 夾脊穴 that is located below the 12th vertebra.

The Yellow Emperor prescribed treatment for pediatric *gān* 疳 dysentery that was unable to be cured after taking various herbs, manifesting with prolapsed rectum, emaciation, desire to drink, and thin weak appearance: Apply three cones of moxibustion on the depression 3 cùn above the coccyx.

Qí Bó said: Bathe children with peach water during the *sān fú* period,[55] apply moxibustion in the sun at noon time, and wipe with green-blue silk cloth; then the *gān* insects seem to come out with sweating. This has divine effects.

---

55. The *sān fú* 三伏 are three ten-day periods that are said to be the hottest time of the year. Each starts with a *gēng* 庚 (yáng metal) stem day. The initial *fú* begins on the third *gēng* day after the *xià zhì* 夏至 summer solstice. The middle *fú* starts ten days later. The final *fú* begins on the first *gēng* day after *lì qiū* 立秋 Autumn Begins (the midpoint between the summer solstice and the autumn equinox).

Children with incessant cold dysentery in the late fall: Apply three cones of moxibustion on the pulsing vessel located two or three cùn below the umbilicus.

婦人水泄痢：灸氣海百壯。泄痢食不消，不作肌膚：灸脾俞隨年壯（《千》）。泄注五利便膿，重下腹痛：灸小腸俞百壯。泄痢不禁，小腹絞痛：灸石門百壯（三報）。久痢百治不瘥：灸足陽明下一寸高骨上陷中，去大指岐三寸，隨年；又臍中二三百壯，又關元三百（十日灸）。赤白下：灸窮骨，多為佳。四肢不舉，多汗洞痢：灸大橫隨年（餘見《千金》）。痢暴下如水云云：氣海百壯（《指》）。

Diarrhea with watery stool in women: Apply a hundred cones of moxibustion on Qì Hǎi 氣海 (Rèn 6).

Diarrhea with undigested food and inability to engender flesh and skin: Apply the same number of cones of moxibustion as the patient's age on Pí Shù 脾俞 (UB 20) (*Qiān* 《千》).

Outpour diarrhea, the five types of diarrhea with stool containing pus, frequent diarrhea, and abdominal pain: Apply a hundred cones of moxibustion on Xiǎo Cháng Shù 小腸俞 (UB 27).

Incessant diarrhea and gripping pain in the smaller abdomen: Apply a hundred cones of moxibustion on Shí Mén 石門 (Rèn 5) (three sessions).

Enduring dysentery which cannot be cured after hundreds of treatments: Apply moxibustion in the depression on the high bone 1 cùn distal to the foot yángmíng 足陽明 (ST 42) and 3 cùn proximal to the junction of the big toe. Burn the same number of cones as the patient's age. Two or three hundred cones of moxibustion can also be applied in the center of the umbilicus; or burn three hundred cones on Guān Yuán 關元 (Rèn 4) (apply moxibustion for ten days).

Red and white diarrhea: Apply moxibustion on Qióng Gǔ 窮骨 (Dū 1). It is better to burn a lot of cones.

Inability to lift the four limbs, profuse sweating, and throughflux diarrhea: Apply the same number of cones of moxibustion as the patient's age on Dà Héng 大橫 (SP 15) (for the rest, see *Qiān Jīn* 《千金》).

Dysentery with violent watery diarrhea (and so forth): Apply a hundred cones of moxibustion on Qì Hǎi (Rèn 6) (*Zhǐ* 《指》).

3.29
Biàn Xuè (Yú Jiàn Lì, Cháng Fēng)

便血（餘見痢　腸風）

Bloody stool
(for the rest, see dysentery and intestinal wind)

復溜 、太衝等（並見痢）、會陽（見瀉）主便血（《千》）。下廉、幽門（《明》同）太白（見吐瀉）治泄利膿血（《銅》）。太白治吐泄膿血（見腹脹）。小腸俞治大便膿血出（《明》同）。下髎治大便下血。腹哀治大便膿血（見腹痛）。《千》又云：寒中，食不化，腹痛。勞宮（見傷寒）治大小便血。

Fù Liū 復溜 (KI 7), Tài Chōng 太衝 (LV 3), and so forth (for all of these, see the section on dysentery), and Huì Yáng 會陽 (UB 35) (see the section on diarrhea) govern bloody stool (*Qiān* 《千》).

Xià Lián 下廉 (ST 39), Yōu Mén 幽門 (KI 21) (*Míng* 《明》 agrees), and Tài Bái 太白 (SP 3) (see the section on vomiting and diarrhea) treat diarrhea with pus and blood (*Tóng* 《銅》).

Tài Bái 太白 (SP 3) treats vomiting and diarrhea with pus and blood (see the section on abdominal fullness).

Xiǎo Cháng Shù 小腸俞 (UB 27) treats stools containing pus and blood (*Míng* agrees).

Xià Liáo 下髎 (UB 34) treats bloody stool.

Fù Āi 腹哀 (SP 16) treats stools containing pus and blood (see the section on abdominal pain). *Qiān* says: It treats cold strike with non-transformation of food and abdominal pain.

Láo Gōng 勞宮 (PC 8) (see the section on cold damage) treats bloody stool and urine.

《陸氏續集驗方》治下血不止：量臍心與脊骨平，於脊骨上灸七壯即止。如再發，即再灸七壯，永除根本。目睹數人有效。予嘗用此灸人腸風，皆除根本，神效無比。然亦須按其骨突處酸疼方灸之，不疼則不灸也。但便血本因於腸風，腸風即腸痔，不可分而為三。或分為三而治之，非也。

253

[Author's notes:] *Lù Shì Xù Jí Yàn Fāng*《陸氏續集驗方》(Sequel to the Collection of Proven Formulas from Master Lù) treats incessant blood in the stool: Measure [from the floor] to the center of the umbilicus and find the site that is level with it on the spine; apply seven cones of moxibustion on the spine [at this level] to stop [incessant blood in the stool]. If it occurs again, burn another seven cones of moxibustion to remove the root. I saw that this method was effective in a lot of people, so I tried treating intestinal wind with this moxibustion; it removes the root [of the disease]. Nothing can compete with it. We should apply this moxibustion on the bony prominence that aches when pressed; don't use moxibustion if there is no pain. Bloody stool originates from intestinal wind, which means intestinal hemorrhoids. We cannot divide this treatment into three sessions; if we divide it into three sessions to treat, it is not correct.

3.30
Zhì (Lòu Lòu, Yú Jiàn Yáng Lòu)

痔（瘻漏　餘見瘍瘻）

Hemorrhoids
(Fistulas,[56] for the rest, see sores and fistulas)

長強治腸風下血，五種痔，疳蝕下部䘌，此痔根本是冷，謹冷食房勞（《銅》與《明》同）。《明下》云：療久痔。會陰治穀道瘙擾，久痔相通者死（《千》云：主痔與陰相通者死）。會陽治久痔。小腸俞治五痔疼（《明》同）。

Cháng Qiáng 長強 (Dū 1) treats intestinal wind with bloody diarrhea, the five types of hemorrhoids, and *gān* 疳 erosion with small insects in the lower body [pelvic area]. The root of these hemorrhoids is cold, so cold food and sexual taxation should be avoided (*Tóng*《銅》and *Míng*《明》agree). *Míng Xià*《明下》says: It treats enduring hemorrhoids.

Huì Yīn 會陰 (Rèn 1) treats itching[57] of the grain duct [anus] and enduring hemorrhoids penetrating to the anus which can make people die (*Qiān*《千》says: It treats hemorrhoids penetrating to the anus which can make people die).

---

56. 瘻 and 漏 are both pronounced *lòu*. *Lòu* 瘻 means fistulas. *Lòu* 漏 literally means leakage and is used in other medical terms, but within the context of this chapter, it also means fistulas. Here, we will translate both terms as fistula.

57. The original text has *sào rǎo* 瘙擾, which means itching and disturbance. It is corrected to *sāo yǎng* 搔癢 (itching) based on *Tóng Rén Tú Jīng*.

Huì Yáng 會陽 (UB 35) treats enduring hemorrhoids.

Xiǎo Cháng Shù 小腸俞 (UB 27) treats pain of the five types of hemorrhoids (*Míng* 《 明 》 agrees).

秩邊治五痔發腫 。復溜治血痔，泄後腫 。飛揚治野雞痔 。承山治久痔腫痛 。扶承治久痔尻臗腫，大便難，陰胞有寒，小便不利 。《 千 》云：療五種痔，瀉鮮血，尻臗中腫，大便難，小便不利 。氣海俞療痔病瀉血（ 《 明 》 ）。

Zhì Biān 秩邊 (UB 54) treats the five types of hemorrhoids with swelling.

Fù Liū 復溜 (KI 7) treats bloody hemorrhoids and swelling after diarrhea.

Fēi Yáng 飛揚 (UB 58) treats wing-necked pheasant hemorrhoids.[58]

Chéng Shān 承山 (UB 57) treats enduring hemorrhoids with swelling and pain.

Fú Chéng 扶承 (UB 36) treats enduring hemorrhoids, swollen sacrum and coccyx, difficult defecation, cold in the uterus, and inhibited urination. *Qiān* 《 千 》 says: It treats the five types of hemorrhoids, with drainage of fresh blood, swelling of the sacrum and coccyx, difficult defecation, and inhibited urination.

Qì Hǎi Shù 氣海俞 (UB 24) cures hemorrhoid diseases with drainage of blood (*Míng*).

飛揚主痔篡傷痛 。商丘 、復溜主痔血，泄後重 。勞宮主熱痔 。承筋 、承扶 、委中 、陽谷主痔痛，掖下腫 。商丘主痔骨蝕（ 《 銅 》云：痔疾，骨疽蝕 ）。支溝 、章門主馬刀腫瘻 。絕骨主瘻，馬刀掖腫 。俠溪 、陽輔（ 《 銅 》同 ）、太衝主掖下腫，馬刀瘻（ 《 銅 》云：太衝 、臨泣治馬刀瘍瘻 ）。

Fēi Yáng (UB 58) governs hemorrhoids and pain of the perineum.

Shāng Qiū 商丘 (SP 5) and Fù Liū (KI 7) govern hemorrhoids with bleeding and rectal heaviness.

Láo Gōng 勞宮 (PC 8) governs hot hemorrhoids.

Chéng Jīn 承筋 (UB 56), Chéng Fú 承扶 (UB 36), Wěi Zhōng 委中 (UB 40), and Yáng Gǔ 陽谷 (SI 5) govern painful hemorrhoids and swollen armpits.

Shāng Qiū (SP 5) governs hemorrhoids and bone erosion (*Tóng* 《 銅 》 says: hemorrhoids and flat-abscess of the bone with erosion).

---

58. Wing-necked pheasant hemorrhoids probably refer to hemorrhoids that appear multicolored.

Zhī Gōu 支溝 (SJ 6) and Zhāng Mén 章門 (LV 13) govern saber lumps with swelling and fistulas.

Jué Gǔ 絕骨 (GB 39) governs fistulas, saber lumps, and swollen armpits.

Xiá Xī 俠溪 (GB 43), Yáng Fǔ 陽輔 (GB 38) (*Tóng*《銅》agrees), and Tài Chōng 太衝 (LV 3) govern armpit swelling, saber lumps, and fistulas (*Tóng* says: Tài Chōng (LV 3) and Lín Qì 臨泣 (GB 41) treat saber lumps, sores, and fistulas).

天突、章門、天池、支溝主漏。天突、天窗主漏頸痛。長強療下漏（《明》見痔。《千》用葶藶子，豉作餅灸漏。《外臺》云：不可灸頭瘡，葶藶氣入腦殺人）。

Tiān Tū 天突 (Rèn 22), Zhāng Mén (LV 13), Tiān Chí 天池 (PC 1), and Zhī Gōu (SJ 6) govern fistulas.

Tiān Tū (Rèn 22) and Tiān Chuāng 天窗 (SI 16) govern fistulas and neck pain.

Cháng Qiáng 長強 (Dū 1) cures fistulas in the lower body (see the section on hemorrhoids in *Míng*《明》. *Qiān*《千》prescribes making cakes with *tíng lì zǐ* 葶藶子 and [*dòu*] *chǐ* 豆豉, then burning moxibustion on the cakes to treat fistulas. *Wài Tái*《外臺》says: Moxibustion is contraindicated on head sores; it will kill the people when qì of *tíng lì* [*zǐ*] 葶藶子 enters the brain.)

灸痔法：疾若未深，尾閭骨下近穀道，灸一穴，便可除去。如《傳信方》先以經年槐枝煎湯洗，後灸其上七壯，大稱其驗。如《本草》祇以馬藍菜根一握、水三碗、煎碗半。乘熱以小口瓦器中熏洗，令腫退，於元生鼠奶根上灸（即不可灸尖頭，恐效遲）。如患深，用湯洗未退，易湯洗令消。然後灸，覺火氣通至胸乃效。病雖深，至二十餘壯，永絕根本。以竹片護四邊肉，仍於天色寒涼時灸，忌毒物（《集效》）。

Moxibustion method for hemorrhoids: For [hemorrhoid] diseases that are not severe, apply moxibustion on a point below the coccyx, close to the grain duct [anus]. The disease will be removed.

Chuán Yán Fāng《傳言方》says to decoct *huái zhī* 槐枝 [sophora twigs] that have been around for one or several years and wash [the hemorrhoids]; then apply seven cones of moxibustion on them. The book says this method is very effective.

The *Běn Cǎo*《本草》only decocts a handful of *mǎ lán cài gēn* 馬藍菜根 [root of Indian Kalimeris Herb] in three bowls of water till 1.5 bowls of the decoction are left. Put the decoction into an earthenware small-mouth bottle, then steam-wash [the hemorrhoids] while the decoction is warm.

To reduce the swelling, apply moxibustion on the root of the "mouse breast"[59] (do not apply moxibustion on the tip, or the effects might be delayed). If the disease is severe and has not receded after washing with a decoction, switch the decoction and wash [again] to make it disappear. Then apply moxibustion; it will be effective when fiery qì passes into the chest. Applying more than twenty cones moxibustion will cut off the root [of the disease] even if it is severe. Use bamboo slices to shield the good flesh around [the hemorrhoids]. Apply moxibustion during cold weather; avoid toxic things (*Jí Xiào* 《集效》).

千金灸漏，更有數穴。

[Author's notes:] *Qiān Jīn* 《千金》 has still more points that can be used for applying moxibustion to treat fistulas.

3.31
Cháng Fēng

腸風

Intestinal wind

脊端窮骨（脊骨盡處），一名龜尾，當中灸三壯，治腸風瀉血即愈。須顛倒身方灸得。久冷五痔便血，脊中百壯（《千翼》）。

Qióng Gǔ 窮骨 [Dū 1] is at the tip of the spine (the end of the spinal bones), and is also named Guī Wěi 龜尾. Apply three cones of moxibustion on it to cure intestinal wind with bloody diarrhea. Moxibustion can be applied with the patient's body turned upside-down.

Burn a hundred cones of moxibustion on Jǐ Zhōng 脊中 (Dū 6) for enduring cold, the five types of hemorrhoids, and bloody stool (*Qiān Yì* 《千翼》).

何教授《湯簿》有此疾積年，皆一灸除根。《湯簿》因傳此法。後觀灸經，此穴療小兒脫肛瀉血，蓋岐伯灸小兒法也。後人因之，以灸大人腸風瀉血爾。蓋大人、小兒之病初不異故也。

---

59. Mouse breast describes the shape of the hemorrhoid.

五痔便血失屎，回氣百壯，在脊窮骨上。赤白下：灸窮骨，惟多為佳。長強治腸風下血（《銅》見痔）。

The five types of hemorrhoids, bloody stool, and fecal incontinence: Apply a hundred cones of moxibustion on Qióng Gǔ 窮骨 (Dū 1) on the spine to return qì.

Red and white diarrhea: Apply moxibustion on Qióng Gǔ (Dū 1); it is better to use a lot of cones.

Cháng Qiáng 長強 (Dū 1) treats intestinal wind and bloody stool (see the section on hemorrhoids in *Tóng* 《銅》).

腸風藥甚眾，多不作效，何也。《本草衍義》曰：腸風乃腸痔，苟知其為痔而治之，無不效矣。若灸腸風，長強為要穴云。近李倉腸風，市醫以杖量臍中於脊骨當臍處灸，即愈。予因此為人灸腸風，皆除根。（陸氏方治下血除根。）

3.32
Cháng Pì

腸澼

Intestinal afflux

復溜（ 見痢 ）、束骨 、會陽（ 見瀉 ）主腸澼（ 《 千 》 ）。中都治腸澼，㿉疝
小腹痛，（ 《 銅 》 ）。四滿治腸澼切痛（ 見積聚 ）。

Fù Liū 復溜 (KI 7) (see dysentery), Shù Gǔ 束骨 (UB 65), and Huì Yáng 會陽 (UB 35) (see diarrhea) govern intestinal afflux (*Qiān* 《 千 》).

Zhōng Dū 中都 (LV 6) treats intestinal afflux, prominent *shàn*-mounting, and pain of the smaller abdomen (*Tóng* 《 銅 》).

Sì Mǎn 四滿 (KI 14) treats intestinal afflux with cutting pain (see accumulations and gatherings).

結積留飲澼囊，胸滿飲食不消：灸通谷五十壯（ 《 千 》 ）。大腸俞主風，腹
中雷鳴，大腸灌沸，腸澼泄痢，食不消化，小腹絞痛，腰脊疼強，大小便
難，不能飲食，灸百壯，三報之 。

Binding accumulations, lodged rheum, and afflux pouch [a pathological accumulation], chest fullness, and non-dispersion of food: Apply fifty cones of moxibustion on Tōng Gǔ 通谷 (KI 20) (*Qiān*).

Dà Cháng Shù 大腸俞 (UB 25) governs wind, thunderous rumbling in abdomen, uproar in the large intestine, intestinal afflux, diarrhea and dysentery, non-transformation of food, gripping pain in the smaller abdomen, stiffness and pain of lower back and spine, difficult defecation and urination, and inability to eat; apply a hundred cones of moxibustion, giving three sessions.

諸結積留飲澼囊，胸滿飲食不消：通谷五十壯，又胃管三百，三報之 。第十
五椎名下極俞，主腹中疾，腰痛，膀胱寒澼，飲注下，隨年壯（ 《 千翼 》 ）
 。會陽主腹中有寒泄注，腸澼便血 。束骨主腸澼泄 。膺窗主腸鳴泄注 。陽綱
主大便不節，小便赤黃，腸鳴泄注 。

All binding accumulations, lodged rheum, afflux pouch [a pathological accumulation], chest fullness, and non-dispersion of food: Apply fifty cones of moxibustion on Tōng Gǔ 通谷 (KI 20), also burn another three hundred cones on Wèi Guǎn 胃管 (Rèn 12 or Rèn 13), giving three sessions.

[The site located] below the fifteenth vertebra is named Xià Jǐ Shù 下脊俞 and it governs diseases of the abdomen, lower back pain, cold afflux in the bladder, rheum, and downpour diarrhea; apply the same number of cones of moxibustion as the patient's age (*Qiān Yì* 《千翼》).

Huì Yáng 會陽 (UB 35) governs cold in the abdomen, outpour diarrhea, intestinal afflux, and bloody stool.

Shù Gǔ 束骨 (UB 65) governs intestinal afflux and diarrhea.

Yīng Chuāng 膺窗 (ST 16) governs rumbling intestines and outpour diarrhea.

Yáng Gāng 陽綱 (UB 48) governs irregular defecation, dark yellow urine, rumbling intestines, and outpour diarrhea.

三焦俞 、小腸俞 、下窌 、意舍 、章門主腸鳴腹脹，欲泄注（《千》）。

Sān Jiāo Shù 三焦俞 (UB 22), Xiǎo Cháng Shù 小腸俞 (UB 27), Xià Liáo 下窌 (UB 34), Yì Shě 意舍 (UB 49), and Zhāng Mén 章門 (LV 13) govern rumbling intestines, abdominal distention, and imminent outpour diarrhea (*Qiān* 《千》).

3.33
Cháng Tòng (Yú Jiàn Cháng Pì)

腸痛（餘見腸澼）

Intestinal pain
(for the rest, see intestinal afflux)

太白主腸痛（《甲》見腸鳴）。陷谷等主腸痛（《千》見腸鳴）。商曲治腸切痛（《銅》見積聚）。建里療腸中疼，嘔逆上氣，心痛身腫（《明》）。氣衝治腸中之熱（《銅》見上氣）。

Tài Bái 太白 (SP 3) governs intestinal pain (see the section on rumbling intestines in *Jiǎ*《甲》).

Xiàn Gǔ 陷谷 (ST 43) and so forth govern intestinal pain (see the section on rumbling intestines in *Qiān*《千》).

Shāng Qū 商曲 (KI 17) treats gripping pain of the intestines (see the section on accumulations and gatherings in *Tóng*《銅》).

Jiàn Lǐ 建里 (Rèn 11) cures pain of the intestines, retching counterflow with qì ascent, heart pain, and generalized swelling (*Míng*《明》).

Qì Chōng 氣衝 (ST 30) treats great heat in the intestines (see the section on qì ascent in *Tóng*).

腸痛亦多端。若疼甚者，乃腸癰：急宜服內補十全散等藥，其它宜隨證灸之。有老嫗大腸中常若里急後重，甚苦之，自言人必無老新婦此奇疾也。為按其大腸俞疼甚，令歸灸之而愈。

[Author's notes:] Intestinal pain has several causes. If there is severe pain, it is intestinal abscess: take *Nèi Bǔ Shí Quán Sǎn* 內補十全散, and so forth immediately; then apply moxibustion for other complications. There was an old lady who had large intestine symptoms such as tenesmus; she suffered a lot and said of herself that soon there will be no old lady. This was a mysterious disease. I pressed her Dà Cháng Shù 大腸俞 (UB 25) and she felt sharp pain, so I told her to apply moxibustion on it and the disease was cured.

癰為病，小腸重，小便數似淋，或繞臍生瘡，或膿從臍出，大便出膿血：屈
兩肘正灸肘頭銳骨各百壯，則下膿止，止瘥。

Intestinal abscess [with the symptoms of] heaviness in the small intestine, frequent urination similar to *lín*-strangury, sores around the umbilicus, or pus exuding from the umbilicus, and defecation
with pus and blood: Apply a hundred cones of moxibustion on the end of the sharp bone when
the patient flexes both elbows. It will stop the diarrhea with pus and cure the disease.

胡權內補十全散治腸癰神效。

[Author's notes:] *Nèi Bǔ Shí Quán Sǎn* 內補十全散 from Hú Quán 胡權[60] treats intestinal
abscess and has miraculous effects.

---

60. Hú Quán 胡權 probably refers the author of *Zhì Yōng Jū Nóng Dú Fāng*《治癰疽膿毒方》
(Formulas for Treating Toxic Diseases with Pus, Welling-Abscesses, and Flat-Abscesses).

3.34
Cháng Míng (Fù Míng)

腸鳴（腹鳴）

Rumbling intestines
(Rumbling abdomen)

不容治腹虛鳴（《銅》見痃癖 ）。三間主胸滿腸鳴（《千》 ）。胃俞主腹滿而鳴（《明下》云：腹中鳴 ）。臍中主腸中常鳴，上衝於心 。天樞主腹脹腸鳴，氣上衝胸（ 又主婦人 ）。陰都主心滿氣逆，腸鳴 。太白、公孫 、大腸俞 、三焦俞等（ 見瀉 ）主腸鳴 。陰交主腸鳴濯濯，有如水聲 。上廉主腸鳴相追逐 。漏谷主腸鳴，強欠，心悲氣逆 。

Bù Róng 不容 (ST 19) treats vacuity rumbling in the abdomen (see the section on strings and aggregations in *Tóng* 《 銅 》).

Sān Jiān 三間 (LI 3) governs chest fullness and rumbling intestines (*Qiān* 《 千 》).

Wèi Shù 胃俞 (UB 21) governs abdominal fullness and rumbling (*Míng Xià* 《 明下 》 says: rumbling in the abdomen).

Qí Zhōng 臍中 (Rèn 8) governs frequent rumbling in the intestines that surges into the heart.

Tiān Shū 天樞 (ST 25) governs abdominal distention, rumbling intestines, qì surging up into the chest (and also governs women's [diseases]).

Yīn Dū 陰都 (KI 19) governs heart fullness, qì counterflow, and rumbling intestines.

Tài Bái 太白 (SP 3), Gōng Sūn 公孫 (SP 4), Dà Cháng Shù 大腸俞 (UB 25), Sān Jiāo Shù 三焦俞 (UB 22) and so forth (see the section on diarrhea) govern rumbling intestines.

Yīn Jiāo 陰交 (Rèn 7) governs rumbling intestines with sounds like water in the intestines.

Shàng Lián 上廉 (ST 37) governs rumbling intestines chasing each other [frequent rumbling].

Lòu Gǔ 漏谷 (SP 7) governs rumbling intestines, belching, sorrowful heart, and qì counterflow.

膺窗主腸鳴泄注。陷谷、溫溜、漏谷、復溜、陽綱主腸鳴而痛。下窌主婦人腸鳴注泄。胸脅脹、腸鳴切痛：太白主之（《甲》）。三里（見胃）、三間、京門（見瀉）關門、（見積氣）、三陰交（見腹脹）、陷谷、水分、神闕（並見水腫）、承滿、溫溜、三焦俞、大腸俞、胃俞（腹脹）、天樞（月事）治腸鳴（《銅》）。

Yīng Chuāng 膺窗 (ST 16) governs rumbling intestines and outpour diarrhea.

Xiàn Gǔ 陷谷 (ST 43), Wēn Liū 溫溜 (LI 7), Lòu Gǔ 漏谷 (SP 7), Fù Liū 復溜 (KI 7), and Yáng Gāng 陽綱 (UB 48) govern rumbling intestines with pain.

Xià Liáo 下窌 (UB 34) governs rumbling intestines in women and outpouring diarrhea.

Tài Bái 太白 (SP 3) governs distention of the chest and rib-sides and rumbling intestines with cutting pain (*Jiǎ*《甲》).

Sān Lǐ 三里 (ST 36) (see the discussion of the stomach ache), Sān Jiān 三間 (LI 3), Jīng Mén 京門 (GB 25) (see the section on diarrhea), Guān Mén 關門 (ST 22) (see the section on accumulation of qì), Sān Yīn Jiāo 三陰交 (SP 6) (see the section on abdominal fullness), Xiàn Gǔ (ST 43), Shuǐ Fēn 水分 (Rèn 9), Shén Quē 神闕 (Rèn 8) (for all, see the section on edema), Chéng Mǎn 承滿 (ST 20), Wēn Liū (LI 7), Sān Jiāo Shù 三焦俞 (UB 22), Dà Cháng Shù 大腸俞 (UB 25), Wèi Shù 胃俞 (UB 21) (see the section on abdominal fullness), and Tiān Shū 天樞 (ST 25) (see the section on menstruation) treat rumbling intestines (*Tóng*《銅》).

章門治腸鳴盈盈然（《千》同），食不化，脅痛不得臥，煩熱口乾，不嗜食，胸脅支滿，喘息心痛，腰（《下經》有背脊）痛不得轉側。上廉治腸鳴，氣走痃痛。商丘治腹脹腸鳴不便，脾虛令人不樂，身寒善太息，心悲氣逆。復溜治腹雷鳴（見鼓脹）。督俞療腹痛雷鳴（《明》見腹痛）。

Zhāng Mén 章門 (LV 13) treats fullness and rumbling in the intestines (*Qiān*《千》agrees), non-transformation of food, pain of the rib-sides, inability to lie down, heat vexation, dry mouth, no desire to eat, propping fullness of the chest and rib-sides, panting, heart pain, low back (*Xià Jīng*《下經》has back and rib-sides) pain, inability to turn to the sides.

Shàng Lián 上廉 (ST 37) treats rumbling intestines and qì infixation pain.[61]

Shāng Qiū 商丘 (SP 5) treats abdominal distention, rumbling intestines and constipation, spleen vacuity that makes people unhappy, cold body with desire to sigh, sorrowful heart, and qì counterflow.

Fù Liū (KI 7) treats thunderous rumbling in the abdomen (see the section on drum distention).

---

61. Infixation pain, indicates pain caused by wind-strike when the constitution is weak.

Dū Shù 督俞 (UB 16) cures abdominal pain and thunderous rumbling in the abdomen (see the section on abdominal pain in *Míng* 《明》).

承滿療腸鳴腹脹，上喘氣逆（《下》）。陽綱療食飲不下，腹中雷鳴，腹滿
膜脹，大便泄，消渴，身熱面目黃，不嗜食，怠惰（《下》）。《千》云：
主腸鳴（見大便不禁）。三焦俞療腹脹腸鳴。

Chéng Mǎn 承滿 (ST 20) cures rumbling intestines, abdominal distention, panting and qì counterflow (*Xià* 《下》).

Yáng Gāng 陽綱 (UB 48) cures difficulty getting food and drink down, thunderous rumbling in the abdomen, abdominal fullness and distention, diarrhea, wasting-thirst, generalized heat, yellow face and eyes, no desire to eat, and fatigue (*Xià*). *Qiān* 《千》 says: It governs rumbling intestines (see the section on fecal incontinence).

Sān Jiāo Shù 三焦俞 (UB 22) cures abdominal distention and rumbling intestines.

腸中雷鳴相逐，痢下：灸承滿五十壯（《千》）。天樞主腹脹，腸鳴，氣上
衝胸，不能久立，腹痛濯濯，冬日重感於寒則泄（見泄瀉）。食不化，嗜食
身腫，夾臍急，腹中雷鳴：灸太衝，無限壯數（《千》見上氣）。

Thunderous rumbling in the intestines chasing each other [frequent rumbling] and diarrhea: Apply fifty cones of moxibustion on Chéng Mǎn (ST 20) (*Qiān*).

Tiān Shū 天樞 (ST 25) governs abdominal distention, rumbling intestines, qì surging upward into the chest, inability to stand for long, abdominal pain with rumbling sounds, diarrhea in the winter due to contraction of cold (see the section on diarrhea).

Non-transformation of food, desire to eat, generalized swelling, tension alongside the umbilicus, thunderous rumbling in the abdomen: Apply moxibustion on Tài Chōng 太衝 (LV 3); the number of the cones is unlimited (see the section on qì ascent in *Qiān*).

3.35

Tuō Gāng

脫肛

Prolapse of the rectum

百會療脫肛（《明》）。《下》云：療大人、小兒脫肛。《銅》云：治小兒脫肛久不瘥。岐伯療小兒瀉血，秋深不較：灸龜尾一壯，脊端窮骨也。黃帝灸小兒疳痢脫肛：小兒痢下脫肛（並見痢），小兒脫肛，灸頂上旋毛中三壯，即入（《千》）；或尾翠骨三壯，或臍中隨年。

Bǎi Huì 百會 (Dū 20) cures prolapse of the rectum (*Míng*《明》). *Xià*《下》 says: It cures prolapse of the rectum in adults and children. *Tóng*《銅》 says: It treats pediatric prolapse of the rectum that does not recover for a long time.

Qí Bó prescribed treatment for pediatric bloody diarrhea in the late fall, which does not recover: Apply one cone of moxibustion on Guī Wěi 龜尾 (Dū 1), which is [also called] Qióng Gǔ 窮骨 (Dū 1) at the tip of the spine.

The Yellow Emperor's moxibustion treatment for pediatric *gān* 疳 dysentery and prolapse of the rectum, dysentery, prolapse of the rectum (for these, see dysentery), and pediatric prolapse of the rectum: Apply three cones of moxibustion at the spinning hair [cowlick] in the center of the vertex. The prolapse will retract right away (*Qiān*《千》); or apply three cones of moxibustion on Wěi Cuì Gǔ 尾翠骨 (Dū 1); or apply moxibustion on the center of the umbilicus using the same number of cones of moxibustion as the patient's age.

寒冷脫肛：灸翠骨七壯立愈，神；又臍中隨年（《千翼》）；橫骨百壯，或龜尾七壯（窮骨）。

Cold feeling with prolapse of the rectum: Apply seven cones of the moxibustion on [Wěi] Cuì Gǔ (Dū 1) to cure the disease immediately; it is a miracle. Or apply the same number of cones as the age of the patient on the center of the umbilicus (*Qiān Yì*《千翼》); or apply a hundred cones of the moxibustion on Héng Gǔ 橫骨 (KI 11); or apply seven cones of the moxibustion on Guī Wěi (Dū 1) [Qióng Gǔ 窮骨].

人有小女患痢脫肛，予傳得一方：用草茶葉一握，薑七片，令煎服而愈。然不知其方所自來也，後閱坡文，始知生薑咬咀煎茶，乃東坡治文潞公痢之方也，故附於此。

[Author's notes:] Someone's daughter suffered dysentery and prolapse of the rectum. A formula had been passed on to me: Decoct a handful of tea leaves with seven slices of ginger and drink it. The disease was cured. But I did not know where the formula came from. Later, when I read the writings of [Sū Dōng] Pō [蘇東]坡, I knew that decocted tea with crushed ginger was the formula [Sū] Dōng Pō used to treat Wén Lùgōng[62] when he had dysentery. So I attach this here.

3.36
Huò Luàn Zhuǎn Jīn (Jīn Huǎn Jí, Yú Jiàn Shǒu Zú Luán)

霍亂轉筋 （筋緩急　餘見手足攣）

Sudden turmoil [cholera] cramping
(Slacking and tension of the sinews; for the rest see hypertonicity of the hands and feet)

凡霍亂，頭痛胸滿，呼吸喘鳴，窘窘不得息：人迎主之（《千》）。巨闕（《明》云：療霍亂不識人）、關衝、支溝、公孫、陰陵泉主霍亂。太陰、大都、金門、僕參主厥逆霍亂。太白主霍亂逆氣。魚際主胃逆霍亂。

Rén Yíng 人迎 (ST 9) governs sudden turmoil [cholera], headache, chest fullness, panting rales, with distress and inability to breathe (*Qiān* 《 千 》).

Jù Quē 巨闕 (Rèn 14) (*Míng* 《 明 》 says: It treats sudden turmoil [cholera] and loss of consciousness), Guān Chōng 關衝 (SJ 1), Zhī Gōu 支溝 (SJ 6), Gōng Sūn 公孫 (SP 4), and Yīn Líng Quán 陰陵泉 (SP 9) govern sudden turmoil [cholera].

Tài Yīn 太陰 (SP 6), Dà Dū 大都 (SP 2), Jīn Mén 金門 (UB 63), and Pū Cān 僕參 (UB 61) govern reverse counterflow and sudden turmoil [cholera].

Tài Bái 太白 (SP 3) governs sudden turmoil [cholera] and counterflow qì.

Yú Jì 魚際 (LU 10) governs stomach counterflow and sudden turmoil [cholera].

---

62. Wén Lùgōng 文潞公 is another name of Wén Yánbó 文彦博, a famous politician and prime minister during the Northern *Sòng* (北宋) Dynasty.

承筋主霍亂脛不仁。承筋、僕參（見尸厥）、解溪、陰陵泉（見疝）治霍亂。金門、僕參、承山、承筋主轉筋霍亂（《千》）。承山治霍亂轉筋，大便難（《銅》）。金門治霍亂轉筋。曲泉（見疝）、懸鐘（見膝攣）、陽輔（見膝痛）、京骨（見足麻）、胃俞治筋攣（見腹脹）。僕參（見足痛）、竅陰（見無子）、至陰（見頭痛）、解溪（見風）、丘墟（見腋腫）治轉筋。髀關治筋絡急（《銅》見膝痛）。

Chéng Jīn 承筋 (UB 56) governs sudden turmoil [cholera] and numbness of the lower legs.

Chéng Jīn (UB 56), Pū Cān 僕參 (UB 61) (see the section on deathlike reversal), Jiě Xī 解溪 (ST 41), and Yīn Líng Quán 陰陵泉 (SP 9) (see the section on prominent *shàn*-mounting) treat sudden turmoil [cholera].

Jīn Mén 金門 (UB 63), Pū Cān (UB 61), Chéng Shān 承山 (UB 57), and Chéng Jīn (UB 56) govern cramping and sudden turmoil [cholera] (*Qiān*《千》).

Chéng Shān (UB 57) treats sudden turmoil [cholera] with cramping, fecal difficulty (*Tóng*《銅》).

Jīn Mén (UB 63) treats sudden turmoil [cholera] with cramping.

Qū Quán 曲泉 (LV 8) (see prominent *shàn*-mounting), Xuán Zhōng 懸鐘 (GB 39) (see the section on hypertonicity of the knees), Yáng Fǔ 陽輔 (GB 38) (see the section on knee pain), Jīng Gǔ 京骨 (UB 64) (see the discussion of foot numbness), and Wèi Shù 胃俞 (UB 21) treat hypertonicity of the sinews (see the section on abdominal fullness).

Pū Cān (UB 61) (see the discussion of foot pain), Qiào Yīn 竅陰 (GB 44) (see the section on infertility), Zhì Yīn 至陰 (UB 67) (see the section on headaches), Jiě Xī 解溪 (ST 41) (see the section on wind [stroke]), and Qiū Xū 丘墟 (GB 40) (see the section on swelling of the axilla) treat cramping.

Bì Guān 髀關 (ST 31) treats tension of the sinews and network vessels (see the section on knee pain in *Tóng*).

浮郄治小腸熱，大腸結，股外經筋急，髀樞不仁。曲池治筋緩，捉物不得，挽弓不開，屈伸難，風臂肘細無力。中瀆治寒氣客於分肉間，痛攻上下，筋痺不仁。承筋治寒搏轉筋支腫，大便難，腳腨酸重，引小腹痛。

Fú Xī 浮郄 (UB 38) treats small intestine heat, large intestine bind, channel-sinew tension of the lateral aspect of the thighs, and numbness of the thigh pivot [great trochanter].

Qū Chí 曲池 (LI 11) treats slack sinews, inability to grab things or draw a bow, difficulty in bending and stretching, and thin weak arms and elbows due to wind.

Zhōng Dú 中瀆 (GB 32) treats cold qì settling between the divisions of the flesh, pain attacking up and down, and sinew *bì*-impediment with numbness.

Chéng Jīn 承筋 (UB 56) treats cold *bì*-impediment,[63] cramping, propping swelling, fecal difficulty, and aching heaviness of the legs and calves that radiates to the smaller abdomen.

委中（見腳弱）、跗陽、承山（見腰腳）療筋急（《明下》）。張仲文灸腳
筋急（見腰腳）。岐伯療腳轉筋發不可忍者：灸腳踝上一壯，內筋急灸內，
外筋急灸外。解溪主膝重腳轉筋濕痹（《千》）。

Wěi Zhōng 委中 (UB 40) (see the section on weak legs), Fū Yáng 跗陽 (UB 59), Chéng Shān 承山 (UB 57) (see the section on low back and leg [pain]) cure sinew tension (*Míng Xià* 《明下》).

Zhāng Zhòngwén had a moxibustion treatment for sinew tension of the legs (see the section on low back and leg [pain]).

Qí Bó prescribed treatment for unbearable leg cramps: Apply one cone of moxibustion on the malleolus; burn moxibustion on the medial malleolus for sinew tension of the medial aspect; burn moxibustion on the lateral malleolus for sinew tension of the lateral aspect.[64]

Jiě Xī 解溪 (ST 41) governs heaviness of the knees, leg cramps, and damp *bì*-impediment (*Qiān* 《千》).

竅陰主四肢轉筋。大淵主眼青轉筋，乍寒乍熱，缺盆中相引痛。丘墟主腳急
腫痛，戰掉不能久立，跗筋足攣。委中、委陽主筋急身熱。肝俞主筋寒熱
痙，筋急手相引。心俞、肝俞主筋急手相引。

Qiào Yīn 竅陰 (GB 44) governs cramping of the four limbs.

Tài Yuān 太淵 (LU 9) governs green-blue color around the eyes, cramping of the sinews, sudden bouts of cold and heat, and pulling pain of the empty basin [supraclavicular fossa].

Qiū Xū 丘墟 (GB 40) governs hypertonicity, swelling and pain of the legs, shaking and inability to stand for long, hypertonicity of the sinews on the dorsum of the feet.

Wěi Zhōng 委中 (UB 40) and Wěi Yáng 委陽 (UB 39) govern sinew tension and generalized heat.

---

63. *Hán bó* 寒搏 (cold contending) is an error and should be *hán bì* 寒痹 (cold *bì*-impediment), based on *Tóng Rén Tú Jīng* 《銅人圖經》.

64. This appears to be related to Yīn Qiāo and Yáng Qiāo vessel pathology and treatment.

Gān Shù 肝俞 (UB 18) governs cold sinews, heat tetany, sinew tension, and contraction of the hands.

Xīn Shù 心俞 (UB 15) and Gān Shù (UB 18) govern sinew tension and contraction of the hands.

轉筋入腹，痛欲死者：使四人捉手足，灸臍左邊二寸十四壯（《備急》）。《千》云：臍上一寸十四壯。轉筋：灸涌泉六七壯（《千》）。轉筋四厥：灸乳根黑白際一壯。若手足厥冷：三陰交二七壯。

Cramps entering the abdomen with such severe pain that the person wants to die: Ask four people to grab his hands and feet, apply fourteen cones of moxibustion on the site 2 cùn lateral to the left side of the umbilicus (*Bèi Jí* 《備急》). *Qiān* 《千》 says: Apply fourteen cones of moxibustion on the site 1 cùn above the umbilicus.

Cramping: Apply six or seven cones of moxibustion on Yǒng Quán 涌泉 (KI 1) (*Qiān*).

Cramping with reversal cold of the limbs: Apply one cone of moxibustion on the border of dark and light skin at the root of the breast.

Reversal cold of the hands and feet: Apply two times seven cones of moxibustion on Sān Yīn Jiāo 三陰交 (SP 6).

霍亂已死有暖氣者：承筋七壯，起死人；又鹽納臍中，灸二七壯。腰背不便，轉筋急痹筋攣：二十一椎隨年。轉筋在兩臂及胸中：灸手掌白肉際七壯；又灸膻中、中府、巨闕、胃管、尺澤，並治筋拘頭足，皆愈。腹脹轉筋：臍上一寸二七壯。

Someone who has already died from sudden turmoil [cholera] but still has warm qì [possibly breath]: Apply seven cones of moxibustion on Chéng Jīn 承筋 (UB 56). It will rescue the dying person. Or put salt in the umbilicus and then apply two times seven cones of moxibustion.

Discomfort of the lower and upper back, cramping, acute *bì*-impediment, and hypertonicity of the sinews: Apply moxibustion on the 21st vertebra. Burn the same number of cones of moxibustion as the patient's age.

Cramping of both arms and the chest: Apply seven cones of moxibustion on the border of white flesh of the palms. In addition, apply moxbustion on Dàn Zhōng 膻中 (Rèn 17), Zhōng Fǔ 中府 (LU 1), Jù Quē 巨闕 (Rèn 14), Wèi Guǎn 胃管 (Rèn 12 or Rèn 13), and Chǐ Zé 尺澤 (LU 5) to cure hypertonicity of the sinews of the head and feet.

Abdominal distention and cramping: Apply two times seven cones of moxibustion on the site 1 cùn above the umbilicus.

人有身屈不可行，亦有膝上腫疼動不得，予為灸陽陵泉皆愈。已救百餘人矣，神效無比（有吐瀉轉筋者，予教灸水分即止）。轉筋十指攣急，不得屈伸，灸腳外踝骨上七壯（餘見千金）。

> [Author's notes:] Some people [with sudden turmoil [cholera] have such severe contraction of the muscles that] their body is bent over and they are unable to walk, or swelling and pain of the knees and inability to move. I apply moxbustion on Yáng Líng Quán (GB 34) to cure [these diseases]. I have saved more than a hundred people already. Nothing can compete against its divine effects (If there is vomiting, diarrhea, and cramping, it will stop after asking the person to apply moxibustion on Shuǐ Fēn 水分 (Rèn 9)).
>
> Cramping with hypertonicity of the ten fingers, inability to bend and stretch: Apply seven cones of moxibustion on the lateral malleolus (for the rest see *Qiān Jīn* 《千金》).

3.37
Huò Luàn Tù Xiè (Yú Jiàn Zhuǎn Jīn)

霍亂吐瀉（餘見轉筋）

Sudden turmoil [cholera], vomiting and diarrhea
(for the rest, see cramping)

凡霍亂泄出不自知：先取太溪，後取太倉之原（《千》）。三里主霍亂，遺矢失氣。期門主霍亂泄注。尺澤主嘔泄上下出，脅下痛。太白主腹脹食不化，喜嘔泄有膿血。關衝治霍亂胸中氣噎，不嗜食，臂肘痛不舉（《銅》）。人迎治吐逆霍亂，胸滿喘呼不得息。

Sudden turmoil [cholera] with uncontrollable diarrhea: treat Tài Xī 太溪 (KI 3) first, then Tài Cāng 太倉 (Rèn 12) (*Qiān*《千》).

Sān Lǐ 三里 (ST 36) governs sudden turmoil [cholera], fecal incontinence, and passing of flatus.

Qī Mén 期門 (LV 14) governs sudden turmoil [cholera] and outpour diarrhea.

Chǐ Zé 尺澤 (LU 5) governs vomiting, diarrhea and pain below the rib-sides.

Tài Bái 太白 (SP 3) governs abdominal distention, non-transformation of food, frequent retching, and diarrhea with pus and blood.

Guān Chōng 關衝 (SJ 1) treats sudden turmoil [cholera], qì blockage in the chest, no desire to eat, and pain of the arms and elbows with inability to raise them (*Tóng*《銅》).

Rén Yíng 人迎 (ST 9) treats vomiting counterflow, sudden turmoil [cholera], and chest fullness with panting and inability to breathe.

期門治胸中煩熱，賁豚上下，目青而嘔，霍亂泄利，腹堅硬，大喘不得臥，脅下積氣。上脘治霍亂吐利，身熱汗不出。隱白治吐泄（見腹脹）。中脘治霍亂出泄不自知。支溝、天樞治嘔吐霍亂（見臍痛）。太白治氣逆霍亂腹痛，又吐泄膿血（見腹脹）。

Qī Mén 期門 (LV 14) treats vexation heat in the chest, upward and downward running piglet, green-blue color around the eyes, vomiting, sudden turmoil [cholera], diarrhea, hardness of the abdomen, severe panting with inability to lie down, and qì accumulation below the rib-sides.

Shàng Wǎn 上脘 (Rèn 13) treats sudden turmoil [cholera], vomiting and diarrhea, and generalized heat with absence of sweating.

Yǐn Bái 隱白 (SP 1) treats vomiting and diarrhea (see the section on abdominal fullness).

Zhōng Wǎn 中脘 (Rèn 12) treats sudden turmoil [cholera] with uncontrollable diarrhea.

Zhī Gōu 支溝 (SJ 6) and Tiān Shū 天樞 (ST 25) treat vomiting and sudden turmoil [cholera] (see the section on umbilical pain).

Tài Bái 太白 (SP 3) treats qì counterflow, sudden turmoil [cholera], abdominal pain, and vomiting and diarrhea with pus and blood (see the section on abdominal fullness).

陰郄治心痛霍亂，胸滿。上管治霍亂心痛，不可臥，吐利（《明》）。巨闕治胸脅滿，霍亂吐利不止，困頓不知人（《下》）。吐逆，霍亂，吐血：灸手心主五十壯（《千》）。凡霍亂先心痛及先吐：灸巨闕七壯。若先腹痛：太倉二七壯。若先下利：灸大腸募（臍旁二寸），男左女右。若吐下不禁，兩手脈疾數：灸蔽骨下三寸，又臍下三寸，各七十壯。若下不止：太都七壯。若泄利傷煩欲死：慈宮二七壯。

Yīn Xī 陰郄 (HT 6) treats heart pain, sudden turmoil [cholera], and chest fullness.

Shàng Guǎn (Rèn 13) cures sudden turmoil [cholera], heart pain, inability to lie down, vomiting, and diarrhea (*Míng*《明》).

Jù Quē 巨闕 (Rèn 14) treats fullness of the chest and rib-sides, sudden turmoil [cholera], incessant vomiting and diarrhea, drowsiness, and loss of consciousness (*Xià*《下》).

Vomiting counterflow, sudden turmoil [cholera], and vomiting blood: Apply fifty cones of moxibustion on Shǒu Xīn Zhǔ 手心主 (PC 7) (*Qiān* 《千》).

Sudden turmoil [cholera] that has heart pain and vomiting first: Apply seven cones of moxibustion on Jù Quē 巨闕 (Rèn 14). If there is abdominal pain first: Apply two times seven cones of moxibustion on Tài Cāng 太倉 (Rèn 12). If there is diarrhea first: Apply moxibustion on the alarm point of the large intestine (2 cùn lateral to the umbilicus) [ST 25]; burn moxibustion on the left side of males and on the right side of females. If there is vomiting and fecal incontinence with a rapid pulse on both hands: Apply seventy cones of moxibustion on the site 3 cùn below the heart-covering bone [xyphoid process] or 3 cùn below the umbilicus. If there is incessant diarrhea: Apply seven cones of moxibustion on Tài Dū 太都 (SP 2). If there is damage from diarrhea, vexation, and the patient is dying: Apply two times seven cones of moxibustion on Cí Gōng 慈宮 (SP 12).

霍亂吐瀉，尤當速治，宜服來復丹、鎮靈丹等藥，以多為貴。尤宜灸
上管、中脘、神關、關元等穴。若水分穴，尤不可緩。蓋水穀不分而
後泄瀉，此穴一名分水，能分水穀故也。或兼灸中管穴，須先中管而
後水分可也。

[Author's notes:] Sudden turmoil [cholera] with vomiting and diarrhea should be treated immediately. It is appropriate to take *Lái Fù Dān* 來復丹 (Return Again Elixir), *Zhèn Líng Dān* 鎮靈丹 (Settle the Spirit Elixir), and so forth; taking a lot is valuable. It is particularly appropriate to apply moxibustion on Shàng Guǎn 上管 (Rèn 13), Zhōng Wǎn 中脘 (Rèn 12), Shén Quē 神關 (Rèn 8) and Guān Yuán 關元 (Rèn 4). Treatment on Shuǐ Fēn 水分 (Rèn 9) cannot be delayed because diarrhea is acquired when water and grain cannot be separated. This point also named Fēn Shuǐ 分水 (Rèn 9), which means it can separate water and grains. Moxibustion can also be applied the on Zhōng Guǎn 中管 (Rèn 12). Zhōng Guǎn (Rèn 12) should go first, then Shuǐ Fēn (Rèn 9).

3.38
Ǒu Tù (Yòu Jiàn Chuǎn Sòu)

嘔吐（又見喘嗽）

Vomiting
(also see the section on panting and cough)

胃俞主嘔吐，筋攣，食不下（《千》）。商丘主脾虛，令人病寒不樂，好太
息，多寒熱，喜嘔。商丘、幽門、通谷主喜嘔。陽陵泉主嘔宿汁，心下澹
澹。天容主咳逆嘔沫。曲澤主逆氣嘔涎。

Wèi Shù 胃俞 (UB 21) governs vomiting, hypertonicity of the sinews, and difficulty getting food down (*Qiān*《千》).

Shāng Qiū 商丘 (SP 5) governs spleen vacuity which makes people suffer coldness and unhappiness, susceptibility to sighing, a lot of [sensations of] cold and heat, and frequent retching.

Shāng Qiū (SP 5), Yōu Mén 幽門 (KI 21), and Tōng Gǔ 通谷 (KI 20) govern frequent retching.

Yáng Líng Quán 陽陵泉 (GB 34) governs vomiting of abiding juices and a rolling sensation[65] below the heart.

Tiān Róng 天容 (SI 17) governs coughing counterflow and vomiting of foam.

Qū Zé 曲澤 (PC 3) governs counterflow qì and retching of drool.

維道主嘔逆不止。大鐘、太溪主煩心滿嘔。絕骨主病熱欲嘔。俞府（《明
下》云不下食）、靈墟、巨闕、率谷、神藏主嘔吐胸滿。胃俞、腎俞、石
門、中庭等（見反胃）、少商、勞宮主嘔吐。隱白主鬲中嘔吐不欲食。

Wéi Dào 維道 (GB 28) governs incessant retching counterflow.

Dà Zhōng 大鐘 (KI 4) and Tài Xī 太溪 (KI 3) govern vexation, fullness of the heart, and vomiting.

---

65. *Dàn dàn* 澹澹 means undulating waves. A rolling sensation in the chest is similiar to palpitations.

Jué Gǔ 絕骨 (GB 39) governs heat disease and desire to vomit.

Shù Fǔ 俞府 (KI 27) (*Míng Xià* 《明下》 says: inability to get food down), Líng Xū 靈墟 (KI 24), Jù Quē 巨闕 (Rèn 14), Shuài Gǔ 率谷 (GB 8), and Shén Cáng 神藏 (KI 25) govern vomiting and chest fullness.

Wèi Shù 胃俞 (UB 21), Shèn Shù 腎俞 (UB 23), Shí Mén 石門 (Rèn 5), Zhōng Tíng 中庭 (Rèn 16) and so forth (see the section on stomach reflux), Shào Shāng 少商 (LU 11), and Láo Gōng 勞宮 (PC 8) govern vomiting.

Yǐn Bái 隱白 (SP 1) governs vomiting from the diaphragm with no desire to eat.

魂門、陽關主嘔吐不住，多涎。巨闕、胸堂主吐食。膈俞主吐食，又灸章門。胃管、魚際療膈虛食欲嘔，身熱汗出，唾嘔，吐血唾血（《明》）。中庭（見反胃）療嘔吐（《明》）。雲門（見上氣）療嘔逆。

Hún Mén 魂門 (UB 47) and Yáng Guān 陽關 (GB 33) govern incessant vomiting and copious drool.

Jù Quē (Rèn 14) and Xiōng Táng 胸堂 (Rèn 17) govern vomiting of food.

Gé Shù 膈俞 (UB 17) governs vomiting of food; also apply moxibustion on Zhāng Mén 章門 (LV 13).

Wèi Guǎn 胃管 (Rèn 12 or Rèn 13) and Yú Jì 魚際 (LU 10) cure diaphragm vacuity, vomiting after eating, generalized heat, sweating, spitting, and retching, vomiting blood, and spitting of blood (*Míng* 《明》).

Zhōng Tíng 中庭 (Rèn 16) (see the section on stomach reflux) cures vomiting (*Míng*).

Yún Mén 雲門 (LU 2) (see the section on qì ascent) cures retching counterflow.

神藏、靈墟治嘔吐胸滿（《銅》見胸脅滿）。承光（見頭痛）、大都（見腹滿）治嘔吐。太衝治嘔逆發寒（見疝）。大鐘治嘔逆多寒（見淋）。勞宮（見傷寒）治氣逆嘔噦。維道治嘔逆不止，三焦不調，水腫，不嗜食。上髎治嘔逆。

Shén Cáng 神藏 (KI 25) and Líng Xū 靈墟 (KI 24) treat vomiting and chest fullness (see the section on fullness of the chest and rib-sides).

Chéng Guāng 承光 (UB 6) (see the section on headaches) and Dà Dū 大都 (SP 2) (see the section on abdominal fullness) treat vomiting.

Tài Chōng 太衝 (LV 3) treats retching counterflow and coldness (see the section on prominent *shàn*-mounting).

Dà Zhōng 大鐘 (KI 4) treats retching counterflow with profuse cold (see the section on dribbling).

Láo Gōng 勞宮 (PC 8) (see the section on cold damage) treats qì counterflow and retching.

Wéi Dào 維道 (GB 28) treats incessant retching counterflow, unregulated sānjiāo, edema, and no desire to eat.

Shàng Liáo 上髎 (UB 31) treats retching counterflow.

膈關治嘔噦多涎唾（見背痛）。率谷治嘔吐不止（見痰）。肺俞治上氣嘔吐（見上氣）。玉堂治嘔吐，寒痰上氣。心俞治嘔吐，不下食（見狂走）。中庭（見胸滿）、俞府（見喘）、意舍（見腹脹）治嘔吐。膈俞治咳逆嘔逆，鬲胃（《明》作上）寒痰，食飲不下，胸滿支腫，脅痛腹脹，胃脘暴痛。

Gé Guān 膈關 (UB 46) treats retching with copious drool and spittle (see the section on back pain).

Shuài Gǔ 率谷 (GB 8) treats incessant vomiting (see the section on phlegm [drool]).

Fèi Shù 肺俞 (UB 13) treats qì ascent and vomiting (see the section on qì ascent).

Yù Táng 玉堂 (Rèn 18) treats vomiting and cold phlegm with qì ascent.

Xīn Shù 心俞 (UB 15) treats vomiting and inability to get food down (see the section on manic walking).

Zhōng Tíng 中庭 (Rèn 16) (see the section on chest fullness), Shù Fǔ 俞府 (KI 27) (see the section on panting), and Yì Shě 意舍 (UB 49) (see the section on abdominal fullness) treat vomiting.

Gé Shù 膈俞 (UB 17) treats coughing counterflow, retching counterflow, cold phlegm in diaphragm and stomach (*Míng* 《明》 says above the diaphragm), difficulty getting food and drink down; chest fullness and propping swelling; rib-side pain, abdominal distention, and violent pain of the stomach duct.

膽俞治嘔則食無所出（見腹脹）。魄戶治嘔吐煩滿（見上氣）。膻中治吐涎。太溪治嘔吐，口中如膠，善噎。顖凶治小兒嘔吐涎沫。瘈脈治小兒嘔吐泄利（並見小兒瘈瘲）。築賓（見狂）、少海治嘔吐涎沫。廉泉療喘息嘔沫（《明》見少氣）。築賓療嘔吐不止。幽門療善吐，食飲不下，兼唾多吐涎，乾噦嘔沫（《下》）。上管療嘔吐食不下，腹脹氣滿，心忪驚悸，時吐嘔血，腹疝痛，痰多吐涎 。

Dǎn Shù 膽俞 (UB 19) treats vomiting but the food is unable to come back up (see the section on abdominal fullness).

Pò Hù 魄戶 (UB 42) treats vomiting, vexation, and fullness (see the section on qì ascent).

Dàn Zhōng 膻中 (Rèn 17) treats vomiting of drool.

Tài Xī 太溪 (KI 3) treats vomiting [with a] gluey sensation in the mouth and frequent belching.

Lú Xìn 顱囟 (SJ 19) treats vomiting of drool and foam in children.

Chì Mài 瘈脈 (SJ 18) treats vomiting and diarrhea in children (for all, see the section on tugging and slackening in children).

Zhù Bīn 筑賓 (KI 9) (see the section on mania) and Shào Hǎi 少海 (HT 3) treat vomiting of drool and foam.

Lián Quán 廉泉 (Rèn 23) cures panting and vomiting of foam (see the section on qì shortage in *Míng* 《明》).

Zhù Bīn (KI 9) cures incessant vomiting.

Yōu Mén 幽門 (KI 21) cures frequent vomiting, difficulty getting food and drink down along with copious spitting and vomiting drool, dry retching, and vomiting foam (*Xià* 《下》).

Shàng Guǎn 上管 (Rèn 13) cures vomiting, difficulty getting food down, abdominal distention, qì fullness, fearful throbbing and palpitations in the heart, occasional vomiting and retching of blood, gripping pain of the abdomen, copious phlegm, and vomiting of drool.

小兒吐奶：灸中庭一壯 。粥食湯藥皆吐不停：灸間使（《千》見乾嘔）。吐逆嘔不得食：灸心俞百壯，或胸堂百壯，或巨闕五十 。嘔吐宿汁，吞酸：灸日月百壯，三報；或鹽半斤炒，故帛裹就熱熨痛處，主嘔吐 。若心腹痛而嘔，此寒熱客於腸胃（云云）：灸中脘（《指》）。三焦俞主飲食吐逆（《千》見勞）。隱白療嘔吐（《明》）。太白治嘔吐 。三焦俞治吐逆（ 並見腹脹 ） 。

Vomiting of milk in children: Apply one cone of moxibustion on Zhōng Tíng 中庭 (Rèn 16).

Incessant vomiting of gruel and herbal decoctions: Apply moxibustion on Jiān Shǐ 間使 (PC 5) (see the section on dry vomiting in *Qiān* 《千》).

Retching counterflow, vomiting, and inability to eat: Apply a hundred cones of moxibustion on Xīn Shù 心俞 (UB 15) or Xiōng Táng 胸堂 (Rèn 17); or burn fifty cones of moxibustion on Jù Quē 巨闕 (Rèn 14).

Vomiting of abiding juices and acid swallowing: Apply a hundred cones of moxibustion on Rì Yuè 日月 (GB 24) in three sessions. Or stir-fry half a *jin*[66] of salt, wrap it in an old silk cloth, and use it to iron the painful area while it is hot. This governs vomiting.

If there is pain of the heart and abdomen with vomiting, it is due to heat and cold settling in the intestines and stomach (and so forth): Apply moxibustion on Zhōng Wǎn 中脘 (Rèn 12) (*Zhǐ* 《指》).

Sān Jiāo Shù 三焦俞 (UB 22) governs vomiting counterflow of food and drink (see the section on taxation in *Qiān* 《千》).

Yǐn Bái 隱白 (SP 1) cures vomiting (*Míng* 《明》).

Tài Bái 太白 (SP 3) treats vomiting.

Sān Jiāo Shù 三焦俞 (UB 22) treats vomiting counterflow (for all these, see the section on abdominal fullness).

---

66. *Jīn* 斤 is a measurement unit of weight. It equaled about 600 grams in past and since 1929 it has equaled 500 grams.

3.39
Gān Ǒu

乾嘔

Dry vomiting

極泉、俠白治心痛，乾嘔煩滿（《銅》）。通谷療乾嘔無所出，又治勞食飲隔結（《明》）。膽俞療胸脅支滿，嘔無所出，口舌乾，飲食不下。幽門療乾噦（《下》見吐）。

Jí Quán 極泉 (HT 1) and Xiá Bái 俠白 (LU 4) treat heart pain, dry vomiting, vexation and fullness (*Tóng*《銅》).

Tōng Gǔ 通谷 (KI 20 or UB 66) cures dry vomiting with nothing coming out; it also treats taxation and food stagnation in the diaphragm (*Míng*《明》).

Dǎn Shù 膽俞 (UB 19) cures propping fullness of the chest and rib-sides, vomiting with nothing coming out, dry tongue and mouth, and difficulty getting drink and food down.

Yōu Mén 幽門 (KI 21) cures dry vomiting (see the section on vomiting in *Xià*《下》).

乾嘔不止，粥食湯藥皆吐不停：灸手間使三十壯。若四厥脈沉絕不至，灸便通，此起死法（《千》）。乾嘔：灸心主，尺澤亦佳，又灸乳下一寸三十壯。霍亂乾嘔：間使七壯，不瘥，更灸。

Incessant dry vomiting or incessant vomiting of gruel and decoctions: Apply thirty cones of moxibustion on Jiān Shǐ 間使 (PC 5). Reversal cold of the limbs with a deep pulse that is about to expire: Applying moxibustion can unblock it. This is the method to rescue the dying (*Qiān*《千》).

Apply moxibustion on Xīn Zhǔ 心主 (PC 7) for dry vomiting; Chǐ Zé 尺澤 (LU 5) also is good. In addition, burn thirty cones of moxibustion on the site 1 cùn below the breast.

Sudden turmoil [cholera] with dry vomiting: Apply seven cones of moxibustion on Jiān Shǐ (PC 5); apply it again if it is not cured.

《千金》言：生薑乃嘔家聖藥，有此疾者，早上宜多用生薑泡湯服，或煨、或生嚼，或取自然汁入酒服，皆效。

> [Author's notes:] *Qiān Jīn* 《千金》says: Fresh ginger is the sage herb for vomiting. When suffering this disease, make soup with ginger and drink it in the morning; or roast it; or chew the fresh; or mix the natural [fresh] juice with liquor and drink it. All these are effective.

隱白主腹滿喜嘔（《千》）。乾嘔：灸心主，尺澤佳，又乳下一寸三十壯。凡噦，令人悁恨：承漿七壯如麥大，又臍下四指七壯。卒噦：膻中、中府、胃管各數十壯，尺澤、巨闕七壯。

Yǐn Bái 隱白 (SP 1) governs abdominal fullness and frequent retching (*Qiān*《千》).

Dry vomiting: Apply moxibustion on Xīn Zhǔ 心主 (PC 7); Chǐ Zé 尺澤 (LU 5) also is good. Thirty cones of moxibustion can be burned on the site 1 cùn below the breast.

For all dry vomiting, making people feel hostile: Apply seven grain-of-wheat size cones of moxibustion on Chéng Jiāng 承漿 (Rèn 24). Or apply seven cones of moxibustion on the site four finger-widths below the umbilicus.

Sudden dry vomiting: Apply tens of cones of moxibustion on Dàn Zhōng 膻中 (Rèn 17), Zhōng Fǔ 中府 (LU 1) and Wèi Guǎn 胃管 (Rèn 12 or Rèn 13); or apply seven cones of moxibustion on Chǐ Zé (LU 5) and Jù Quē 巨闕 (Rèn 14).

3.40
Yī

噫

Belching

蠡溝主數噫，恐悸，氣不足（《千》）。陷谷主腹大滿，喜噫。鳩尾主噫喘，胸滿咳嘔。少海主氣逆呼吸，噫，噦嘔。勞宮主氣逆噫不止。咳唾，噫，善咳，氣無所出：先取三里，後取太白、章門。

Lí Gōu 蠡溝 (LV 5) governs frequent belching, fear with palpitations, and qì insufficiency (*Qiān* 《千》).

Xiàn Gǔ 陷谷 (ST 43) governs severe abdominal fullness and frequent belching.

Jiū Wěi 鳩尾 (Rèn 15) governs belching, panting, chest fullness, cough, and vomiting.

Shào Hǎi 少海 (HT 3) governs qì counterflow when breathing, belching, and retching.

Láo Gōng 勞宮 (PC 8) governs qì counterflow and incessant belching.

Coughing up spittle, belching, and frequent coughing when qì has nowhere to go: treat Sān Lǐ 三里 (ST 36) first, then Tài Bái 太白 (SP 3) and Zhāng Mén 章門 (LV 13).

大敦主噦噫，又灸石關。太溪（見吐）治善噫（《銅》）。蠡溝治數噫（見疝）。神門治數噫，恐悸（見心煩）。陷谷（見水腫）、期門治產後善噫（見心痛）。太淵治噫氣噦逆。少商治煩心善噦，心下滿，汗出而寒，咳逆。

Dà Dūn 大敦 (LV 1) governs retching and belching; moxibustion can also be applied on Shí Guān 石關 (KI 18).

Tài Xī 太溪 (KI 3) (see the section on vomiting) treats frequent belching (*Tóng* 《銅》).

Lí Gōu (LV 5) treats frequent belching (see the section on prominent *shàn*-mounting).

Shén Mén 神門 (HT 7) treats frequent belching and fear with palpitations (see the section on vexation of the heart).

Xiàn Gǔ 陷谷 (ST 43) (see the section on edema) and Qī Mén 期門 (LV 14) treat frequent belching after childbirth (see the section on heart pain).

Tài Yuān 太淵 (LU 9) treats belching and retching counterflow.

Shào Shāng 少商 (LU 11) treats vexation of the heart, frequent hiccups, fullness below the heart, sweating while feeling cold, and coughing counterflow.

太淵治善噦嘔（ 見胸痹 ）。溫溜治傷寒，噦逆 。噫噦，鬲中氣閉寒：灸腋下聚毛下附肋宛宛中五十壯（ 《 千 》 ）。噫噦，嘔逆：灸石關百壯 。

Tài Yuān (LU 9) treats frequent hiccups and retching (see the section on chest *bì*-impediment).

Wēn Liū 溫溜 (LI 7) treats cold damage and retching counterflow.

Belching and retching counterflow with qì blockage due to cold in the diaphragm: Apply fifty cones of moxibustion in the depression where the hair below the armpits attaches to the ribs (*Qiān* 《 千 》).

Belching, retching, and vomiting counterflow: Apply a hundred cones of moxibustion on Shí Guān 石關 (KI 18).

3.41
Shāng Hán Ǒu Yuě (Zhū Yuě)

傷寒嘔噦（諸噦）

Cold damage and retching
(All types of retching)

巨闕主傷寒煩心喜嘔（《千》）。《甲》云：主心腹脹噫，煩熱善嘔，鬲中
不利。間使主熱病煩心喜噦，胸中澹澹。溫溜主傷寒，寒熱頭痛，噦衄。百
會主汗出而嘔痙。商丘主寒熱好嘔。大椎主傷寒，熱盛煩嘔。腎俞主頭身熱
赤欲嘔（並《千》）。勞宮主熱病煩滿，欲嘔噦（《甲》）。曲澤主傷寒逆
氣嘔唾（《千》）。

Jù Quē 巨闕 (Rèn 14) governs cold damage, vexation of the heart, and frequent retching (*Qiān*
《千》). *Jiǎ* 《甲》 says: It governs distention of the heart [region] and abdomen, belching,
vexation heat with frequent vomiting, and inhibited diaphragm.

Jiān Shǐ 間使 (PC 5) governs heat disease, vexation of the heart, frequent retching, and a rolling
sensation in the chest.

Wēn Liū 溫溜 (LI 7) governs cold damage, [sensations of] cold and heat, headaches, and retching
of blood.

Bǎi Huì 百會 (Dū 20) governs sweating, vomiting, and tetany.

Shāng Qiū 商丘 (SP 5) governs [sensations of] cold and heat and frequent vomiting.

Dà Zhuī 大椎 (Dū 14) governs cold damage, exuberant heat, vexation, and vomiting.

Shèn Shù 腎俞 (UB 23) governs heat and redness of the head and body with desire to vomit (all
in *Qiān*).

Láo Gōng 勞宮 (PC 8) governs heat disease, vexation and fullness, and desire to retch (*Jiǎ*).

Qū Zé 曲澤 (PC 3) governs cold damage, qì counterflow, vomiting, and spitting (*Qiān*).

《必用方》論噦者，俗云克逆也，針灸者當以此求之。

[Author's notes:] *Bì Yòng Fāng* 《必用方》 says that vomiting is commonly called coughing counterflow.[67] The acupuncturist should pursue the treatment based on this.

若氣自腹中起，上築咽喉，逆氣連屬不能出，或至數十聲上下不得喘息，此由寒傷胃脘，腎氣先虛，逆氣上乘於胃，與氣相并不止者，難治。謂之噦，宜茱萸丸；灸中脘、關元百壯。未止，灸腎俞百壯（《指》）。

If qì arises from within the abdomen, pounds up into the throat, and the counterflow qì continues without being able to exit, perhaps accumulating tens of times, it then causes inability to breathe. It is caused by cold damaging the stomach duct after kidney qì was already vacuous, so counterflow qì runs upward and overwhelms the stomach. If [cold] keeps combining with [counterflow] qì, it is difficult to treat. This is also called retching and it is appropriate to use *Zhū Yú Wán* 茱萸丸 (Evodia Pill) or apply a hundred cones of moxibustion on Zhōng Wǎn 中脘 (Rèn 12) and Guān Yuán 關元 (Rèn 4). If it does not stop, apply a hundred cones of moxibustion on Shèn Shù 腎俞 (UB 23) (*Zhǐ* 《指》).

---

67. *Ké nì* 咳逆 (coughing counterflow) is corrected from *kè nì* 克逆 (restrain and resist) based on *Pǔ Jì Fāng* 《普濟方》 (Universal Salvation Formulary).

3.42
Tuò

唾

Spitting

肺氣
412
胸脅
476
癭
301
癇
357
逆氣
420
悲愁
331

中府治咳唾濁涕（《銅》見肺氣）。庫房治多唾濁沫膿血。周榮治咳唾稠膿（並見胸脅滿）。少商治腹滿唾沫（見癭）。百會（見癇）治唾沫。石關治多唾嘔沫（《明下》）。

Zhōng Fǔ 中府 (LU 1) treats coughing and spitting of turbid snivel (see the section on lung qì in *Tóng* 《銅》).

Kù Fáng 庫房 (ST 14) treats frequent spitting of turbid foam, pus, and blood.

Zhōu Róng 周榮 (SP 20) treats coughing and spitting of thick pus (for all these, see the section on fullness of the chest and rib-sides).

Shào Shāng 少商 (LU 11) treats abdominal fullness and spitting of foam (see the section on malaria).

Bǎi Huì 百會 (Dū 20) (see the section on withdrawal and epilepsy) treats spitting of foam.

Shí Guān 石關 (KI 18) cures frequent spitting and vomiting of foam (*Míng Xià* 《明下》).

庫房治肺寒咳嗽唾膿（見逆氣）。幽門（見同）治嘔沫吐涎，喜唾（《銅》）。石關治脊強不開，多唾。日月治多唾（見悲愁）。天井治心胸痛，咳嗽上氣，吐膿，不嗜食。紫宮治吐血，及唾如白膠（《明》）。曲澤主傷寒逆氣嘔唾（《千》）。

Kù Fáng (ST 14) treats cold in the lungs and coughing and spitting of pus (see the discussion of counterflow qì).

Yōu Mén 幽門 (KI 21) (see the same [the discussion of counterflow qì]) treats vomiting of foam, vomiting of drool, and frequent spitting (*Tóng* 《銅》).

Shí Guān 石關 (KI 18) treats stiff spine with inability to open up and frequent spitting.

Rì Yuè 日月 (GB 24) treats frequent spitting (see the section on sorrow [of the heart]).

Tiān Jǐng 天井 (SJ 10) treats pain of the chest and heart, cough with qì ascent, spitting of pus, and no desire to eat.

Zǐ Gōng 紫宮 (Rèn 19) cures vomiting blood and spittle that looks like white glue (*Míng*《明》).

Qū Zé 曲澤 (PC 3) governs cold damage, counterflow qì, vomiting, and spitting (*Qiān*《千》).

名醫賈祐錄云：積主臟病，聚主腑病。積者，是飲食包結不消；聚者，是伏痰結而不化。痰伏在上鬲，主頭目眩痛，多自涎唾，或致潮熱。用平胃散、烏金散治之。其論有理，故載之。

> [Author's notes:] A famous doctor, Jiǎ Yòulù said: Accumulations govern diseases of the viscera; gatherings govern diseases of the bowels. Accumulations are caused by food and drink enveloping and binding, unable to be dispersed; gatherings are caused by deep-lying phlegm binding, unable to be transformed. Phlegm hides above the diaphragm, so it causes dizziness and pain of the head and eyes, uncontrollable drooling and spitting, or tidal heat. Use *Píng Wèi Sǎn* 平胃散 (Stomach-Calming Powder) and *Wū Jīn Sǎn* 烏金散 (Black Gold Powder) to treat it. The discussion is reasonable, so I attach it here.

3.43
Wèi Tòng (Hán Rè)

胃痛（寒熱）

Stomach ache
(Cold or heat)

魚際療胃氣逆（《明》）。分水治胃脹不調（見腹痛）。《銅》云：胃虛脹不嗜食。膈俞治胃脘暴痛（《銅》見嘔吐）。

Yú Jì 魚際 (LU 10) cures qì counterflow (*Míng* 《明》).

Fēn Shuǐ 分水 (Rèn 9) cures distention and irregularities of the stomach (see the section on abdominal pain). *Tóng* 《銅》 says: It cures vacuity distention of the stomach with no desire to eat.

Gé Shù 膈俞 (UB 17) treats violent pain of the stomach duct (see the section on vomiting in *Tóng*).

下管治腹胃不調，腹痛（《明》見腹堅）。腎俞主胃寒脹（《千》見食多）。胃俞治胃中寒（《銅》見腹脹）。水分治胃虛脹（見水腫）。三里治胃中寒，心腹脹滿，胃氣不足，惡聞食臭，腸鳴腹痛，食不化（《明下》同）。下廉（見飧泄）、懸鐘治胃熱不嗜食。

Xià Guǎn 下管 (Rèn 10) cures irregularities of the abdomen and stomach and abdominal pain (see the section on hardness of the abdomen in *Míng*).

Shèn Shù 腎俞 (UB 23) governs cold distended stomach (see the section on overeating in *Qiān* 《千》).

Wèi Shù 胃俞 (UB 21) treats cold in the stomach (see the section on abdominal fullness in *Tóng*).

Shuǐ Fēn 水分 (Rèn 9) treats vacuity distention in the stomach (see the section on edema).

Sān Lǐ 三里 (ST 36) treats cold in the stomach, distention and fullness of the heart and abdomen, insufficiency of stomach qì, aversion to the smell of food, rumbling intestines, abdominal pain, and non-transformation of food (*Míng Xià* 《明下》 agrees).

Xià Lián 下廉 (ST 39) (see the section on swill diarrhea) and Xuán Zhōng 懸鐘 (GB 39) treat stomach heat with no desire to eat.

心俞療胃中弱，食不下（《明下》）。太淵（《千》見心痛）療胃氣上逆，唾血。治胃補胃：胃俞百壯。主胃寒不能食，食多身瘦，腸鳴腹滿胃脹。胃熱：三里三十壯。反胃，食即吐，上氣：灸兩乳下各一寸（以瘥為期）；又臍上一寸二十壯；又內踝下三指稍斜向前穴三壯（《外臺》云一指。《千翼》）。

Xīn Shù 心俞 (UB 15) cures weak stomach and difficulty getting food down (*Míng Xià* 《明下》).

Tài Yuān 太淵 (LU 9) (see the section on heart pain in *Qiān* 《千》) cures stomach qì counterflowing upward and spitting of blood.

To treat and supplement the stomach: Apply a hundred cones of moxibustion on Wèi Shù 胃俞 (UB 21). This governs stomach cold, inability to eat, eating excessively with emaciated body, rumbling intestines, abdominal fullness, and stomach distention.

Stomach heat: Apply thirty cones of moxibustion on Sān Lǐ 三里 (ST 36).

Stomach reflux, vomiting right after eating, and qì ascent: Apply moxibustion on the site 1 cùn below the two breasts (use recovery as the length of treatent); or apply twenty cones of moxibustion on the site 1 cùn above the umbilicus; or three cones of moxibustion on the point that is located three finger-breadths below the medial malleolus and slightly anterior (*Wài Tái* 《外臺》 says: one finger-breadth. *Qiān Yì* 《千翼》).

3.44
Fǎn Wèi

反胃

Stomach reflux

凡食飲不化，入腹還出：先取下管，後取三里瀉之。章門主食飲不化，入腹還出（見不嗜食）。中庭、中府主鬲寒，食不下，嘔吐還出，又主嘔逆吐食不得出。中庭療胸脅支滿，心下滿（《銅》、《明下》同），食不下嘔逆，吐食還出。

Non-transformation of food; the food enters the abdomen then comes back out: drain Xià Guǎn 下管 (Rèn 10) first, then Sān Lǐ 三里 (ST 36).

Zhāng Mén 章門 (LV 13) governs non-transformation of food; the food enters the abdomen then comes back out (see the section on no desire to eat).

Zhōng Tíng 中庭 (Rèn 16) and Zhōng Fǔ 中府 (LU 1) governs cold in the diaphragm, difficulty getting food down, and vomiting. It also cures retching counterflow and vomiting but the food is [stuck and] unable to come back out.

Zhōng Tíng (Rèn 16) cures propping fullness of the chest and rib-sides, fullness below the heart (*Tóng* 《銅》 and *Míng Xià* 《明下》 agree), difficulty getting food down, retching counterflow, and vomiting of food.

三里療胃氣不足，反胃。胃俞（見不能食）療吐食。意舍療吐食不留住（下見背痛）。吐逆食不住：胃管百壯（《千》）。吐嘔逆不得下食，今日食、明日吐：灸膈俞百壯。

Sān Lǐ (ST 36) cures insufficiency of stomach qì and stomach reflux.

Wèi Shù 胃俞 (UB 21) (see the section on inability to eat) cures vomiting of food.

Yì Shě 意舍 (UB 49) cures vomiting of food; the food cannot remain [in the stomach] (see the section on back pain in *Xià* 《下》).

Incessant vomiting of food: Apply a hundred cones of moxibustion on Wèi Guǎn 胃管 (Rèn 12 or Rèn 13) (*Qiān*《千》).

Vomiting, retching counterflow, inability to get food down, vomiting tomorrow what was eaten today: Apply a hundred cones of moxibustion on Gé Shù 膈俞 (UB 17).

有人久患反胃，予與鎮靈丹服，更令服七氣湯，遂能立食。若加以著艾，尤為佳也。有老婦人患反胃，飲食至晚即吐出，見其氣繞臍而轉，予為點水分、氣海並夾臍邊兩穴。他歸，只灸水分、氣海即愈，神效。

[Author's notes:] Someone suffered stomach reflux for a long time. I gave him *Zhèn Líng Dān* 鎮靈丹 (Settle Spirit Elixir), also asked him to take *Qī Qì Tāng* 七氣湯 (Seven Qì Decoction). He could eat immediately. If moxibustion is added, it is even better. An old lady suffered stomach reflux and vomiting when she ate late in the evening; I also could see qì rotating around the umbilicus. I pressed Shuǐ Fēn 水分 (Rèn 9), Qì Hǎi 氣海 (Rèn 6), and points located lateral to the umbilicus. She returned, and I only applied moxibustion on Shuǐ Fēn (Rèn 9) and Qì Hǎi (Rèn 6). She was cured; this has divine effects.

3.45
Shí Bù Xià (Bù Huà)

食不下（不化）

Difficulty getting food down
(Non-transformation [of food])

魂門治飲食不下，腹中雷鳴（《銅》）。三焦俞治吐逆飲食不下（見腹脹）。胃倉、意舍（見腹脹）、膈關治食飲不下（見背痛）。胃俞主嘔吐筋攣，食不下（《千》）。大腸俞、周榮主食不下，喜飲。中庭、中府主鬲寒食不下（見反胃）。陽綱、期門、少商、勞宮主飲食不下。

Hún Mén 魂門 (UB 47) treats difficulty getting drink and food down and thunderous rumbling in the abdomen (*Tóng* 《銅》).

Sān Jiāo Shù 三焦俞 (UB 22) treats vomiting counterflow difficulty getting drink and food down (see the section on abdominal fullness).

Wèi Cāng 胃倉 (UB 50), Yì Shě 意舍 (UB 49) (see the section on abdominal fullness), and Gé Guān 膈關 (UB 46) treat difficulty getting food and drink down (see the section on back pain).

Wèi Shù 胃俞 (UB 21) governs vomiting, hypertonicity of the sinews, and difficulty getting food down (*Qiān* 《千》).

Dà Cháng Shù 大腸俞 (UB 25) and Zhōu Róng 周榮 (SP 20) govern difficulty getting food down and desire to drink [fluids].

Zhōng Tíng 中庭 (Rèn 16) and Zhōng Fǔ 中府 (LU 1) govern cold in the diaphragm and difficulty getting food down (see the section on stomach reflux).

Yáng Gāng 陽綱 (UB 48), Qī Mén 期門 (LV 14), Shào Shāng 少商 (LU 11), and Láo Gōng 勞宮 (PC 8) govern difficulty getting drink and food down.

三焦俞主傷寒頭痛，食不下。心俞治胃弱，食飲不下（《明下》）。膈俞治鬲寒食飲不下，腹脅滿，胃弱、食少，嗜臥怠惰，不欲動，身溫不能食。《千》云：主吐食（見嘔）。陽綱治食不下，腹中雷鳴，大小便不節，黃水（《明》）。

Sān Jiāo Shù 三焦俞 (UB 22) governs cold damage, headache, and difficulty getting food down.

Xīn Shù 心俞 (UB 15) cures weak stomach and difficulty getting food and drink down (*Míng Xià* 《明下》).

Gé Shù 膈俞 (UB 17) treats cold in the diaphragm, difficulty getting food and drink down, fullness of the abdomen and rib-sides, weak stomach, eating less, somnolence with fatigue, no desire to move, warm body,[68] and inability to eat. *Qiān*《千》says: It governs vomiting of food (see the section on vomiting).

Yáng Gāng 陽綱 (UB 48) cures difficulty getting food down, thunderous rumbling in the abdomen, irregular urination and defecation, and yellow watery [stool] (*Míng*《明》).

紫宮（見煩心）、中庭（見反胃）、膽俞（見嘔）治飲食不下。三里（見胃）、大腸俞、三陰交（並見腹脹）、下脘（見腹痛）、三焦俞、懸樞（見瀉）、梁門（見積氣）治穀不化。

Zǐ Gōng 紫宮 (Rèn 19) (see the section on vexation of the heart), Zhōng Tíng 中庭 (Rèn 16) (see the section on stomach reflux), and Dǎn Shù 膽俞 (UB 19) (see the section on vomiting) treat difficulty getting drink and food down.

Sān Lǐ 三里 (ST 36) (see the section on stomachache), Dà Cháng Shù 大腸俞 (UB 25), Sān Yīn Jiāo 三陰交 (SP 6) (for all, see the section on abdominal fullness), Xià Wǎn 下脘 (Rèn 10) (see the section on abdominal pain), Sān Jiāo Shù (UB 22), Xuán Shū 懸樞 (Dū 5) (see the section on diarrhea), and Liáng Mén 梁門 (ST 21) (see the section on accumulation of qì) treat non-transformation of grains [food].

天樞（見瀉）、志室（見脊痛）、腎俞（見勞）治食不化。腹哀治寒中食不化。三焦俞治水穀不消，腹脹腰痛，吐逆（《明》）。腹哀（《銅》同）、太白（見瀉）主食不化（《千》）。凡食飲不化，入腹還出：先取下管，後取三里瀉之。石門主不欲食，穀入不化。

Tiān Shū 天樞 (ST 25) (see the section on diarrhea), Zhì Shì 志室 (UB 52) (see the section on pain of the spine), and Shèn Shù 腎俞 (UB 23) (see the section on taxation) treat non-transformation of food.

Fù Āi 腹哀 (SP 16) treats cold strike and non-transformation of food.

Sān Jiāo Shù (UB 22) cures non-dispersion of food, abdominal distention, lower back pain, and vomiting counterflow (*Míng*《明》).

---

68. This text has *shēn wēn* 身溫 (warm body) but *Tóng Rén Tú Jīng*《銅人圖經》and *Shèng Jì Zǒng Lù*《聖濟總錄》(Sage's Salvation Records, 1111-1117, Government Publication of the *Sòng* (宋) Dynasty) have *shēn shī* 身濕 (moist body) in the same passage.

Fù Āi 腹哀 (SP 16) (*Tóng* 《銅》 agrees) and Tài Bái 太白 (SP 3) (see the section on diarrhea) govern non-transformation of food (*Qiān* 《千》).

Non-transformation of food with food entering the abdomen then coming back out: Drain Xià Guǎn 下管 (Rèn 10) first, then Sān Lǐ 三里 (ST 36).

Shí Mén 石門 (Rèn 5) governs no desire to eat and non-transformation of food.

天樞、厲兌、內庭主食不化，不嗜食，夾臍痛。章門主食飲不化（見不嗜食）。上管、中管主寒中傷飽，食飲不化。中庭治胸脅滿，食不下（見反胃）。胃管、三焦俞主小腹積聚，堅大如盤，胃脹食不消（《千》）。

Tiān Shū 天樞 (ST 25), Lì Duì 厲兌 (ST 45), and Nèi Tíng 內庭 (ST 44) govern non-transformation of food, no desire to eat, and pain around the umbilicus.

Zhāng Mén 章門 (LV 13) governs non-transformation of food (see the section on no desire to eat).

Shàng Guǎn 上管 (Rèn 13) and Zhōng Guǎn 中管 (Rèn 12) govern cold strike, damage from overeating, and non-transformation of food.

Zhōng Tíng 中庭 (Rèn 16) treats fullness of the chest and rib-sides and difficulty getting food down (see the section on stomach reflux).

Wèi Guǎn 胃管 (Rèn 13) and Sān Jiāo Shù 三焦俞 (UB 22) govern accumulations and gatherings in the smaller abdomen which are as hard and big as a plate; stomach distention, and non-dispersion of food (*Qiān*).

志室（《明》見腹痛）療食不下。太白、公孫（見腹脹）主食不化。中府、胃倉、承滿（見腹脹）、魚際（見腹痛）、周榮（見胸滿）治食不下。中管（腹脹）、三陰交（見腹脹）治食不化。

Zhì Shì 志室 (UB 52) (see the section on abdominal pain in *Míng* 《明》) cures difficulty getting food down.

Tài Bái 太白 (SP 3) and Gōng Sūn 公孫 (SP 4) (see the section on abdominal fullness) cure non-transformation of food.

Zhōng Fǔ 中府 (LU 1), Wèi Cāng 胃倉 (UB 50), Chéng Mǎn 承滿 (ST 20) (see the section on abdominal fullness), Yú Jì 魚際 (LU 10) (see the section on abdominal pain), and Zhōu Róng 周榮 (SP 20) (see the section on chest fullness) treat difficulty getting food down.

Zhōng Guǎn (Rèn 12) (abdominal distention) and Sān Yīn Jiāo 三陰交 (SP 6) (see abdominal distention) treat non-transformation of food.

3.46
Bù Néng Shí

不能食

Inability to eat

然谷治腦痛不能食（《銅》見痰）。豐隆主不能食。中極主飢不能食。胃俞主嘔吐筋攣，食不下，不能食。維道主三焦有水氣，不能食。膈俞主傷寒嗜臥，怠惰不欲動，身濕不能食（《銅》同）。石門主不欲食，穀入不化。率谷主醉酒，風熱發，不能飲食，嘔吐（《甲》）。

Rán Gǔ 然谷 (KI 2) treats brain pain and inability to eat (see the section on phlegm in *Tóng*《銅》).

Fēng Lóng 豐隆 (ST 40) governs inability to eat.

Zhōng Jí 中極 (Rèn 3) governs hunger with inability to eat.

Wèi Shù 胃俞 (UB 21) governs vomiting, hypertonicity of the sinews, difficulty getting food down, and inability to eat.

Wéi Dào 維道 (GB 28) governs water qì in the sānjiāo and inability to eat.

Gé Shù 膈俞 (UB 17) governs cold damage, somnolence, fatigue with no desire to move, moist body, and inability to eat (*Tóng* agrees).

Shí Mén 石門 (Rèn 5) governs no desire to eat and non-transformation of grains.

Shuài Gǔ 率谷 (GB 8) governs drunkenness, occurrence of wind-heat, inability to eat, and vomiting (*Jiǎ*《甲》).

少商療不能食，腹中氣滿，吃食無味（《明》）。分水（見腹痛）療不能食。胃俞療煩滿吐食，腹脹不能食。《下》云：療胃中寒氣不能食，胸脅滿，身瘦。

Shào Shāng 少商 (LU 11) cures inability to eat, qì fullness of the abdomen, and inability to taste food when eating (*Míng*《明》).

Fēn Shuǐ 分水 (Rèn 9) (see the section on abdominal pain) cures inability to eat.

Wèi Shù 胃俞 (UB 21) cures vexation and fullness, vomiting of food, abdominal distention, and inability to eat. *Xià* 《下》 says: It cures cold qì in the stomach with inability to eat, fullness of the chest and rib-sides, and emaciated body.

不能食，胸滿，鬲上逆氣悶熱：灸大腸俞二七壯，小兒減之（《千》）。三里療腹滿不能食，胃氣不足，反胃（《明》：不能飲食（見腸澼），臟腑積聚及飲食不消（見寒熱））。涌泉主心痛不嗜食，咽中痛不可內食（見虛勞）。脾俞、胃俞治不嗜食。

Inability to eat, chest fullness, counterflow qì above the diaphragm, oppression and heat: Apply two times seven cones of moxibustion on Dà Cháng Shù 大腸俞 (UB 25); reduce the number of cones on children (*Qiān* 《千》).

Sān Lǐ 三里 (ST 36) cures abdominal fullness, inability to eat, insufficiency of stomach qì, stomach reflux (*Míng* 《明》 says: It treats inability to eat (see the section on intestinal afflux), accumulations and gatherings in the viscera, and non-dispersion of food (see the section on [sensations of] cold and heat).

Yǒng Quán 涌泉 (KI 1) governs heart pain, no desire to eat, sore pharynx, and inability to eat (see the section on vacuity taxation).

Pí Shù 脾俞 (UB 20) and Wèi Shù 胃俞 (UB 21) treat no desire to eat

3.47
Bù Shì Shí

不嗜食

No desire to eat

凡不嗜食：刺然谷多見血，使人立飢（《千》）。隱白（見吐）、然谷、脾俞、內庭主不嗜食。天樞、厲兌、內庭主食不化，不嗜食，夾臍急。中封主身黃有微熱，不嗜食。章門主食飲不化，入腹還出，熱中不嗜食，苦吞而聞食臭傷飽，身黃酸疼羸瘦。肺俞治上氣嘔吐，支滿不嗜食（《銅》）。

No desire to eat: prick Rán Gǔ 然谷 (KI 2) to let blood. This makes people feel hungry immediately (*Qiān* 《千》).

Yǐn Bái 隱白 (SP 1) (see the section on vomiting), Rán Gǔ (KI 2), Pí Shù 脾俞 (UB 20), and Nèi Tíng 內庭 (ST 44) govern no desire to eat.

Tiān Shū 天樞 (ST 25), Lì Duì 厲兌 (ST 45), and Nèi Tíng (ST 44) govern non-transformation of food, no desire to eat, and tension around the umbilicus.

Zhōng Fēng 中封 (LV 4) governs yellow body with mild fever and no desire to eat.

Zhāng Mén 章門 (LV 13) governs non-transformation of food, food entering the abdomen and coming back out, heat strike, no desire to eat, bitter swallowing, not feeling hungry when smelling food, yellow body, aching body, and emaciation.

Fèi Shù 肺俞 (UB 13) treats qì ascent with vomiting, propping fullness, and no desire to eat (*Tóng* 《銅》).

胃俞、脾俞治腹痛不嗜食（見腹脹）。地機、陰陵泉、水分（並見水腫）、幽門（見胸痛）、小腸俞（見香港腳）治不嗜食。下脘治六腑氣寒不嗜食（見腹痛）。下廉（見飧泄）、懸鐘治胃熱不嗜食（見膝攣）。

Wèi Shù 胃俞 (UB 21) and Pí Shù (UB 20) treat abdominal pain and no desire to eat (see the section on abdominal fullness).

Dì Jī 地機 (SP 8), Yīn Líng Quán 陰陵泉 (SP 9), Shuǐ Fēn 水分 (Rèn 9) (for all, see the section on edema), Yōu Mén 幽門 (KI 21) (see the section on chest pain), and Xiǎo Cháng Shù 小腸俞 (UB 27) (see the section on leg qì) treat no desire to eat.

Xià Wǎn 下脘 (Rèn 10) treats cold qì in six bowels with no desire to eat (see the section on abdominal pain).

Xià Lián 下廉 (ST 39) (see the section on swill diarrhea) and Xuán Zhōng 懸鐘 (GB 39) treat stomach heat and no desire to eat (see the section on hypertonicity of the knees).

陰蹻療病飢不欲食（《明》）。懸鐘療腹滿，中焦客熱不嗜食（《明下》）。又云：心腹脹滿，胃熱不嗜食。陽綱（見腸鳴）療不嗜食。分水治胃虛脹不嗜食（《銅》）。

Yīn Qiāo 陰蹻 (KI 6 or KI 8) cures hunger but no desire to eat (*Míng* 《明》).

Xuán Zhōng (GB 39) cures abdominal fullness, heat settling in middle *jiāo* and no desire to eat (*Míng Xià* 《明下》). It also says: distention and fullness of the heart and abdomen, stomach heat, and no desire to eat.

Yáng Gāng 陽綱 (UB 48) (see the section on rumbling intestines) cures no desire to eat (*Tóng* 《銅》).

Fēn Shui 分水 (Rèn 9) treats vacuity distention in the stomach, and no desire to eat.

不嗜食有數端：有三焦客熱不嗜食；有胃熱不嗜食；有胃寒不嗜食；有六腑氣寒不嗜食。固當隨證用藥治之，而針灸者亦當知補瀉之法可也。

《史記》：陽虛侯病甚，眾醫皆以為蹶。太倉公診脈以為痹，根在右脅下，大如覆杯，令人喘，逆氣不能食，病得之內。即以火齊粥且飲六日，氣下即令更服圓藥出入六日，病已。然則人之不能食，亦有患痹而得者。概曰胃有寒熱，則不可也。

[Authors' notes:] There are several reasons for no desire to eat: heat settling in the sānjiāo with no desire to eat; stomach heat with no desire to eat; stomach cold with no desire to eat, and cold qì of the six bowels with no desire to eat. It should be treated with herbs according to the pattern; the acupuncturist should also know supplementing and draining techniques so he can [treat it properly].

中風
379
無子
721

Shǐ Jì 《史記》 says: Marques Yáng Xū[69] was seriously ill; all the doctors thought it was a falling-down disease. Master Tài Cāng read the pulse and said it was *bì*-impediment, and the root was in the right rib-sides, large as an overturned cup. This causes people to have panting, qì counterflow, and inability to eat. The disease was acquired internally. Tài Cāng gave him *Huǒ Jì* 火齊 gruel[70] for six days; after qì descended he then asked him to take pills for another six days. The disease was cured. So no desire to eat can also develop from *bì*-impediment. It is not appropriate to say the disease is always caused by cold and heat in the stomach.

扁鵲曰：凡人心風：灸心俞 。肝俞主心風腹脹滿，食不消化，四肢羸露不欲食（ 見中風 ）。曲泉主不嗜食（ 見無子 ）。

Biǎn Què said: For heart wind, apply moxibustion on Xīn Shù 心俞 (UB 15) and Gān Shù 肝俞 (UB 18). They govern heart wind, abdominal distention and fullness, non-transformation of food, emaciation of the four limbs, and no desire to eat (see wind stroke).

Qū Quán 曲泉 (LV 8) governs no desire to eat (see infertility).

---

69. Marques Yáng Xū refers a ruler of Qí State during the *Hàn* (漢) Dynasty.

70. *Huǒ Jì Zhōu* 火齊粥 was an herbal porridge used in ancient China to treat *bì*-impediment. The ingredients are unknown.

3.48
Shí Qì (Wú Wèi)

食氣（無味）

Consumption of qì[71]
(Inability to taste food)

三里治食氣惡聞食臭（ 見胃 ）。大杼（ 見勞 ）治食氣。百會（ 見風癇 ）、少商（ 見不能食 ）療吃食無味（《 明 》）。凡身重不得食，食無味，心下虛滿，時時欲下喜臥：皆針胃管 、太倉，服建中湯及平胃丸 。

Sān Lǐ 三里 (ST 36) treats consumption of qì and aversion to the smell of food (see the section on stomachache).

Dà Zhù 大杼 (UB 11) (see the section on taxation) treats consumption of qì.

Bǎi Huì 百會 (Dū 20) (see the section on wind epilepsy) and Shào Shāng 少商 (LU 11) (see the section on inability to eat) cure inability to taste food (*Míng* 《 明 》).

Generalized heaviness, inability to eat, inability to taste food, vacuity fullness under the heart, frequent defecation, and somnolence: Needle Wèi Guǎn 胃管 (Rèn 12 or Rèn 13) and Tài Cāng 太倉 (Rèn 12); drink *Jiàn Zhōng Tāng* 建中湯 (Center-Fortifying Decoction) and *Píng Wèi Wán* 平胃丸 (Stomach-Calming Pill).

有鑽胃丸溫中開胃， 病患覷飲食不得， 三五服即思食。破故紙半兩、肉豆蔻四枚為末， 蒸棗肉， 丸梧子大， 空心米飲三十九。

[Author's notes:] *Zuān Wèi Wán* 鑽胃丸 (Dig Into the Stomach Pill) can warm the center and open the stomach. If the patient looks at the food without desire to eat, take three or five doses of the pill. Then he will have a desire to eat. Powder 0.5 *liǎng* of *pò gù zhǐ* 破故紙 [psoralea fructus] and 4 pieces of *ròu dòu kòu* 肉豆蔻 [nutmeg, myristicae semen], steam with dates, and make pills the size of phoenix tree seeds [firmiana seeds]. Take thirty pills with rice on an empty stomach.

---

71. *Consuming qì* is also a name for a Daoist ascetic practice, but here this must refer to a disease with loss of appetite, food is unappealing, and probably results in emaciation.

3.49
Shí Duō

食多

Eating a lot
(Over-eating)

脾俞治食飲多身瘦（《銅》見腹脹 ）。腎俞療食多身瘦（《明下》見勞 ）。
胃俞、腎俞主胃中寒脹，食多身瘦。脾俞、大腸俞主食多身瘦（ 見腹脹 ）。

Pí Shù 脾俞 (UB 20) treats eating and drinking a lot but [the patient becomes] emaciated (see the section on abdominal fullness).

Shèn Shù 腎俞 (UB 23) cures eating a lot but emaciated (see the section on taxation in *Míng Xià* 《明下》).

Wèi Shù 胃俞 (UB 21) and Shèn Shù (UB 23) govern cold distention of the stomach and eating a lot but emaciated.

Pí Shù (UB 20) and Dà Cháng Shù 大腸俞 (UB 25) govern eating a lot but emaciated (see the section on abdominal fullness).

舍侄偶食罷即飢，再食又飢。自碎生薑，濃泡二碗，服愈。

[Author's notes:] Occasionally, my nephew used to feel hungry right after eating, yet still felt hungry after eating more. He crushed and soaked fresh ginger to make two bowls of highly concentrated juice. The disease was cured after he drank it.

3.50
Nüè (Pí Hán)

瘧（脾寒）

Malaria
(Cold in the spleen)

《千金》云：夫瘧皆生於風，夏傷於暑，秋為痎（痎同）瘧。（《素問》云：痎，老也，亦瘦也。楊上善云：二日一發為痎瘧。其說與《素問》、《千金》異）。瘧有數名：先寒後熱曰寒瘧；先熱後寒曰溫瘧；熱而不寒曰癉瘧；多寒曰牡瘧；久不瘥曰勞瘧（久不斷曰老瘧）；時行後變成瘧曰瘴瘧；病結為癥瘕曰瘧母，以至肝肺脾腎心胃亦皆有瘧。或每日發，或間日發，或作稍益晏，或作日益早。《素問》、《千金》等方論之詳矣。治瘧之方甚多，惟小金丹最佳，予嘗以予人皆效。然人豈得皆有此藥哉，此灸之所以不可廢也。鄉居人用旱蓮草椎碎，置在手掌上一夫（四指間也），當兩筋中，以古文錢壓之，繫之以故帛，未久即起小泡，謂之天灸，尚能愈瘧。況於灸乎，故詳著之。

[Author's notes:] *Qiān Jīn*《千金》 says: All malaria comes from wind. When there is damage from summer heat in the summer, *jiē* 痎 malaria will form in the fall. (*Sù Wèn*《素問》 says: *jiē* means old; it also means thin. Yáng Shàngshàn said: Disease that occurs once every two days is *jiē* malaria. His discussion is different than *Sù Wèn* and *Qiān Jīn*). Malaria has several names: cold first and heat later is called cold malaria; heat first and cold later is called warm malaria; heat only without cold is *dàn* 癉 malaria [pure-heat malaria]; more cold is called *mǔ* 牡 malaria [male malaria]; enduring malaria that cannot recover is called taxation malaria (enduring malaria without end is called old malaria); malaria formed after seasonal epidemics is called miasmic malaria; when the disease binds into concretions and conglomerations, it is called mother-of-malaria; liver, lung, spleen, kidney, heart and stomach all can have malaria. Malaria can occur every day, or every other day, or manifest a little later, or manifest a little earlier.[72] *Sù Wèn* and *Qiān Jīn* both discussed

72. *Sù Wèn·Nüè Lùn*《素問·瘧論》 (Plain Questions·Treatise on Malaria), Chapter 35 states: Defense qì circulates inside the body and meets at Fēng Fǔ 風府 (Dū 16) each day in the early morning. When evil qì attacks the body, it settles in Fēng Fǔ 風府 (Dū 16), then flows downward along the spine, one vertebra lower each day. So malaria occurs later each day. The evil qì finally reaches the sacral region in 25 days and enters into spine in the 26th day; it flows upward again and comes out in the empty basin [supraclavicular fossa]. Then the malaria occurs at an earlier time each day.

this in detail. There are lots of formulas to treat malaria, but *Xiǎo Jīn Dān* 小金丹 (Minor Golden Elixir) is the best. I have given it to people, and it is always effective. But how can everyone get this medicine? That is why moxibustion cannot be abandoned. People living in the countryside beat and crush *hàn lián cǎo* 旱蓮草 (Eclipta Herba) with a mallet, and put it on the site that is a hands-width (four fingers distance) above the palm, between the two sinews. It is then pressed with an ancient coin, and wrapped in old cloth. A small blister will occur after a while. This is called heavenly moxibustion.[73] Even this method can cure malaria, not to mention moxibustion. So I attach it here in detail.

譩譆治溫瘧、寒瘧。（《明下》云：療瘧久不愈。腰俞、中管治溫瘧痎瘧。膈俞（見痰）、命門（見頭疼）、太溪（見咳逆）療痎瘧。陰蹻治暴瘧。上廉治寒瘧。三間治瘧寒熱，唇口乾，身熱喘，目急痛。至陰治瘧發寒熱，頭重煩心（《下》）。

Yī Xī 譩譆 (UB 45) treats warm malaria and cold malaria. *Míng Xià* 《明下》 says: It treats enduring malaria that cannot recover.

Yāo Shù 腰俞 (Dū 2) and Zhōng Guǎn 中管 (Rèn 12) treat warm malaria and chronic malaria.

Gé Shù 膈俞 (UB 17) (see the section on phlegm), Mìng Mén 命門 (Dū 4) (see the section on headaches), and Tài Xī 太溪 (KI 3) (see the section on coughing counterflow) cure chronic malaria.

Yīn Qiāo 陰蹻 (KI 6 or KI 8) treats violent malaria.

Shàng Lián 上廉 (ST 37 or LI 9) treats cold malaria.

Sān Jiān 三間 (LI 3) treats malaria with [sensations of] cold and heat, dry mouth and lips, generalized heat and panting, and acute pain of the eyes.

Zhì Yīn 至陰 (UB 67) treats malaria with [sensations of] cold and heat, heaviness of the head, and vexation of the heart (*Xià* 《下》).

液門、合谷、陷谷、天池治寒熱痎瘧。偏歷治發寒熱，瘧久不愈，目視䀮䀮。大椎治瘧久不愈。

Yè Mén 液門 (SJ 2), Hé Gǔ 合谷 (LI 4), Xiàn Gǔ 陷谷 (ST 43), and Tiān Chí 天池 (PC 1) treat cold-heat malaria and chronic malaria.

---

73. While the practice was described in earlier books, this is the first usage of the term *tiān jiǔ* 天灸 (heavenly moxibustion) that we have received. Heavenly moxibustion is the application of warm acrid herbs to acupuncture points in order to cause an irritation or blister. This continually stimulates the point until it heals. While no fire is used, it is considered moxibustion since it is an external heat therapy applied to a point.

Piān Lì 偏歷 (LI 6) treats malaria with fever and chills, enduring malaria that is unable to recover, and blurred vision.

Dà Zhuī 大椎 (Dū 14) treats enduring malaria that is unable to recover.

少府治痎瘧久不愈者，煩滿少氣，悲恐畏人，臂酸掌熱，手握不伸。陶道治痎瘧，寒熱洒淅。命門治寒熱痎瘧，腰腹相引痛。足臨泣治瘧日西發（《千》同，《銅》云：治瘧日發）。療小兒瘧久不愈：灸足大指次指外間陷中，各一壯（並《下》）。

Shào Fǔ 少府 (HT 8) treats enduring malaria that is unable to recover, vexation and fullness, qì shortage, sadness and fear of people, sore arms, hot palms, and clenched hands that cannot be stretched.

Táo Dào 陶道 (Dū 13) treats old malaria and [sensations of] cold and heat as if after soaked in the rain.

Mìng Mén 命門 (Dū 4) treats cold-heat malaria and pulling pain between the low back and abdomen.

Zú Lín Qì 足臨泣 (GB 41) cures malaria that occurs at dusk (*Qiān* 《千》 agrees). *Tóng* 《銅》 says: It treats malaria that occurs every day). To treat enduring malaria that is unable to recover in children: Apply one cone of moxibustion in the depression lateral to the second toe (*Xià* 《下》 agrees).

太溪、（見心痛）照海、中渚治久瘧。丘墟治久瘧振寒（《千》同）。陷谷治瘧。中封、治痎瘧，色蒼蒼（《千》云太息），振寒，小腹腫，食快快繞臍痛，足逆冷，不嗜食，身體不仁。液門治痎瘧寒熱，目眩頭痛，暴得耳聾。腕骨治痎瘧頭痛煩悶。

Tài Xī 太溪 (KI 3) (see the section on heart pain), Zhào Hǎi 照海 (KI 6), and Zhōng Zhǔ 中渚 (SJ 3) treat enduring malaria.

Qiū Xū 丘墟 (GB 40) treats enduring malaria and quivering with cold (*Qiān* agrees).

Xiàn Gǔ 陷谷 (ST 43) treats malaria.

Zhōng Fēng 中封 (LV 4) treats malaria, pale complexion (*Qiān* says sighing), quivering with cold, swelling of the smaller abdomen, discontented eating, pain around the umbilicus, reversal cold of the feet, no desire to eat, and numbness of the body.

Yè Mén 液門 (SJ 2) treats malaria with [sensations of] cold and heat, dizzy vision, headache, and sudden deafness.

Wàn Gǔ 腕骨 (SI 4) treats malaria, headache, vexation and oppression.

商陽治寒熱痎瘧，口乾。《明下》云：治瘧口乾。譩譆（見肩背痛）、中脘、白環俞治溫瘧（見腰脊）。上髎、偏歷治寒熱瘧。三間治寒瘧，唇焦口乾，氣喘。脾俞治痎瘧，寒熱。

Shāng Yáng 商陽 (LI 1) treats cold-heat malaria and dry mouth. *Míng Xià* 《明下》 says: It treats malaria and dry mouth.

Yī Xǐ 譩譆 (UB 45) (see the section on shoulder and back pain), Zhōng Wǎn 中脘 (Rèn 12), and Bái Huán Shù 白環俞 (UB 30) treat warm malaria (see the section on [pain of the] low back and spine).

Shàng Liáo 上髎 (UB 31) and Piān Lì 偏歷 (LI 6) treat cold-heat malaria.

Sān Jiān 三間 (LI 3) treats cold malaria, parched lips and dry mouth, and qì panting.

Pí Shù 脾俞 (UB 20) treats malaria with [sensations of] cold and heat.

有人患久瘧，諸藥不效，或教之以灸脾俞，即愈。更一人亦久患瘧，聞之，亦灸此穴而愈。蓋瘧多因飲食得之，故灸脾俞作效。

[Author's notes:] Someone was suffering enduring malaria. No medicine was effective. He was taught to apply moxibustion on Pí Shù (UB 20) and the disease was cured. There was another who suffered malaria for a long time. I heard it and also had him apply moxibustion on this point Pí Shù (UB 20); the disease also was cured. This is because malaria usually is caused by food and drink, so it is effective to apply moxibustion on Pí Shù (UB 20).

內庭、厲兌（面腫）、公孫治寒瘧不嗜食。京骨治瘧寒熱，喜驚不欲食（《明下》同）。神門治瘧，心煩甚，欲得飲冷，惡寒則欲處溫中，咽乾不嗜食。合谷、陽溪、後溪、陽池、陰都治身寒熱瘧（《明下》云：痎瘧），病心下煩滿氣逆。天樞治寒瘧。列缺治寒瘧嘔沫，善笑縱唇口（《明下》云：瘧面色不定）。

Nèi Tíng 內庭 (ST 44), Lì Duì 厲兌 (ST 45) (facial swelling), and Gōng Sūn 公孫 (SP 4) treat cold malaria with no desire to eat.

Jīng Gǔ 京骨 (UB 64) treats malaria with [sensations of] cold and heat, susceptibility to fright, and no desire to eat (*Míng Xià* agrees).

Shén Mén 神門 (HT 7) treats malaria, severe vexation of the heart, desire for cold drinks, aversion to cold and desire to stay warm, dry throat, and no desire to eat.

Hé Gǔ 合谷 (LI 4), Yáng Xī 陽溪 (LI 5), Hòu Xī 後溪 (SI 3), Yáng Chí 陽池 (SJ 4), and Yīn Dū 陰都 (KI 19) treat generalized cold-heat malaria (*Míng Xià* 《明下》 says: *jiē* 痎 old malaria), falling sick with vexation and fullness under the heart, and qì counterflow.

Tiān Shū 天樞 (ST 25) treats cold malaria.

Liè Quē 列缺 (LU 7) treats cold malaria, vomiting of foam, tendency to laugh, and slack lips (*Míng Xià* says: unstable facial complexion from malaria).

少商治痎瘧振寒，腹滿（《明下》有煩心善噦），唾沫，唇乾，引飲不下膨膨，手攣指痛，寒栗鼓頷，喉鳴。經渠治瘧寒熱，胸背拘急，胸滿膨膨（《明》同）。大椎、腰俞治溫瘧痎瘧（《明》同）。大杼療瘧頸項強，不可俯仰，頭痛振寒。前谷、風池、神道（見頭痛）、百會治痎瘧。上星治痎瘧，振寒，熱汗不出。

Shào Shāng 少商 (LU 11) treats old malaria and quivering with cold, abdominal fullness (*Míng Xià* has vexation of the heart, frequent hiccups), spitting of foam, dry lips, inability to get drinks down, feeling of inflation, hypertonicity of the hands, finger pain, shivering and chattering of the jaws,[74] and throat rales.

Jīng Qú 經渠 (LU 8) treats malaria with [sensations of] cold and heat, hypertonicity of the chest and back, chest fullness, and feeling of inflation (*Míng* 《明》 agrees).

Dà Zhuī 大椎 (Dū 14) and Yāo Shù 腰俞 (Dū 2) treat warm malaria and malaria (*Míng* agrees).

Dà Zhù 大杼 (UB 11) cures malaria, stiffness of the neck and nape, inability to bend forward and backward, headache, and quivering with cold.

Qián Gǔ 前谷 (SI 2), Fēng Chí 風池 (GB 20), Shén Dào 神道 (Dū 11) (see the section on headaches), and Bǎi Huì 百會 (Dū 20) treat malaria.

Shàng Xīng 上星 (Dū 23) treats malaria and quivering with cold, fever with absence of sweating.

偏歷主風瘧汗不出（《千》）。少澤（《明》云：頭痛，《銅》云：寒熱）、復溜、崑崙主瘧寒汗不出。衝陽主瘧先寒洗淅，甚久而熱，熱去汗出。然谷、崑崙主瘧多汗。《甲》云：主瘧多汗，腰痛不可俯仰，目如脫，項如拔。列缺、後溪、少澤、前谷主瘧寒熱。太泉、太溪、經渠主瘧咳逆，心悶不得臥，寒熱。大陵、腕骨、陽谷、少衝主午寒乍熱，瘧。天樞主瘧振寒，熱甚狂言。太鐘主瘧，多寒少熱。《甲》云：瘧悶嘔甚，熱多寒少，欲閉戶而處，寒厥足熱。

---

74. Chattering of the jaws: In English we say chattering of teeth; this is due to the coldness.

Piān Lì 偏歷 (LI 6) governs wind malaria with absence of sweating (*Qiān* 《 千 》).

Shào Zé 少澤 (SI 1) (*Míng* 《 明 》 says: headaches; *Tóng* 《 銅 》 says: [sensations of] cold and heat), Fù Liū 復溜 (KI 7), and Kūn Lún 崑崙 (UB 60) govern cold malaria with absence of sweating.

Chōng Yáng 衝陽 (ST 42) governs malaria, at first with aversion to cold as if after soaking in the rain; [the cold] stays for quite a long time and then it becomes heat with sweating after the heat goes away.

Rán Gǔ 然谷 (KI 2) and Kūn Lún (UB 60) cure malaria with profuse sweating. *Jiǎ* 《 甲 》 [75] says: This governs malaria with profuse sweating, lower back pain with inability to bend forward and backward. The eyes feel like they are about to burst from their sockets and the nape feels dislocated.

Liè Quē 列缺 (LU 7), Hòu Xī 後溪 (SI 3), Shào Zé (SI 1), and Qián Gǔ 前谷 (SI 2) govern malaria with [alternating sensations of] cold and heat.

Tài Quán 太泉 (LU 9), Tài Xī 太溪 (KI 3), and Jīng Qú 經渠 (LU 8) govern malaria, coughing counterflow, heart oppression with inability to lie down, and [sensations of] cold and heat.

Dà Líng 大陵 (PC 7), Wàn Gǔ 腕骨 (SI 4), Yáng Gǔ 陽谷 (SI 5), and Shào Chōng 少衝 (HT 9) govern sudden bouts of [sensations of] cold and heat as well as malaria.

Tiān Shū 天樞 (ST 25) governs malaria and quivering with cold, severe heat, and manic raving.

Tài Zhōng 太鐘 (KI 4) governs malaria with more pronounced cold than heat. *Jiǎ* [76] says: It treats malaria with oppression and severe vomiting, more pronounced heat than cold, desire to shut the door and stay inside, and cold reversal with hot feet.

商丘主寒瘧腹痛。少海主瘧背振寒。《 甲 》云：項痛引肘掖，腰痛引少腹，四肢不舉。陽溪主瘧甚苦，寒咳嘔沫。厲兌、內庭主瘧不嗜食，惡寒。少商主瘧振栗鼓頷。商丘、神庭、上星、百會、完骨、風池、神道、液門、前谷、光明、至陰、大杼主瘧熱。陰都、少海、商陽、三間、中渚主瘧身熱。

Shāng Qiū 商丘 (SP 5) governs cold malaria and abdominal pain.

Shào Hǎi 少海 (HT 3) governs malaria and quivering with cold. *Jiǎ* says: It governs nape pain that radiates to the elbows and armpits, lower back pain radiating to the smaller abdomen, and inability to lift four limbs.

---

75. The passage here is erroneously attributed to *Jiǎ* 《 甲 》; it is modified from a discussion in the *Qiān Jīn Yào Fāng* 《 千金要方 》 under the section for Kūn Lún 崑崙 (UB 60).

76. The passage here is also erroneously attributed to *Jiǎ* 《 甲 》; it is actually from a footnote under the section for Tài Xī 太溪 (KI 3) in *Qiān Jīn Yào Fāng* 《 千金要方 》. It is wrongly attributed to *Jiǎ* 《 甲 》 and placed under Tài Zhōng 太鐘 (KI 4).

Yáng Xī 陽溪 (LI 5) governs malaria with severe suffering, cold cough, and vomiting of foam.

Lì Duì 厲兌 (ST 45) and Nèi Tíng 內庭 (ST 44) govern malaria, no desire to eat, and aversion to cold.

Shào Shāng 少商 (LU 11) governs malaria, shivering, and chattering of the jaws.

Shāng Qiū 商丘 (SP 5), Shén Tíng 神庭 (Dū 24), Shàng Xīng 上星 (Dū 23), Bǎi Huì 百會 (Dū 20), Wán Gǔ 完骨 (GB 12), Fēng Chí 風池 (GB 20), Shén Dào 神道 (Dū 11), Yè Mén 液門 (SJ 2), Qián Gǔ 前谷 (SI 2), Guāng Míng 光明 (GB 37), Zhì Yīn 至陰 (UB 67), and Dà Zhù 大杼 (UB 11) govern malaria with heat.

Yīn Dū 陰都 (KI 19), Shào Hǎi (HT 3), Shāng Yáng 商陽 (LI 1), Sān Jiān 三間 (LI 3), and Zhōng Zhǔ 中渚 (SJ 3) govern malaria with generalized heat.

列缺主瘧甚熱。陽谷主瘧，脅痛不得息。俠溪主瘧，足痛。衝陽、束骨主瘧從腳起。陽谷主瘧，脅痛不得忍。飛揚主狂瘧，頭眩痛，痙反折。溫溜主瘧，面赤腫。天井主瘧，食時發，心痛，悲傷不樂。天府主瘧病。譩譆、支正、小海主風瘧。三里、陷谷、俠溪、飛揚主痎瘧少氣。

Liè Quē 列缺 (LU 7) governs malaria with severe heat.

Yáng Gǔ 陽谷 (SI 5) governs malaria, pain of the rib-sides, and inability to breathe.

Xiá Xī 俠溪 (GB 43) governs malaria and foot pain.

Chōng Yáng 衝陽 (ST 42) and Shù Gǔ 束骨 (UB 65) govern malaria which starts from the lower legs.

Yáng Gǔ (SI 5) governs malaria and intolerable pain of the rib-sides.

Fēi Yáng 飛揚 (UB 58) governs mania and malaria, dizziness and headaches, and arched-back tetany.

Wēn Liū 溫溜 (LI 7) governs malaria and red swollen face.

Tiān Jǐng 天井 (SJ 10) governs malaria which occurs when eating, heart pain, and sadness.

Tiān Fǔ 天府 (LU 3) governs malaria.

Yī Xī 譩譆 (UB 45), Zhī Zhèng 支正 (SI 7), and Xiǎo Hǎi 小海 (SI 8) govern wind malaria.

Sān Lǐ 三里 (ST 36), Xiàn Gǔ 陷谷 (ST 43), Xiá Xī (GB 43), and Fēi Yáng (UB 58) govern malaria and qì shortage.

大附子一枚炮末，薑兩半取自然汁，丸如小豆大，每十五九空心熱酒
吞下，老少加減。川客治瘧，只二三服皆愈。云兼治脾胃，愈於薑附
湯，故附此。

[Author's notes:] Get one big piece of *fù zǐ* 附子 (Aconiti Radix Lateralis Praeparate), blast-fry
and powder it; and the fresh juice from 1.5 *liǎng* of ginger. Make this into pills the size of a small
bean. Swallow fifteen pills with hot liquor on an empty stomach. Cut the dosage for the elderly and
young people. People from Sìchuān take two or three doses of these to cure malaria. It is said that
to simultaneously treat the spleen and stomach, take *Jiāng Fù Tāng* 薑附湯 (Ginger and Aconite
Decoction), so I attached this here.

3.51
Pí Téng (Yú Jiàn Xīn Fù Tòng)

脾疼（餘見心腹痛）

Spleen pain
(for the rest, see the section on heart and abdominal pain)

府舍治疝癖，脾中急痛，循脅上下搶心，腹滿積聚，厥氣兩乳（《銅》）。商丘治脾虛令人不樂（見腸鳴，《千》見吐）。三陰交治脾病身重（見腹脹）。

Fǔ Shě 府舍 (SP 13) treats *shàn*-mounting aggregations, acute pain of the spleen that runs upward along the rib-sides and prods the heart, abdominal fullness, accumulations and gatherings, and reversal qì of the two breasts[77] (*Tóng*《銅》).

Shāng Qiū 商丘 (SP 5) treats spleen vacuity that makes people unhappy (see the section on rumbling intestines; see the section on vomiting in *Qiān*《千》).

Sān Yīn Jiāo 三陰交 (SP 6) treats spleen disease with generalized heaviness (see the section on abdominal fullness).

予嘗久患脾疼，服治脾藥，反膨脹不得已，依耆域方用面裹火炮蓬莪茂末，水與酒醋煎服，立愈。已而告人，人亦云高良薑末米飲調服，亦作效。後鄭教授傳一方云：草果、延胡索、靈脂並沒藥酒調三兩錢，一似手拈却。草果子、苓脂四味等分為末，此亦平穩藥也，有此疾者宜服之。或不吐不瀉，心中疼甚，日輕夜甚者，用乾鹽梅並茶煎服，神效。若灸者，宜上管、中管、下管、脾俞、三陰交等穴。

[Author's notes:] I have suffered spleen pain for a long time. After I took herbs for the spleen, I had unceasing inflation. Then based on *Qí Yù Fāng* 耆域方 (Formula from Qí Yù) [I tried the following]: Wrap powdered *péng é mào* 蓬莪茂 [*é zhú* 莪術] [curcumae rhizome] with flour [paste] and blast-fry it with fire. Decoct it in water with liquor and vinegar, and take it. The disease was cured immediately. I told other people about it after it was cured. Someone also said it is effective to

77. In *Tóng Rén Tú Jīng*《銅人圖經》, this passage says *huò luàn* 霍亂 (cholera [sudden turmoil]) instead of *liǎng rǔ* 兩乳 (the two breasts).

mix powdered *gāo liáng jiāng* 高良薑 [alpiniae officnarum rhizome] with rice and drank it. Later, Education Officer Zhèng gave me a formula: Stir 2 to 3 *qián* of powdered *cǎo guǒ* 草果 [lanceae fructus], *yán hú suǒ* 延胡索 [corydalis rhizome], *líng zhǐ* 苓脂 [*wǔ líng zhǐ* 五靈脂 [trogopteri faeces frictum] and *mò yào* 沒藥 [myrrha] into liquor; [the effect] is just like using the fingers to pick up things.[78] Powder equal portions of [the above] four herbs: *cǎo guǒ zǐ* 草果子 [lanceae fructus], *líng zhǐ* [*wǔ líng zhǐ* [trogopteri faeces frictum], etc. This is a gentle formula. It is appropriate to drink it when suffering this disease. If there is no vomiting or diarrhea, but there is severe pain of the heart that is better in the daytime and worse at night, decoct [the formula] with dried salty plum and tea. It is divinely effective. It is appropriate to apply moxibustion on Shàng Guǎn 上管 (Rèn 13), Zhōng Guǎn 中管 (Rèn 12), Xià Guǎn 下管 (Rèn 10), Pí Shù 脾俞 (UB 20), Sān Yīn Jiāo 三陰交 (SP 6), and so forth.

---

78. This is a colloquial Chinese saying with a similar meaning to 'as easy as pie' in English.

Zhēn Jiǔ Zī Shēng Jīng
Appendix

References cited in
Zhēn Jiǔ Zī Shēng Jīng 《針灸資生經》

Zhēn Jiǔ Zī Shēng Jīng 《針灸資生經》 Life-Promoting Classic of Acupuncture frequently quotes the following literature:

Title English Author	Dynasty and/or Date
Běn Cǎo Yǎn Yì 《本草衍義》	Sòng (宋) 1116
Amplification of the Materia Medica	
Compiled by Kòu Zōngshì 寇宗奭	
Běn Shì Fāng 《本事方》	
See Pǔ Jì Běn Shì Fāng 《普濟本事方》	
Bì Yòng Fāng 《必用方》	Sòng (宋) 1078-1085
Formulas of Necessity	
Possibly by Chū Yúshì 初虞世	
Bì Yòng 《必用》	
Parts of Bì Yòng Fāng were cited in Pǔ Jì Běn Shì Fāng 《普濟本事方》 (Skillful Formulas for Universal Salvation).	
Chǎn Lùn 《產論》	Sòng (宋) 1078-1085
Discussion on Childbirth	
Possibly Yáng Zǐjiàn 杨子建	
Cháo Yě Qiān Zǎi 《朝野僉載》	Táng (唐)
Combined Chronicle of the Government and the Public	
By Zháng Zhuó 張鷟	
A series of novels.	
Dān Fāng Gē 《單方歌》	unknown
Single Formula Rhymes	
unknown	
Dān Fāng 《單方》	
Hǎi Shàng Xiān Míng Fāng 《海上仙名方》	Sòng (宋)
Famous Formulas from Immortals who Live at the Sea	
By Qián Yú 錢竽, using Sūn Sīmiǎo's 孫思邈 name	
Hǎi Shàng Fāng 《海上方》	
Discusses treatment of over 120 different diseases	

Huáng Dì Míng Táng Jiǔ Jīng 《黃帝明堂灸經》	*Táng* (唐)

The Yellow Emperor's Moxibustion Classic of the Bright Hall

> unknown

Jiǔ Jīng 《灸經》

> The Classic of Moxibustion

Huáng Dì Nèi Jīng 《黃帝內經》	Spring and Autumn Period through the Warring States Period (1st century BCE)

The Yellow Emperor's Inner Classic

> unknown

Nèi Jīng 《內經》 has two parts: See also *Sù Wèn* 《素問》 (Plain Questions) and *Líng Shū* 《靈樞》 (Magic Pivot)

Nèi Jīng 《內經》

Jí Xiào Fāng 《集效方》	unknown

Collections of Effective Formulas

> unknown

Jí 《集》

> Two volumes. The first is a collection of simple empirical folk formulas; the second is a collection of formulas for several diseases. The total number of formulas is around 400.

Jì Xiào Fāng 《既效方》	*Yuán* (元)

Already Effective Formulas

> By Wáng Zhízhōng 王執中 (the author of this book)

Wáng collected the formulas from other people. After trying them on himself, he put the effective ones together into this book. It has been lost since the *Yuán* (元) Dynasty.

Jiǎ 《甲》

> *Jiǎ Yǐ* 《甲乙》
>
> *Jiǎ Yǐ Jīng* 《甲乙經》
>
> See *Zhēn Jiǔ Jiǎ Yǐ Jīng* 《針灸甲乙經》

Jīn Guì Yào Luè 《金匱要略》	Eastern *Hàn* Dynasty (東漢)

Essential Prescriptions of the Golden Cabinet

> By Zhāng Zhòngjīng 張仲景

Jīn Guì 《金匱》

Jīng Fāng Xiǎo Pǐn 《經方小品》	Between 454-473, the *Nán běi cháo* (南北朝) (Southern and Northern Dynasties, 420-589)

Short Sketches of Classical Formulas

> By Chén Yánzhī 陳延之

Xiǎo Pǐn Fāng 《小品方》

Xiǎo Pǐn 《小品》

> Short Sketches of Formulas

Jiǔ Jīng 《灸經》

> The Classic of Moxibustion
>
> See *Huáng Dì Míng Táng Jiǔ Jīng* 《黃帝明堂灸經》

Jiǔ Yōng Jū Fāng 《灸癰疽方》   unknown

    Applying Moxibustion for Welling- and Flat-Abscesses

        By Líu Héshū 劉和叔

    The dates are unknown, but Wáng wrote a preface for it so it was probably written in his lifetime.

Jú Fāng 局方

    See *Tài Píng Huì Mín Hé Jì Jú Fāng* 《太平惠民和劑局方》

Liáng Fāng 《良方》

    See *Sū Shěn Liáng Fāng* 《蘇沈良方》

Liè Zǐ 《列子》(Master Liè)   Western scholars believe it was compiled around the 4th century CE.

    Honorifically entitled the *Chōng Xū Zhēn Jīng* 《衝虛真經》

      True Classic of Simplicity and Vacuity, also known as the Classic of the Perfect Emptiness.

      A Dàoist book of philosophy.

Líng Shū 《靈樞》   Spring and Autumn Period through the Warring States Period (1st century BCE)

    Magic Pivot

        unknown

    Zhēn Jīng 《針經》

    Acupuncture Classic

    Part of *Huáng Dì Nèi Jīng* 《黃帝內經》(The Yellow Emperor's Inner Classic)

Lù Shì Xù Jí Yàn Fāng 《陸氏續集驗方》   Southern *Sòng* (南宋) 1180

    Sequel to the Collection of Proven Formulas from Master Lù

        By Lù Yóu 陸游

    It was written after *Lù Shì Xù Jí Yàn Fāng* 《陸氏集驗方》by Lù Zhí 陸贄 during the *Táng* (唐) Dynasty.

Lù Yàn Fāng 《錄驗方》   *Táng* (唐)

    Records of Effective Formulas

        By Zhēn Lìyán 甄立言

    This book has been lost.

Mài Jué 《脈訣》   *Sòng* (宋)

    Rhymed Songs of Pulse

        By Cuī Jiāyán 崔嘉言

Míng Táng 《明堂》   edited during the Western and Eastern *Hàn* (西東漢) (between 138 B.C.E.-106 C.E.)

    Bright Hall

        unknown

    The first book to systematically discuss acupuncture points. The original book has been lost, but its material was include in *Tài Píng Shèng Huì Fāng* (See also that entry).

Míng Táng Jīng 《明堂經》

    Bright Hall Classic

Míng Táng Shàng Jīng 《明堂上經》

    Upper Canon of the Bright Hall Classic

Míng Shàng 《明上》

Shàng 《上》

    Volume 99 of *Tài Píng Shèng Huì Fāng* 《太平聖惠方》 (Sage-like Prescriptions of *Tài Píng* Era). (See also *Míng Táng* 《明堂》.)

Míng Táng Xià Jīng 《明堂下經》

    Lower Canon of the Bright Hall

Míng Xià 《明下》

Xià 《下》

    Volume 100 of *Tài Píng Shèng Huì Fāng* 《太平惠方》 (Sage-like Prescriptions of Tài Píng Era) (See also *Míng Táng* 《明堂》.)

Míng Shàng 《明上》

    See *Míng Táng Shàng Jīng* 《明堂上經》

Míng Xià 《明下》

    See *Míng Táng Xià Jīng* 《明堂下經》

Nàn Jīng 《難經》   Late *Hàn* (漢)

    Classic of Difficulties

            unknown

Nàn 《難》

Nàn Jīng Shū 《難經疏》   *Sòng* (宋)

    Explanation of the Classic of Difficulties

        By Hóu Zìrán 候自然

Nàn Shū 《難疏》

    It had 13 volumes, but the book has been lost.

Nèi Jīng 《內經》

    See *Huáng Dì Nèi Jīng* 《黃帝內經》

Pǔ Jì Běn Shì Fāng 《普濟本事方》   *Sòng* (宋) Dynasty (1132)

    Skillful Formulas for Universal Salvation

        Compiled By Xǔ Shūwēi 許叔微, also known as Xǔ Zhīkě 許知可

Běn Shì Fāng 《本事方》

Pǔ Jì Fāng 《普濟方》

Qiān 《千》

    Qiān Jīn 《千金》

    See *Qiān Jīn Yào Fāng* 《千金要方》 or *Qiān Jīn Yì Fāng* 《千金翼方》; these could refer to either one.

Qiān Jīn Yào Fāng 《千金要方》   *Táng* (唐)

    Prescriptions Worth a Thousand Pieces of Gold

        By Sūn Sīmiǎo 孫思邈

Qiān Jīn Yì Fāng 《千金翼方》   *Táng* (唐)

    Appendix to Prescriptions Worth a Thousand Pieces of Gold

        By Sūn Sīmiǎo 孫思邈

Qiān Jīn 《千金》

Qiān 《 千 》

Shàng 《 上 》

See *Míng Táng Shàng Jīng* 《 明堂上經 》

Quán Shēng Zhǐ Mí Fāng 《 全生指迷方 》   *Sòng* (宋), 1119-1125

> Formulas of Comments on Confusion to Rescue Life
>
> > By Wáng Kuàng 王貺

Zhǐ 《 指 》

Zhǐ Mí 《 指迷 》

Shén Yìng Zhēn Jīng Yào Jué 《 神應針經要訣 》   Northern *Sòng* (宋)

> The Acupuncture Classic of Essential Rhymed Songs of Wondrous Response
>
> > By Xǔ Xī 許希

Zhēn Jīng 《 針經 》

> The Acupuncture Classic

Shǐ Jì 《 史記 》   *Hàn* (漢) 91 B.C.E.

> The Records of the Grand Historian
>
> > By Sīmǎ Qiān 司馬遷
>
> An important history book. It recounts Chinese history from the time of the Yellow Emperor to King Wǔ 武 of the *Hàn* Dynasty, covering about 3000 years.

Shí Liáo Běn Cǎo 《 食療本草 》   *Táng* (唐)

> Herbal Foundation of Dietary Therapy
>
> > By Mèng Shēn 孟詵

Shuō Wén Jiě Zì 《 說文解字 》   Eastern *Hàn* Dynasty (漢) (early 2nd century CE)

> Explaining and Analyzing Characters
>
> > By Xǔ Shèn 許慎

Shuō Wén 《 說文 》

> A dictionary of Chinese characters.

Sù 《 素 》

See *Sù Wèn* 《 素問 》

Sù Nǚ Lùn 《 素女論 》   unknown

> Statements of the *Sù Nǚ*
>
> > unknown

Sù Nǚ 《 素女 》

> An ancient sexology book. It was lost after the *Táng* Dynasty. But it was partially recorded in the *Yī Xīn Fāng* 《 醫心方 》, Volume 28, by Dān Bō Kāng Lài 丹波康賴 in 982. This is a famous Japanese book called Ishimpo in Japanese. *Sù Nǚ* was a goddess of ancient China. She was skilled in music and lived in the same era as Huáng Dì (the Yellow Emperor).

Sū Shěn Liáng Fāng 《蘇沈良方》   *Sòng* (宋)

    Good Formulas from Masters Sū and Shěn

       unknown

   Liáng Fāng 《良方》

    This book is a combination of *Shěn Shì Liáng Fāng* 《沈氏良方》 (Good Formulas from Master Shěn) by Shěn Kuò 沈括 and *Sū Xué Shì Fāng* 《蘇學士方》 (Good Formulas from Master Sū) by Sū Shì 蘇軾. It discusses pulse diagnoses, internal organs, moxibustion, herbology and the treatment of different diseases.

Sù Wèn 《素問》   Spring and Autumn Period through the Warring States Period (1st century BCE)

    Plain Questions

       unknown

   Sù 《素》

    Part of *Huáng Dì Nèi Jīng* 《黃帝内經》 (The Yellow Emperor's Inner Classic)

Sù Wèn Zhù 《素問注》   *Sòng* (宋)

    Annotations to Plain Questions

       By Wáng Bīng 王冰

   Sù Zhù 《素注》

    These are Wáng Bing's 王冰 annotations on *Sù Wèn* 《素問》

Tài Píng Huì Mín Hé Jì Jú Fāng 《太平惠民和劑局方》

    Imperial Grace Pharmacy Formulas

       Compiled by the *sòng tài yī jú biān* 宋太醫局編   *Sòng* (宋) (1078-85)
       Sòng Imperial Medical Bureau

   Jú Fāng 局方

    The official *Sòng* (宋) Dynasty government-published formulary.

Tài Píng Shèng Huì Fāng 《太平聖惠方》   *Sòng* (宋), 992

    Sage-like Prescriptions of Tài Píng Era

       By Wáng Huáiyǐn 王懷隱

Tāng Bù 《湯簿》

    Book of Decoctions

Tóng Rén Shū Xuè Zhēn Jiu Tú Jīng 《銅人腧穴針灸圖經》   *Sòng* (宋), 1027

    The Bronze Statues Illustrated Classic of Acupuncture Points

       By Wáng Wéiyī 王維一

   Tóng 《銅》

   Tóng Rén 《銅人》

Wài Tái Mì Yào 《外臺秘要》   *Táng* (唐), 752

    Essential Secrets from Outside of the Metropolis

       By Wàng Tāo 王燾

   Wài Tái 《外臺》

Xià 《下》

    See *Míng Táng Xìa Jīng* 《明堂下經》

Xīn Jiào Zhèng 《 新校正 》   *Sòng* (宋)

New Annotations and Corrections [*of Sù Wèn* (Plain Questions]

Lín Yì 林億 (editor)

A later edited edition of *Sù Wèn* 《 素問 》 (Plain Questions) with *Sù Wèn Zhù* 《 素問注 》 (Annotations to Plain Questions) (Also see these)

Xiǎo Pǐn Fāng 《 小品方 》

See *Jīng Fāng Xiǎo Pǐn* 《 經方小品 》

Yīn Yáng Shū 《 陰陽書 》   Warring State Period

Book of Yīn and Yáng

By Zhōu Yán 周衍 and Zhōu Shì 周奭

A book of calendars, divination, and constellations.

Yù Piān 《 玉篇 》   *Liáng* 梁 (519-581) circa 543 CE

Jade Chapters

Edited by Gù Yěwáng 顧野王

A Chinese dictionary.

Zhēn Jīng 《 針經 》

Acupuncture Classic

Unfortunately, this could be one of three things. See also 1. *Líng Shū* 《 靈樞 》; 2. *Zhēn Jīng Chāo* 《 針經鈔 》; or 3. *Shén Yìng Zhēn Jīng Yào Jué* 《 神應針經要訣 》

Zhēn Jīng Chāo 《 針經鈔 》   *Táng* (唐)

Copy of the Acupuncture Classic

By Zhēn Quán 甄權

Zhēn Jīng 《 針經 》

Lost.

Zhēn Jiǔ Jiǎ Yǐ Jīng 《 針灸甲乙經 》

The Systematic Classic of Acupuncture and Moxibustion   282 C.E.

By Huángfǔ Mì 皇甫謐

Jiǎ Yǐ Jīng 《 甲乙經 》

Jiǎ Yǐ 《 甲乙 》

Jiǎ 《 甲 》

Zhì Yōng Jū Nóng Dú Fāng 《 治癰疽膿毒方 》   unknown

Formulas for treating toxic diseases with pus, welling-abscesses, and flat-abscesses

By Hú Quán 胡權

This book is lost. More information on Hú Quán and when the book was written is not available.

Zhóu Hòu Bèi Jí Fāng 《 肘後備急方 》   *Jìn* (晉)

Emergency Standby Remedies

By Gě Hóng 葛洪

Zhóu Hòu Fāng 《 肘後方 》

It mainly discusses the treatment of emergency cases.

Zuǒ Zhuàn 《 左傳 》

> Commentary of Mr. Zuǒ

>> Attributed to Zuǒ Qīumíng 左丘明

Zhuàn 《 傳 》

Among the earliest Chinese works of narrative history, covering the period from 722 to 468 BCE. It is one of the most important sources for understanding the history of the Spring and Autumn Period (*Chūn Qiū* 春秋).

People

Texts

Extra Points

Regular Points

Zhōng Fǔ 中府 LU 1	**68**–69, 156–157, 239, 270, 280, 285, 289, 291, 293
Yún Mén 雲門 LU 2	34, **68**, 275
Tiān Fǔ 天府 LU 3	**97**, 102–103, 157, 307
Xiá Bái 俠白 LU 4	**97**, 279
Chǐ Zé 尺澤 LU 5	**96**–97, 102–103, 270–271, 279–280
Kǒng Zuì 孔最 LU 6	**96**
Liè Quē 列缺 LU 7	**95**, 202, 227, 232, 305–307
Jīng Qú 經渠 LU 8	**95**, 305–306
Tài Yuān 太淵 LU 9	**94**–95, 160, 184, 269, 282, 288
Yú Jì 魚際 LU 10	**94**, 206, 267, 275, 287, 293
Shào Shāng 少商 LU 11	**93**, 96, 100, 102–103, 110, 113–115, 124, 275, 282, 285, 291, 294, 299, 305, 307
Shāng Yáng 商陽 LI 1	**98**, 304, 307
Èr Jiān 二間 LI 2	**98**
Sān Jiān 三間 LI 3	**98**, 159, 244, 263–264, 302, 304, 307
Hé Gǔ 合谷 LI 4	**99**, 127, 302, 305
Yáng Xī 陽溪 LI 5	**100**, 305, 307
Piān Lì 偏歷 LI 6	**100**, 303–304, 306
Wēn Liū 溫溜 LI 7	**100**, 264, 282–283, 307
Xià Lián 下廉 LI 8	**100**, 130–131, 160, 190, 193, 210, 229, 231, 246, 253, 288, 297
Shàng Lián 上廉 LI 9	100–**101**, 130–132, 134, 160, 184, 229–230, 246, 263–264, 302
Sān Lǐ 三里 LI 10	**101**, 133, 160, 188, 227
Qū Chí 曲池 LI 11	101–**102**, 195, 268
Zhǒu Liáo 肘髎 LI 12	102
Wǔ Lǐ 五里 LI 13	**102**–103, 109, 120, 160, 228
Bì Nào 臂臑 LI 14	**103**
Jiān Yú 肩髃 LI 15	**35**–36, 103, 160–161
Jù Gǔ 巨骨 LI 16	**33**–34
Tiān Dǐng 天鼎 LI 17	**59**, 160
Fú Tū 扶突 LI 18	59–**60**
Hé Liáo 禾髎 LI 19	**23**–24, 30, 160
Yíng Xiāng 迎香 LI 20	**23**
Chéng Qì 承泣 ST 1	**24**
Sì Bái 四白 ST 2	**25**
Jù Liáo 巨髎 ST 3	**22**–23
Dì Cāng 地倉 ST 4	**25**
Dà Yíng 大迎 ST 5	**26**
Jiá Chē 頰車 ST 6	**31**
Xià Guān 下關 ST 7	**28**–30

A-Z

accumulations and gatherings that are hard as a stone	*jī jù jiān rú shí*	積聚堅如石	209
accumulations govern diseases of the viscera	*jī zhǔ zàng bìng*	積主臟病	286
accumulations in the abdomen	*fù zhōng yǒu jī*	腹中有積	236
aching body	*suān téng*	酸疼	296
aching heaviness of the legs and calves	*jiǎo shuàn suān zhòng*	腳腨酸重	269
aching pain of the legs and knees	*tuǐ xī suān tòng*	腿膝酸痛	125
aching pain of the knees and lower legs	*tuǐ xī suān tòng*	腿膝酸痛	132
acid swallowing	*tūn suān*	吞酸	278
acute *bì*-impediment	*jí bì*	急痹	270
acute fullness and obstruction below the umbilicus	*qí xià jí mǎn bù tōng*	臍下急滿不通	201
acute pain of the eyes	*mù jí tòng*	目急痛	302
acute pain of the spleen	*pí zhōng jí tòng*	脾中急痛	309
acute swelling of the smaller abdomen	*xiǎo fù jí zhǒng*	小腹急腫	244
adhering	*zhuó*	著	70–71
adults	*dà rén*	大人	258, 266
afflux pouch [a pathological accumulation]	*pì náng*	澼囊	259–260
aggregations			132, 166, 186, 190, 193, 200, 204, 220–221, 228, 263, 309
alarm point of small intestine	*xiǎo cháng zhī mù*	小腸之募	78
alarm point of the gall bladder	*dǎn zhī mù*	膽之募	88
alarm point of the heart	*xīn zhī mù*	心之募	72
alarm point of the kidneys	*shèn zhī mù*	腎之募	91
alarm point of the large intestine	*dà cháng zhī mù*	大腸之募	86, 273
alarm point of the liver	*gān zhī mù*	肝之募	88
alarm point of the lungs	*fèi zhī mù*	肺之募	68
alarm point of the spleen	*pí zhī mù*	脾之募	91
alarm point of the stomach	*wèi zhī mù*	胃之募	73–74
all diseases of the genitals	*yīn zhōng zhū bìng*	陰中諸病	203
all *lín*-stranguries	*zhū lín*	諸淋	223, 225
all *shàn qì*	*zhū shàn qì*	諸疝氣	213
alternating [sensations of] cold and heat	*hán rè wǎng lái*	寒熱往來	192
amaranth	*xiàn cài*	莧菜	54
anger	*huì nù*	恚怒	77, 169, 179
angle of the mandible	*qū hàn*	曲頷	26
angry	*dà nù*	大怒	152
anterior to the ear	*ěr qián*	耳前	14, 23, 28–32
anuria	*bù niào*	不尿	198, 201
anxiety	*yōu chóu*	憂愁	169, 182
apply moxibustion in summer if the disease improves in the spring	*chūn jiào xià jiǔ*	春較夏灸	216
arched-back tetany	*jìng fǎn zhé*	痙反折	307

bitter swallowing	*kǔ tūn*	苦吞	296
bitter taste in the mouth	*kǒu kǔ*	口苦	179
black	*hēi*	黑	24–25, 78, 168, 229, 286
black eyes	*mù wū sè*	目烏色	24–25
bladder qì	*páng guāng qì*	膀胱氣	204–205, 213
bladder qì surging upward and attacking both rib-sides	*páng guāng qì gōng chōng liǎng xié*	膀胱氣攻衝兩脅	204
bled, blood-letting	*chū xuè*	出血	3–4, 137
bleeding a lot	*duō chū xuè*	多出血	17
bleed it	*duō chū xuè*	多出血	21, 94, 136–137
blind	*mù wú suǒ jiàn*	目無所見	26
blockage of the bladder	*bāo bì sè*	胞閉塞	201, 222
blockage of the throat	*hóu zhōng bì sè*	喉中閉塞	94
blockage of the water passages	*shuǐ dào bù tōng*	水道不通	227, 229
blood	*xuè*	血	17, 67, 71, 78, 132, 137, 166, 168, 170–171, 181, 184, 186, 188, 191, 193, 207, 216, 220–221, 224, 229–230, 249–251, 253–255, 262, 271–273, 275, 277, 283, 285–286, 288, 296
blood avoidance	*xuè jì*	血忌	170–171
blood branch	*xuè zhī*	血支	170–171
blood disease	*xuè bìng*	血病	46, 184
blood inside the bladder	*bāo zhōng yǒu xuè*	胞中有血	220
blood stasis in the chest	*xiōng zhōng yū xuè*	胸中瘀血	132
blood vessels	*xuè mài*	血脈	20, 151, 166
bloody dribbling block	*xuè lóng*	血癃	223, 227
bloody hemorrhoids	*xuè zhì*	血痔	255
bloody *lín*-strangury	*xuè lín*	血淋	222
bloody stool	*biàn xuè*	便血	208, 210, 245, 253–254, 257–258, 260
bloody stool and urine	*dà xiǎo biàn xuè*	大小便血	253
bloody urine	*nì xuè*	溺血	190, 230–233
blurred vision	*mù bù míng*	目不明	22, 132, 190, 303
Bó Jǐng vessel	*bó jǐng mài*	髆井脈	32
body arched backwards	*shēn fǎn zhé*	身反折	179
body hair	*máo*	毛	151
body heat with shivering	*shēn rè zhèn lì*	身熱振栗	190
body heat	*shēn rè*	身熱	189–190, 215
body pain	*tǐ tòng*	體痛	244
bone disease	*gǔ bìng*	骨病	186
bones and marrow	*gǔ suǐ*	骨髓	151–152
both testicles retracted upward into the smaller abdominal with pain	*liǎng wán shàng rù xiǎo fù tòng*	兩丸上入小腹痛	215

desire to stay warm	*yù chǔ wēn zhōng*	欲處溫中	304
desire to vomit	*yù ǒu*	欲嘔	275, 283
deviation of the mouth	*kǒu zhuǎn wāi*	口轉喎	26
diaphragm vacuity	*gé xū*	膈虛	275
diarrhea	*xiè xiè*	泄瀉	171, 176, 179–180, 188, 190, 210, 215–216, 220, 227, 239, 241–255, 257–260, 262–266, 271–273, 277, 288, 292–293, 297, 310
diarrhea in the winter due to contraction of cold	*dōng rì zhòng gǎn yú hán zé xiè*	冬日重感於寒則泄	265
diarrhea with mixed red and white stool	*xiè lì chì bái*	泄痢赤白	250
diarrhea with pus and blood	*xiè lì nóng xuè*	泄利膿血	253, 271–272
diarrhea with rectal heaviness	*xiè lì hòu zhòng*	泄痢後重	250
diarrhea with watery stool	*xiè shuǐ*	泄水	252
diarrhea with watery stool in women	*fù rén shuǐ xiè lì*	婦人水泄痢	252
die young	*yāo*	夭	6, 63, 72
difficult defecation and urination	*bù de dà xiǎo biàn*	不得大小便	193, 203, 224, 259
difficult defecation	*dà biàn nán*	大便難	180, 188, 193, 203, 224, 227, 235–237, 255, 259
difficult painful urination	*xiǎo biàn nán ér tòng*	小便難而痛	220
difficult urination	*xiǎo biàn nán*	小便難	203–205, 211, 215, 223, 226–230, 232–233, 237–238, 241
difficult urination and defecation	*dà xiǎo biàn nán*	大小便難	205, 237–238
difficult urination with turbid urine	*xiǎo biàn zhuó nán*	小便濁難	232
difficulty getting drink and food down	*yǐn shí bù xià*	飲食不下	279, 291–292
difficulty getting food down	*shí bù xià*	食不下	195, 274, 277, 288–289, 291–294
difficulty in bending and stretching	*qū shēn nán*	屈伸難	268
difficulty standing or sitting	*qǐ zuò nán*	起坐難	125
difficulty swallowing food	*bù kě nà shí*	不可內食	180
dim vision	*mù bù míng*	目不明	2, 179, 215
discharge the water completely	*chū shuǐ jìn*	出水盡	19
discomfort in the umbilicus and abdomen	*qí fù zhōng yì yì bù lè*	臍腹中悒悒不樂	219
discomfort of the lower and upper back	*yāo bèi bú biàn*	腰背不便	270
discontented eating	*shí yàng yàng*	食怏怏	303
diseases of qi	*qì bìng*	氣病	64, 184
diseases of the abdomen	*fù zhōng jí*	腹中疾	260
diseases of the blood	*xuè bìng*	血病	184
diseases of the bones	*gǔ bìng*	骨病	184
diseases of the bowels	*fǔ bìng*	腑病	74, 184, 286
diseases of the marrow	*suǐ bìng*	髓病	184
diseases of the sinews	*jīn bìng*	筋病	124, 184
diseases of the vessels	*mài bìng*	脈病	95, 184

dribbling qì block	*qì lóng*	氣癃	222
dribbling red urine	*xiǎo biàn chì lín*	小便赤淋	217
dribbling urinary block	*lóng bì*	癃閉	200, 202, 215, 218, 222–224, 226, 237
dribbling urination	*xiǎo biàn lín lì*	小便淋瀝	188, 201, 223, 225, 230, 233
drink and food both accumulate here	*yǐn shí xù jī*	飲食蓄積	74
drinking alcohol	*yǐn jiǔ*	飲酒	169
drinking water	*yǐn shuǐ*	飲水	169, 196
drinking water without limit	*kě yǐn shuǐ wú dù*	渴飲水無度	196
drowsiness	*kùn dùn*	困頓	272
drum distention	*gǔ zhàng*	鼓脹	132, 199, 264
drunk	*jiǔ zuì*	酒醉	3, 152
drunkenness	*zuì jiǔ*	醉酒	137, 196, 294
dry eyes	*mù sè*	目澀	29–30
dry lips	*chún gān*	唇乾	246, 305
dry mouth	*kǒu gān*	口乾	189, 264, 302, 304
dry mouth and lips	*chún kǒu gān*	唇口乾	302
dry retching	*gān yuě*	乾噦	277
dry vomiting	*gān yuě*	乾噦	277, 279–280
dry stool	*dà biàn gān*	大便乾	235
dry throat	*yàn gān*	咽乾	195, 218, 230, 304
dry throat with tendency to drink [fluids]	*yì gān shàn kě*	嗌乾善渴	195
dry tongue	*shé gān*	舌乾	196, 224, 279
dry tongue and mouth	*kǒu shé gān*	口舌乾	279
dry vomiting	*gān ǒu*	乾嘔	277, 279–280
dry vomiting with nothing coming out	*gān ǒu wú suǒ chū*	乾嘔無所出	279
dū mài	*dū mài*	督脈	7, 42, 79
during pregnancy	*huái tāi*	懷胎	78, 99, 127, 201
dysentery	*lì*	痢	241, 247, 249–253, 259, 266–267
dysentery with violent watery diarrhea	*lì bào xià rú shuǐ*	痢暴下如水	252
dysentery with white stool	*lì bái sè*	痢白色	249

E

earth	*tǔ*	土	93, 102, 104, 109–110, 115, 117, 124, 126, 132, 137, 146, 170, 195, 197
earth cannot overcome the water	*tǔ bù néng shèng shuǐ*	土不能勝水	197
easy to treat	*yì zhì*	易治	216
eating a lot but emaciated	*shí duō shēn shòu*	食多身瘦	300
eating a lot	*shí duō*	食多	180, 190, 300
eats a lot	*shí duō*	食多	192
eating and drinking a lot [but the patient becomes] emaciated	*shí yǐn duō shēn shòu*	食飲多身瘦	300
eating but without engendering flesh	*shí bù shēng jī*	食不生肌	251

F

heat reversal in the feet	*zú rè jué*	足熱厥	146
heat settling in middle jiāo	*zhōng jiāo kè rè*	中焦客熱	297
heat strike	*rè zhòng*	熱中	296
heat tetany	*rè jìng*	熱痙	270
heat vexation	*fán rè*	煩熱	264
heavenly moxibustion	*tiān jiǔ*	天灸	302
heavenly virtue	*tiān dé*	天德	171
heaviness in the small intestine	*xiǎo cháng zhòng*	小腸重	262
heaviness of the head	*tóu zhòng*	頭重	190, 245, 302
heaviness of the knees	*xī zhòng*	膝重	269
heaviness of the lower back	*yāo zhòng*	腰重	125
heavy body	*tǐ zhòng*	體重	180
heavy rain	*měng yǔ*	猛雨	172
heel bone	*gēn gǔ*	跟骨	137, 143
hemilateral wind	*piān fēng*	偏風	35, 96, 130, 132
hemilateral wind and paralysis	*piān fēng bù suì*	偏風不遂	35
hemilateral withering	*piān kū*	偏枯	211
hemiplegia	*bàn shēn bù suì*	半身不遂	4
hemorrhoid diseases	*zhì bìng*	痔病	255
hemorrhoids	*zhì*	痔	42, 238, 254–258
hemorrhoids and bone erosion	*zhì gǔ shí*	痔骨蝕	255
hemorrhoids with bleeding and rectal heaviness	*zhì xuè，xiè hòu zhòng*	痔血，泄後重	255
hé-sea points	*hé*	合	229
hip joint	*bì shū*	髀樞	124, 244
holding in urination during sexual activity	*rěn xiǎo biàn rù fáng*	忍小便入房	201
holding in urine after eating	*bǎo shí qì rěn xiǎo biàn*	飽食訖忍小便	201
hostile	*wǎn hèn*	惋恨	280
hot body	*tǐ rè*	體熱	190
hot clothing	*rè yī*	熱衣	1
hot feet	*zú rè*	足熱	137, 306
hot food	*rè shí*	熱食	1
hot hemorrhoids	*rè zhì*	熱痔	255
hot noodles	*rè miàn*	熱面	169
hot painful urination	*xiǎo biàn rè tòng*	小便熱痛	227
hot palms	*zhǎng rè*	掌熱	303
hot qì	*rè qì*	熱氣	2, 21, 35, 44, 185, 205
hot qì in the sānjiāo, urinary bladder and kidneys	*sānjiāo、páng guāng、shèn zhōng rè qì*	三焦、膀胱、腎中熱氣	185, 205
hot red urine	*xiǎo biàn chì rè*	小便赤熱	203, 207
hot water washing from the medial aspect of the genitals to the low back	*tāng wò gǔ nèi zhì yāo*	湯沃股內至腰	220

I

N

nape feels dislocated	*xiàng rú bá*	項如拔	306
nape pain that radiates to the elbows and armpits	*xiàng tòng yĭn zhŏu yè*	項痛引肘掖	306
nasal congestion	*bí sāi*	鼻塞	5, 11, 13, 174
neck pain	*jĭng tòng*	頸痛	256
neck stiffness	*xiàng qiáng*	項強	189
needle for a long time	*jiŭ liú zhēn*	久留針	22, 51
needle is retained			28
needle gently	*wēi cì*	微刺	67, 134
needles pricking [a sensation during urination]	*zhēn cì*	針刺	207
needling is contraindicated	*jìn zhēn*	禁針	1, 6, 24–25, 28, 34, 46, 62–63, 68, 75, 77–78, 87, 102, 114, 145–146
needling is not recommended	*bù yí zhēn*	不宜針	17, 68
needling to overcome [evil] qì	*shèng qì zhēn*	勝氣針	94
network [point] of the hand yángmíng	*shŏu yáng míng luò*	手陽明絡	100, 103
network vessel of the hand shàoyáng	*shàoyáng luò*	少陽絡	114
network vessels	*luò*	絡	17, 125, 151, 268
network with the liver and spleen	*luò gān pí*	絡肝脾	89
never have heart strength	*yŏng wú xīn lì*	永無心力	166
night sweating	*duō dào hàn*	多盜汗	191
no desire to eat	*yĭn shí bù sī*	飲食不思	174, 180–181, 220, 243, 246, 264–265, 272, 275–276, 286–289, 293–298, 303–304, 307
no desire to move	*bù yù dòng*	不欲動	292, 294
noble woman	*mìng fù*	命婦	205, 217
non-dispersion of food	*shí bù xiāo*	食不消	259–260, 292–293, 295
non-transformation of food	*bù huà*	不化	178–179, 190, 243–244, 247, 249, 253, 259, 264–265, 271, 287, 289, 292–293, 296, 298
non-transformation of grains	*gŭ rù bù huà*	穀入不化	292, 294
non-transformation of grains [food]	*gŭ bù huà*	穀不化	243, 292
non-transformation of grains and water [food]	*shuĭ gŭ bù huà*	水穀不化	244
nostrils	*bí kŏng*	鼻孔	22–23, 30
not feeling hungry when smelling food	*wén shí chòu shāng bǎo*	聞食臭傷飽	296
nourish the heart	*yǎng xīn*	養心	182, 195, 234
nourish the qì and blood	*zī yǎng qì xuè*	滋養氣血	168
numbness from the low back down to the feet	*yāo xià zhì zú bù rén*	腰下至足不仁	217
numbness of the body	*shēn tǐ bù rén*	身體不仁	303
numbness of the feet and lower legs	*jiǎo jìng má*	腳脛麻	125
numbness of the lower back, hands and feet	*yāo tuǐ shŏu zú bù rén*	腰腿手足不仁	132
numbness of the lower legs	*jìng bù rén*	脛不仁	268

Q

scab over	*jiā hòu*	痂後	168
scant semen	*jīng shǎo*	精少	203, 206–207
scant semen with dampness in the scrotum	*jīng shǎo náng shī*	精少囊濕	207
sea of blood	*xuè hǎi*	血海	176
sea of marrow	*suǐ hǎi*	髓海	176
sea of original qì	*yuán qì zhī hǎi*	元氣之海	77, 176
sea of qì	*qì zhī hǎi*	氣之海	63, 77, 176
sea of vital qì in males	*nán zǐ shēng qì zhī hǎi*	男子生氣之海	76
seasonal qì	*shí qì*	時氣	171
seeing dimly afar [nearsightedness]	*yuǎn shì máng máng*	遠視䀮䀮	93
seminal emission with dreaming	*mèng shī jīng*	夢失精	232, 234
seminal emissions with dreams	*mèng yí*	夢遺	194
seminal loss	*chū jīng*	出精	52, 178, 182, 184–185, 190, 209, 223, 232–234
seminal loss and infertility	*shī jīng jué zǐ*	失精絕子	178, 209
seminal loss and retracted genitals	*shī jīng yīn suō*	失精陰縮	232
seminal loss while dreaming	*mèng zhōng shī jīng*	夢中失精	52, 185, 190
seminal spillage	*jīng yì*	精溢	198, 233
sensations of cold and heat in the bones	*gǔ hán rè*	骨寒熱	
seven damages	*qī shāng*	七傷	132, 179, 182, 188, 190, 203, 206–207
seventh vertebra	*qī zhuī*	七椎	40, 45–46, 54, 153, 232, 236
severe abdominal fullness	*fù dà mǎn*	腹大滿	281
severe drunkenness	*yǐn jiǔ dà zuì*	飲酒大醉	137
severe heat	*rè shèn*	熱甚	306–307
severe marked emaciation	*xī xī léi shòu*	翕翕羸瘦	191
severe pain	*dà tòng*	大痛	42, 194, 261, 270, 310
severe panting with inability to lie down	*dà chuǎn bù dé wò*	大喘不得臥	272
severe suffering	*shèn kǔ*	甚苦	307
severe swelling of the knees	*xī zhǒng shèn*	膝腫甚	136
severe vexation of the heart	*xīn fán shèn*	心煩甚	304
severe vomiting	*ǒu shèn*	嘔甚	306
sexual taxation	*fáng láo*	房勞	42, 50, 169, 254
shaking	*zhàn diào*	戰掉	17, 269
shàn-mounting	*shàn*	疝	165
shàn-mounting accumulations	*shàn jī*	疝積	221
shàn-mounting aggregations	*shàn pǐ*	疝癖	309
shàn-mounting and accumulations under the umbilicus	*qí xià shàn jī*	臍下疝積	220
shàn-mounting and conglomerations	*shàn jiǎ*	疝瘕	220–221, 246
shàn-mounting and conglomerations in women	*fù rén shàn jiǎ*	婦人疝瘕	220
shàn-mounting in women	*nǚ zǐ shàn*	女子疝	214, 216

small intestine diarrhea	*xiǎo cháng xiè*	小腸泄	249
small intestine heat	*xiǎo cháng rè*	小腸熱	229, 268
small intestine qì	*xiǎo cháng qì*	小腸氣	193–194, 218
snowstorms	*xuě*	雪	172
someone eats a lot, but has marked emaciation	*shí huì*	食晦	192
someone who suffers severe wind	*dà huàn fēng*	大患風	13
somnolence	*dú wò*	獨臥	190, 209, 211, 219, 224, 292, 294, 299
somnolence with fatigue	*shì wò dài duò*	嗜臥怠惰	292
sore arms	*bì suān*	臂酸	303
sore lower legs with difficulty bending and stretching	*jìng suān qū shēn nán*	脛酸屈伸難	219
sore pharynx	*yān zhōng tòng*	咽中痛	180, 295
soreness and weakness of the low back and four limbs	*yāo zhōng sì zhī yín luò*	腰中四肢淫濼	190
sores around the umbilicus	*rào qí shēng chuāng*	繞臍生瘡	262
sores erupt	*chuāng fā*	瘡發	167–168
sorrowful heart	*xīn bēi*	心悲	263–264
sorrowful speech and weeping	*yǔ bēi qì*	語悲泣	181
space below the heart and above the diaphragm	*huāng*	肓	53, 185
sparrow droppings	*què fèn*	雀糞	19
sparrow vision	*què mù*	雀目	22
spermaturia	*niào jīng*	尿精	232, 234
spillage rheum	*yì yǐn*	溢飲	227
spirit exhaustion	*jīng shén kùn dùn*	精神困頓	191
spirit scatters	*shén qù*	神去	182
spitting	*tuò*	唾	211, 275, 277, 283, **285–286**
spitting of blood	*tuò xuè*	唾血	181, 191, 224, 275, 288
spitting of foam	*tuò mò*	唾沫	285, 305
spitting of pus	*tǔ nóng*	吐膿	285–286
spitting of thick pus	*tuò chóu nóng*	唾稠膿	285
spittle that looks like white glue	*tuò rú bái jiāo*	唾如白膠	286
spleen and kidney disease	*pí shèn bìng*	脾腎病	174
spleen debilitation	*pí shuāi*	脾衰	197
spleen diarrhea	*pí xiè*	脾泄	242, 249
spleen does not grind	*pí bù mó*	脾不磨	181
spleen is not vigorous	*pí bù zhuàng*	脾不壯	181
spleen vacuity	*pí xū*	脾虛	264, 274, 309
spleen vacuity that makes people unhappy	*pí xū lìng rén bù lè*	脾虛令人不樂	264, 309
spleen was extremely large	*pí jí jù*	脾極巨	197
spontaneous bleeding of the brain	*nǎo nǜ*	腦衄	174

the four limbs	*sì zhī*	四肢	164–165, 179, 211, 215, 219, 225, 243, 252, 269, 298
the fourth toe	*zú xiǎo zhǐ cì zhǐ*	足小指次指	121–122
the hundred diseases also arise out of the kidneys	*bǎi bìng jiē shēng yú shèn*	百病皆生於腎	194
the hundred diseases are all governed	*bǎi bìng jiē zhǔ*	百病皆主	4
the hundred diseases arise out of the heart	*bǎi bìng jiē shēng yú xīn*	百病皆生於心	194
the middle finger	*shǒu zhōng zhǐ*	手中指	32, 44, 109–110, 125, 133, 156–158, 187
the nail	*zhuǎ jiǎ*	爪甲	93, 98, 104, 107, 109, 113, 117, 121, 126, 129, 141, 158, 219, 242
the palm	*zhǎng*	掌	95, 97, 104–106, 109–111, 302
the qì meets in the sānjiāo	*qì huì sān jiāo*	氣會三焦	64
the qì spreads the yīn and yáng	*qì bù yīn yáng*	氣布陰陽	63
the qì surges upward into the eyes	*qì shàng chōng mù*	氣上衝目	133, 179
the ring finger	*wú míng zhǐ*	無名指	109–110, 113
the root of hemorrhoids	*zhì gēn běn*	痔根本	42
the root of the disease	*bìng gēn*	病根	163
the same number of cones of moxibustion as the age of the patient	*suí nián*	隨年	47–48, 192, 216, 224, 240
the second toe	*zú dà zhǐ cì zhǐ*	足大指次指	117, 129, 193, 303
the sharp bone [the styloid process of the ulna]	*duì gǔ*	兌骨	104
the size of the cone cannot be large	*ài zhù bù yòng dà*	艾炷不用大	28
the size of the leg of a thick hairpin	*zhù rú cū chāi jiǎo dà*	炷如粗釵腳大	25
the stool comes out directly [incontinence]	*dà biàn zhí chū*	大便直出	241
The Transverse Three Cùn Method	*Héng Sān Jiān Cùn*	橫三間寸	159
the triangle	*sān jiǎo*	三角	7
the two yīn [anus and genitals]	*liǎng yīn*	兩陰	79
thigh	*gǔ*	股	120, 124, 147, 214, 217, 228, 268
thigh bone	*bì gǔ*	髀骨	124
thin	*jí*	瘠	2–3, 16, 21, 35, 143, 158, 161, 164–166, 180–181, 191, 251, 268, 301
thin muscles	*jī shòu*	肌瘦	191
thin weak appearance	*xíng róng shòu cuì*	形容瘦悴	251
thin weak arms and elbows due to wind	*fēng bì zhǒu xì wú lì*	風臂肘細無力	268
thin weak extremities	*sì zhī xì ér wú lì*	四肢細而無力	164
thinning of the arms	*shǒu bì xì*	手臂細	35
thirst	*dà kě*	大渴	40, 152, 193, 195–197, 211, 231, 265
thirst with desire for cold or hot drinks	*hán rè kě*	寒熱渴	195
thirsty drinking	*yǐn kě*	飲渴	195
thirty-six diseases below the umbilicus	*qí xià sān shí liù jí*	臍下三十六疾	222

Formulas

Medicinals

The Chinese Medicine Database

www.cm-db.com

The Chinese Medicine Database has been organized around one central principle -- translation of Classical Chinese texts, and dissemination of that information.

There are thousands of Chinese medicine texts that have never been translated. We have compiled a small list on our website of the ones that we have found, but we believe that there are tens of thousands of documents that span from the *Hàn* Dynasty to pre-Republican times. Most of these documents will never be read by people in the West, simply because of lack of translation.

We have created a vehicle, that allows interested practitioners, students, institutions, and scholars to help support and fund the translation of these documents, and then mine and synthesize the data that is gained from these texts.

The Database contains:

Monographs on:
690 Single Herbs
1510 Formulas
Mayway's Patents
ITM's Formulations
Golden Flowers Formulations
Classical Pearls Formulations by Heiner Fruehauf
OBGYN Modifications to Formulas
Single Points: the 361 Regular Points
Time Line of the History of Chinese Medicine

Beer Hall Lecture Series
Watch videos from our monthly Beer Hall lecture series with guest speakers such as: Arnaud Versluys, Subhuti Dharmananda, Jason Robertson, Craig Mitchell, Michael Max, Lorraine Wilcox, and Ed Neal.

Play STORT
Play our free online game STORT where you can learn Chinese while having a bit of fun (www.cm-db.com/stort).

15,000 Western Diagnoses with ICD-9 Codes

A Chinese-English dictionary:
Containing over 102,271 terms, including the Eastland and the WHO term sets.

A Western Book search containing:
Fenner's Complete Formulary
    by B. Fenner
The 1918 Dispensatory of the United States of America
    Edited by Joseph P. Remington, Horatio C. Woods and others

The Eclectic Materia Medica, Pharmacology and Therapeutics
by Harvey Wickes Felter, M.D.

A Personal Dashboard, which allows users to:
Blog
Take notes on any monograph.
Search for other users by city, state, country and name.
Make friends all around the world.
Share and compare notes with friends.
Personalize your dashboard by adding photos, and information about your practice.

Translations:

Shāng Hán Lái Sū Jí	傷寒來蘇集	Renewal of Treatise on Cold Damage
Qí Jīng Bā Mài Kǎo	奇經八脈考	Explanation of the Eight Vessels of the Marvellous Meridians
Shāng Hán Míng Lǐ Lùn	傷寒明理論	Treatise on Enlightening the Principles of Cold Damage
Wú Jū Tōng Yī Àn	吳鞠通医案	Case Studies of Wú Jūtōng
The Nàn Jīng	難經	The Classic of Difficulties
The Zàng Fǔ Biāo Běn Hán Rè Xū Shí Yòng Yào Shì	臟腑標本寒熱虛實用藥式	Viscera and Bowels, Tip and Root, Cold and Heat, Vacuity and Repletion Model for Using Medicinals
Wēn Rè Lún	温熱論	Treatise on Warm Heat Disease
Shāng Hán Shé Jiàn	傷寒舌鑒	Tongue Mirror of Cold Damage
Xǔ Shì Yī Àn	許氏醫案	Case Histories of Master Xǔ
Fǔ Xìng Jué Zāng Fǔ Yòng Yào Fǎ Yào	輔行決臟腑用藥法要	Secret Instructions for Assisting the Body:Essential Methods for the Application of Drugs to the Viscera & Bowels
Biāo Yōu Fù	標幽賦	Indicating the Obscure
Liú Juān Zǐ Guǐ Yí Fāng	劉涓子鬼遺方	Liu Juanzi's Formulas Inherited from Ghosts
Shèn Jí Chú Yán	慎疾芻言	Precautions in Illness: My Humble Thoughts
Yào Zhèng Jì Yí	藥症忌宜	Medicinals & Patterns Contraindications & Appropriate [Choices]
Fù Kē Wèn Dá	婦科問答	Questions and Answers in Gynecology
Nèi Jīng Zhī Yào	內經知要	Essential Knowledge from the Nèijīng

Benefits:
Subscribers to the Database receive a 10% discount on our published books when they are in pre-release.

We translate texts as often, and in quantities that reflect our user base. The larger amount of subscribers that we have, the more translation that we can accomplish.

Published Books:

2010 Zhēn Jiǔ Dà Chéng 針灸大成: The Great Compendium of Acupuncture & Moxabustion vol. I by Yáng Jìzhōu 楊繼洲
Translated by Sabine Wilms.
ISBN 978-0-9799552-2-8

2010 Zhēn Jiǔ Dà Chéng 針灸大成: The Great Compendium of Acupuncture & Moxabustion vol. V by Yáng Jìzhōu 楊繼洲
Translated by Lorraine Wilcox.
ISBN 978-0-9799552-4-2

2010 Jīn Guì Fāng Gē Kuò 金匱方歌括: Formulas from the Golden Cabinet with Songs vol. I - III by Chén Xiūyuán 陳修園
Translated by Sabine Wilms.
ISBN 978-0-9799552-5-9

2011 Zhēn Jiǔ Dà Chéng 針灸大成: The Great Compendium of Acupuncture & Moxabustion vol. VIII by Yáng Jìzhōu 楊繼洲
Translated by Yue Lu.
ISBN 978-0-9799552-7-3

2011 Zhēn Jiǔ Dà Chéng 針灸大成: The Great Compendium of Acupuncture & Moxabustion vol. IX by Yáng Jìzhōu 楊繼洲
Translated by Lorraine Wilcox.
ISBN 978-0-9799552-6-6

2012 Raising the Dead and Returning Life: Emergency Medicine of the Qīng Dynasty by Bào Xiāng'áo 鮑相璈
Translated by Lorraine Wilcox.
ISBN 978-0-9799552-3-5

2014 Zhēn Jiǔ Zī Shēng Jīng 針灸資生經: The Classic of Supporting Life with Acupuncture and Moxibustion vol. I-III by Wáng Zhízhōng 王執中
Translated by Yue Lu.
ISBN 978-0-9799552-1-1

2014 Jīn Guì Fāng Gē Kuò 金匱方歌括: Formulas from the Golden Cabinet with Songs vol. IV - VI by Chén Xiūyuán 陳修園
Translated by Eran Even.
ISBN 978-0-9799552-8-0

www.ingramcontent.com/pod-product-compliance
Lightning Source LLC
Chambersburg PA
CBHW080656220326
41598CB00033B/5226